ROBERT J. WALTER, Ph.

LEUKOCYTE CHEMOTAXIS:
METHODS, PHYSIOLOGY,
AND CLINICAL IMPLICATIONS

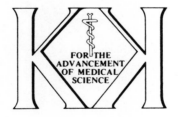

FOR THE
ADVANCEMENT
OF MEDICAL
SCIENCE

Leukocyte Chemotaxis: Methods, Physiology, and Clinical Implications

Edited by

John I. Gallin, M.D.
Laboratory of Clinical Investigation
National Institute of Allergy and
*   Infectious Diseases*
National Institutes of Health
Bethesda, Maryland

Paul G. Quie, M.D.
Department of Pediatrics
University of Minnesota
*   Medical School*
Minneapolis, Minnesota

Raven Press ▪ New York

Raven Press, 1140 Avenue of the Americas, New York, New York 10036

Made in the United States of America

Library of Congress Cataloging in Publication Data

Main entry under title:

Leukocyte chemotaxis

    (Kroc Foundation; v. 9)
    Papers presented at a conference jointly sponsored by the National Institute of Allergy and Infectious Diseases and the Kroc Foundation, and held Jan. 1977, Santa Ynez, California.

    Includes bibliographical references and index.
    1. Leukocytes–Congresses. 2. Chemotaxis–Congresses.
I. Gallin, John I. II. Quie, Paul G.
III. United States. National Institute of Allergy and Infectious Diseases. IV. Kroc Foundation. V. Series: Kroc Foundation. Kroc Foundation series; v. 9
QP95.L644   599'.01'13   76-58053
ISBN 0-89004-198-9

Preface

Appreciation of the central role of the phagocytic system in host defense against microbial diseases has led to a virtual explosion of new knowledge about the functions of phagocytic cells. Locomotion is one of the functions that is of great current interest, and therefore a conference on leukocyte chemotaxis was planned by John I. Gallin, Paul G. Quie, Ralph Snyderman, Peter A. Ward, and Ralph C. Williams, Jr. The program was divided into three areas of discussion: methodology, physiology, and clinical implications. The several methods that are currently being used for evaluation of leukocyte locomotion and chemotactic response were described, and detailed descriptions of methodology are included in this volume. The chapters by Wilkinson, Nelson, Maderazo, and Zigmond contain descriptions of methods for evaluation of leukocyte locomotion and response. There are other methods including "modified Boyden," "chromium label," and "leading front," which are described in detail as an appendix to the methods section. The "open discussion" at the end of the section provides frank exchange about the techniques among the investigators. It is expected that this volume will serve as a reference on chemotaxis methodology for scientists interested in establishing chemotaxis assays in their laboratories.

The physiology of leukocyte locomotion is much better understood by application of new techniques and new reagents. For example, experiments with synthetic peptides have brought out more exact definition of receptors and the processes of activation and deactivation. Light and electron microscope techniques have provided additional understanding of cellular orientation and internal reorganization in response to chemotactic stimulation. Ion flux studies with isotope tracers and electrophysiological techniques have demonstrated changes in membrane permeability to ions during leukocyte activation by chemotactic factors. The isolation of actin and myosin from leukocytes has provided certain analogies between leukocyte locomotion and muscle contraction. These physiological studies provide a beginning to our understanding of how leukocytes carry out their complicated functions. Our understanding of the physiology of leukocyte function should grow rapidly.

Leukocyte locomotion is modulated by multiple factors during immunologic and hypersensitivity reactions. Chemotaxis, therefore, appears to be regulated by a highly complex system. Lymphocytes, platelets, neutrophils, monocytes and plasma factors are all involved in this system for attraction, immobilization and inhibition of phagocytic cells at inflammatory-immune sites.

Clinical conditions with disordered leukocyte locomotion are usually associated with increased susceptibility to recurrent pyogenic infections. Of particular interest were the observations by Snyderman of abnormal chemotaxis in patients with cancer and the possibility that neoplasms themselves may produce factors which subvert monocyte-macrophage function. There was classification of clinical conditions associated with disorders of chemotaxis and attempts to define a relationship between cellular dysfunction and diseases. The remarkable advances in the understanding of regulatory mechanisms and physiology of leukocyte locomotion discussed at this meeting give reality to an expectation that disorders of chemotaxis may soon be effectively treated.

John I. Gallin
Paul G. Quie

Contents

Acknowledgments

The conference on which this volume is based was jointly supported by The National Institute of Allergy and Infectious Diseases and the Kroc Foundation and was held January 1977 at the J and R Double Arch Ranch, Santa Ynez, California.

Contributors

Robert B. Allan
Department of Bacteriology and
   Immunology
University of Glasgow, Western Infirmary
Glasgow G11 6NT Scotland

Leonard C. Altman
Department of Medicine
University of Washington
Seattle, Washington 98105

S. Awanikumar
Laboratory of Developmental Biology
   and Anomalies
National Institute of Dental Research
National Institutes of Health
Bethesda, Maryland 20014

John Baum
Clinical Immunology Unit
University of Rochester
School of Medicine and Dentistry
Rochester, New York 14642

Elmer L. Becker
Department of Pathology
University of Connecticut
   Health Center
Farmington, Connecticut 06032

John P. Bronza
Department of Pathology
University of Connecticut
   Health Center
Farmington, Connecticut 06032

K. Lynn Cates
Department of Pediatrics
University of Minnesota
School of Medicine
Minneapolis, Minnesota 55455

George Cianciolo
Department of Microbiology
University of Miami School of Medicine
Miami, Florida 33152

Richard A. F. Clark
Department of Dermatology
Massachusetts General Hospital
Boston, Massachusetts 02114

Robert A. Clark
Department of Medicine
University of Washington
Seattle, Washington 98105

B. A. Corcoran
Laboratory of Developmental Biology and
   Anomalies
National Institute of Dental Research
National Institutes of Health
Bethesda, Maryland 20014

Eva B. Cramer
Department of Anatomy
Downstate Medical Center
Brooklyn, New York 11203

Violet Esquenazi
Department of Microbiology
University of Miami
School of Medicine
Miami, Florida 33152

Vance D. Fiegel
Department of Surgery
University of Minnesota Medical School
Minneapolis, Minnesota 55455

Elaine K. Gallin
Division of Experimental Hematology
Armed Forces Radiobiology Research
   Institute
Bethesda, Maryland 20014

John I. Gallin
Laboratory of Clinical Investigation
National Institute of Allergy and Infectious Diseases
National Institutes of Health
Bethesda, Maryland 20014

Edward J. Goetzel
Harvard Medical School
Robert Breck Brigham Hospital
Parker Hill Avenue
Boston, Massachusetts 02120

Harry R. Hill
University of Utah
College of Medicine
1400 East 2nd South
Salt Lake City, Utah 84132

Joerg A. Jensen
Department of Microbiology
University of Miami
School of Medicine
Miami, Florida 33152

Allen P. Kaplan
Clinical Physiology Section
National Institute of Allergy and Infectious Diseases
National Institutes of Health
Bethesda, Maryland 20014

John P. Leddy
Department of Medicine
and Microbiology
University of Rochester
School of Medicine
Rochester, New York 14642

William S. Lynn
Department of Biochemistry
Duke University Medical Center
Durham, North Carolina 27710

Eufronio G. Maderazo
Department of Medicine
Hartford Hospital
Hartford, Connecticut 06115

Harry L. Malech
Laboratory of Clinical Investigation
National Institute of Allergy and Infectious Diseases
National Institutes of Health
Bethesda, Maryland 20014

Robert T. McCormack
Department of Pediatrics
University of Minnesota Medical School
Minneapolis, Minnesota 55455

Michael E. Miller
Department of Pediatrics
Harbor General Hospital
1000 West Carson Street
Torrance, California 90509

Paul H. Naccache
Department of Pathology
University of Connecticut Health Center
Farmington, Connecticut 06032

Robert D. Nelson
Department of Surgery and
Laboratory-Medicine-Pathology
University of Minnesota Hospital
Minneapolis, Minnesota 55455

Marilyn C. Pike
Division of Rheumatic and Genetic
* Diseases*
Duke University Medical Center
Durham, North Carolina 27710

Paul G. Quie
Department of Pediatrics
University of Minnesota Medical School
Minneapolis, Minnesota 55455

Casann E. Ray
Department of Pediatrics
University of Minnesota School of
* Medicine*
Minneapolis, Minnesota 55455

Stephen I. Rosenfeld
Clinical Immunology Unit
University of Rochester
School of Medicine and Dentistry
Rochester, New York 14642

Saura Sahu
Department of Biochemistry
Duke University Medical Center
Durham, North Carolina 27710

Elliott Schiffmann
Laboratory of Developmental Biology and
* Anomalies*
National Institute of Dental Research
National Institutes of Health
Bethesda, Maryland 20014

Jeff Selph
Department of Biochemistry
Duke University Medical Center
Durham, North Carolina 27710

Ramadan Sha'afi
Department of Pathology
University of Connecticut Health Center
Farmington, Connecticut 06032

Henry J. Showell
Department of Pathology
University of Connecticut Health Center
Farmington, Connecticut 06032

Ralph Snyderman
Duke University School of Medicine
Department of Immunology
Durham, North Carolina 27710

R. S. N. Somayajalulu
Department of Biochemistry
Duke University Medical Center
Durham, North Carolina 27710

Thomas P. Stossel
Medical Oncology Unit
Massachusetts General Hospital
Boston, Massachusetts 02114

Stephen R. Turner
Duke University Medical Center
Department of Medicine
Durham, North Carolina 27710

Dennis Van Epps
Department of Medicine
University of New Mexico
Albuquerque, New Mexico 87131

Peter A. Ward
University of Connecticut Health Center
Department of Pathology
Farmington, Connecticut 06032

Peter C. Wilkinson
Department of Bacteriology and
* Immunology*
University of Glasgow, Western Infirmary
Glasgow G11 6NT Scotland

Ralph C. Williams, Jr.
Department of Medicine
University of New Mexico
School of Medicine
Albuquerque, New Mexico 87106

Charles L. Woronick
Medical Research Laboratory
Division of Infectious Diseases
Department of Medicine
Hartford Hospital
Hartford, Connecticut 06115

Daniel G. Wright
Laboratory of Clinical Investigation
National Institute of Allergy and Infec-
* tious Diseases*
National Institutes of Health
Bethesda, Maryland 20014

Sally H. Zigmond
Department of Biology
University of Pennsylvania
Philadelphia, Pennsylvania 19174

Leukocyte Chemotaxis, edited by John I. Gallin
and Paul G. Quie. Raven Press, New York
© 1978.

Assay Systems for Measuring Leukocyte Locomotion: An Overview

Peter C. Wilkinson and Robert B. Allan

Department of Bacteriology and Immunology, University of Glasgow, Western Infirmary, Glasgow G11 6NT, Scotland

The most useful research techniques are those that allow rigorous and thorough testing of hypotheses. They should permit, not only experiments that merely corroborate hypotheses, but also those that test them to the core, those which Karl Popper (20) has described as "falsifying experiments" and which he considers to be the most fruitful. Joseph Black, the discoverer of latent heat, and Professor of Chemistry as well as of Botany and of the Practice of Medicine in the University of Glasgow in the mid-eighteenth century, put his finger on a weakness of much scientific methodology. "A nice adaptation of conditions," he wrote, "will make almost any hypothesis agree with the phenomena. This will please the imagination but does not advance our knowledge" (5). We should therefore ask ourselves to what extent present techniques for measuring leukocyte chemotaxis merely allow "a nice adaptation of conditions," and to what extent they allow real advances in understanding to be made.

FORMS OF LEUKOCYTE LOCOMOTION

To avoid confusion in the subsequent discussion, it is important and timely to begin by discussing briefly the nature of leukocyte locomotion and its modification by chemical substances. In the past few years, a number of workers in the field have found the loose use of the word *chemotaxis* to describe any migration of cells in the presence of an attractant increasingly unsatisfactory and confusing. It is now apparent that chemical attractants can influence not only the direction in which cells move but also their rate of locomotion (24,34,41). Substances that cause directional migration of cells in a gradient to the source of the gradient will lead the cells to accumulate at the source, since movement against the gradient will be inhibited. Substances that only increase the rate of locomotion without influencing direction, however, may not cause cell accumulation because, once the cells reach the source, there is no force preventing them from moving away again. To understand the behavior of cells in inflammation, it is clearly necessary to distinguish between these two forms of response. Proposals for definitions of terms used in reference to cell locomotion are in press (17), and some important points from these proposals are summarized below.

1

The term *random locomotion* refers to locomotion in which the axis of the moving cell is not orientated in relation to any stimulus and in which the cell shows no preference for, or avoidance of, a particular direction. The term does not cover or define the effects of chemical attractants on the locomotor reactions of cells.

Chemokinesis is a reaction by which the *speed* or frequency of locomotion and/or the frequency and magnitude of turns of cells is determined by substances in their environment. Chemokinetic responses may change the velocity of cells moving at random.

Chemotaxis is a reaction by which the *direction* of locomotion of cells is determined by substances in their environment.

Directional locomotion is not synonymous with chemotaxis. It may be chemotactic but may also result from other types of tactic influence or from contact guidance. Leukocytes have not, however, been shown to move directionally by mechanisms other than chemotaxis.

As mentioned earlier, attractants may cause chemokinetic reactions in leukocytes. The velocity of migration is determined by the absolute concentration of the attractant in the absence of a gradient. The same substances may also be chemotactic when cells are placed in a gradient. This dual effect must be evaluated in measuring cellular responses to chemoattractants.

Bearing these remarks in mind, it is apparent that migration of cells through a filter toward a stimulus on the other side, or accumulation of cells in a skin window or other inflammatory site, does not, in itself, constitute a demonstration of chemotaxis, and the word chemotaxis should be avoided unless a directional reaction has been demonstrated.

CATEGORIES OF CHEMOTAXIS METHODS

Techniques for studying locomotion of leukocytes fall into two categories. First are those in which the locomotion of individual cells is observed and analyzed and the influence of chemoattractants on this locomotion studied. This is usually achieved by time-lapse cinematography of cells on a warmed slide-and-coverslip preparation. Second are those in which the migration of a sample of a cell population is measured and, again, the influence of chemoattractants can be studied. The most popular method of this type in use at present is the Boyden chamber micropore filter method. These two approaches examine cell locomotion from different viewpoints and give information which, although there is some overlap, is of a different nature. Both have advantages and disadvantages which are discussed below.

DIRECT OBSERVATIONS OF CELLS IN LOCOMOTION

It is not difficult to set up and examine slide-and-coverslip preparations of leukocytes under a microscope using a warm stage. With patience, the locomotion of cells can be followed visually. With a time-lapse camera, a film can be taken and analyzed later. The most difficult part comes in extracting meaningful information from these observations and analyses.

Leukocytes, particularly neutrophils, are relatively fast-moving cells compared, for instance, with fibroblasts, and there are now a number of excellent descriptions of the morphology of leukocytes in locomotion (2,7,18,23,41). Most authors agree that the first event in the moving cell is the appearance of a veil-like flattened hyaline membrane or lamellipodium at the anterior end of the cell which may show considerable ruffling. Initially, this does not contain cytoplasmic organelles, which remain in the more sharply delineated posterior portion of the cell. There may be a tail with or without retraction fibers. During locomotion, this orientated morphology is retained. The cell elongates as the lamellipodium spreads forward and the cytoplasmic contents stream forward into the anterior part of the cell. On glass, neutrophils glide over the substratum, making transient and, judged by interference-reflection microscopy (2), fairly light adhesions as compared with the stronger, more permanent, adhesions made by fibroblasts. Occasionally, however, leukocytes may become firmly adherent by their tails, sufficiently so to inhibit forward movement, and then the contractile anterior portion may pull forward sufficiently to break completely away from the adherent tail fibers. It has not been easy to study the effects of chemotactic factors on these events, chiefly because of the difficulty of setting up stable gradients in slide-and-coverslip preparations. This has been achieved using a solid source such as a clump of bacteria in a serum medium (18,21). On the basis of studies using serum media, it has been stated that chemoattractants do not increase the speed of migration of leukocytes but only influence their direction of locomotion. These studies, however, ignored the pronounced chemokinetic effect of serum itself, which is sufficient to obscure analysis. If better-defined attractants are used, effects on both rate and direction can be observed (41).

McCutcheon (18) plotted the paths that leukocytes took when exposed to a chemotactic gradient. He quantified the directional response of cells in such gradients by determining the "chemotactic ratio," defined as the ratio of the net distance traveled by a cell toward or away from the test object to the total distance traveled by the cell. The limiting values for this ratio were +1.0 for movement in a straight line toward the object and −1.0 for movement in a straight line away from the object. McCutcheon thus showed that the presence of a chemotactic gradient caused the cells to show considerable net displacement toward the gradient source. This was confirmed by Zigmond and Hirsch (41). Zigmond (40) made the important observation that cells placed in gradients became oriented toward the gradient source before they began translocation, suggesting that the cells were able to detect the gradient across their own length. This argues against a "temporal" sensing system where the cell orients itself by sampling the gradient at different times, since this would require the cell to move before detecting the gradient. It is consistent with a "spatial" sensing system in which the cell compares concentrations of attractants at different points on its own surface and can thus detect differences in concentration between its front and its back. Zigmond's analysis of the paths taken by leukocytes moving in gradients indicated that an important action of the gradient was to determine the direction of turn of cells. Cells moving at an angle of more than 30° away from the gradient source were highly likely to make their next turn toward the source.

Visual Assay of Chemotaxis Using *Candida albicans*

We have recently been engaged in developing direct visual assays of leukocyte locomotion for use in parallel with micropore filter assays. The most promising of these assays, the full details of which are in preparation for publication, measures the response of leukocytes in plasma to a gradient diffusing from blastospores of *Candida albicans.* Purified human blood neutrophils (2×10^6/ ml) were allowed to settle on a glass surface and rinsed to remove erythrocytes and debris. To them was added a suspension of 2×10^5/ml blastospores of *C. albicans* (from a 48-hr dextrose-peptone agar culture) in 50% normal human plasma in Gey's solution. The preparation was sealed under a coverslip and filmed at 37°C on a warm stage. A typical response is shown in Fig. 1, in which a group of neutrophil leukocytes from normal human blood rapidly detected a gradient set up by Candida in plasma. The cells oriented toward the yeast, migrated directly toward it, and ingested it within a minute. Having ingested a group of yeasts, neutrophils were often seen, after a brief period of less than a minute, to migrate directionally toward another clump of yeasts and thus rapidly to ingest ten or more spores per cell. The phenomenon was plasma- or serum-dependent. Little chemotaxis toward yeasts or phagocytosis of yeasts was seen in the absence of plasma. Normal human sera contain antibody to Candida, and we have not established whether this chemotaxis was a result of yeast-bound antibody-induced complement fixation, of alternate pathway activation by yeast cell wall saccharides, or of other mechanisms.

We have tracked the paths followed by cells migrating toward *C. albicans* under various experimental conditions. In these assays, the neutrophils before they moved were usually quite a short distance (about 50 μm) from the nearest yeast. Table 1 shows results obtained with a single cell batch. Normal neutrophils followed rather straight paths toward Candida spores with mean McCutcheon chemotactic ratios higher than +0.9. Table 1 also shows the effects of colchicine on neutrophil chemotaxis. Observation of these cells showed that colchicine treatment caused the cell to become more plastic and irregular in morphology and to follow more irregular paths with occasional sharp turns away from the yeast, usually followed by corrections at the next turn. Analysis of the turns made by colchicine-treated cells showed that the major effect of the drug was on the direction of turning of neutrophils. Normal neutrophils migrating toward Candida did not deviate sharply from their paths, and most of the turns made were at an angle of less than 25° from the line of the path they were following before turning (76% in Table 1). Table 1 shows that colchicine treatment caused an increase in the mean angle of turn of cells migrating in the gradient. This was reflected in a drop in the McCutcheon chemotactic ratio but the cells still reached and ingested the Candida. The mean velocity of neutrophils untreated with colchicine in this experiment was 15.6 μm per min with very marked differences between different cells (some moving at up to 70 μm per min for short periods). Velocity was not altered by colchicine treatment in these experiments nor was the frequency of turning of the cells altered. Cells incubated immediately with colchicine showed normal behavior and incoordination increased slowly (Table 1), which is consistent with the idea that colchicine affects locomotion by an action inside the cell, e.g., as an inhibitor of microtubule polymerization.

Visual Assay of Chemokinesis

The behavior of leukocytes exposed to uniform concentrations of an attractant without any gradient source, i.e., under chemokinetic conditions, was studied by filming cells migrating in a uniform concentration of casein (1 mg/ml). Cells in Gey's solution without casein showed almost no displacement. Addition of casein caused a chemokinetic reaction, since the cells showed an acceleration of locomotion. Cells observed during the first 400 sec after beginning filming moved with a mean velocity of 12 μm per min. During the second 400 sec, their mean velocity had dropped to 10.8 μm per min, and during the third 400 sec, to 9 μm per min. The paths taken by individual cells were tracked and analyzed by plotting mean square displacement against time, as described for fibroblasts by Gail (10) and Gail and Boone (11). If the cells were to show pure random-walk locomotion, this plot should be a straight line passing through the origin. The plot actually obtained was very similar to that obtained for fibroblasts by Gail (10) (Fig. 2). It is linear except near the origin, and the straight line extrapolates not to zero but to the time intercept. Neutrophils moving in a given direction tend to persist in that direction and not to make sharp turns away from it (P. C. Wilkinson, *unpublished data*), and, as in fibroblasts, it is probably this "persistent random-walk" locomotion that accounts for nonlinearity near the origin in Fig. 2. Slowing of the cells as the experiment proceeded, the cause for which is not known, may account for the flattening of the top of the curve in Fig. 2.

Visual Assay of Chemotaxis Using Soluble Attractants Diffusing From Beads of Sephadex

A serious limitation to visual assays is that, so far, to study chemotaxis, it has proved necessary to use a solid object, e.g., a clump of bacteria, a damaged erythrocyte (4), or a yeast, as the gradient source. This has excluded study of

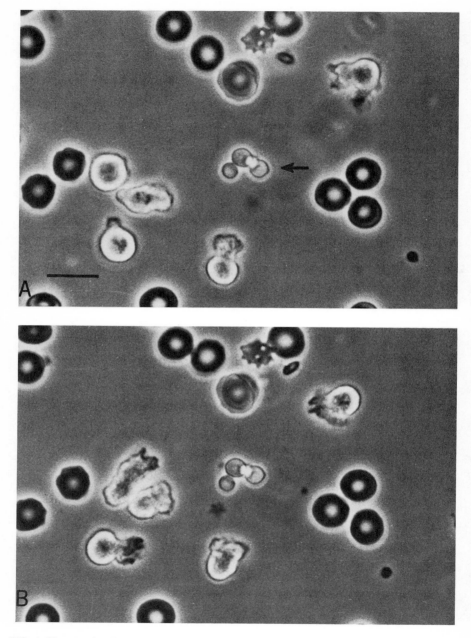

FIG. 1. Chemotaxis of human blood neutrophils to *Candida albicans* followed by phagocytosis (in sequence). **A.** A group of *Candida albicans* blastospores is seen in the center of the field *(arrow)*. The behavior of nearby neutrophils is shown in **A** to **D.** There is an interval of about 45 sec between **A** and **D.** The cells and yeasts are in Gey's solution + 20% normal

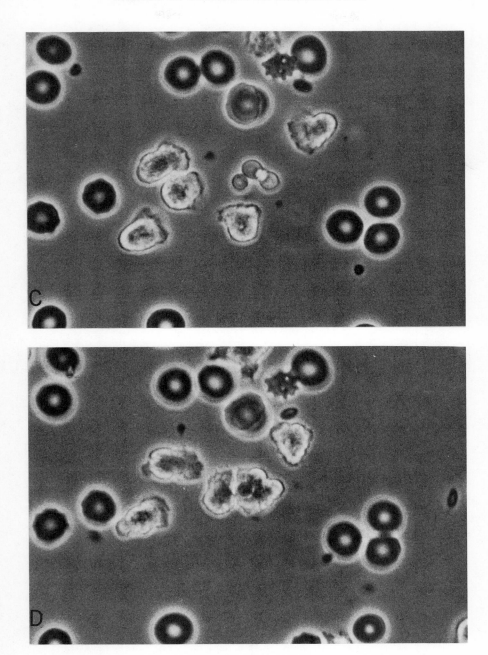

human plasma at 37°C. Note the orientation of the cells toward the Candida, followed by chemotaxis in a near-straight-line path, and engulfment **(D)** of the whole group of blastospores. (From Wilkinson et al., ref. 39, with permission). The bar represents 10 μm.

TABLE 1. *Chemotactic ratios and turning behavior of human blood neutrophils moving toward* Candida albicans *with and without treatment with colchicine*

Treatment of cells with	Conditions of treatment	Number of cells observed	Mean chemotactic ratio[a] ± SEM	Turning Behavior	
				Number of turns observed	Percentage of turns through an angle less than 25°
No treatment	No pretreatment Cells observed in first 15 min. after adding drug	28	+0.96 ± 0.007	130	76
Colchicine 5 × 10⁻⁴ M	No pretreatment Cells observed in first 15 min. after adding drug	7	+0.92 ± 0.03	40	64
Colchicine 5 × 10⁻⁴ M	No pretreatment Cells observed 15 to 25 min. after adding drug	9	+0.83 ± 0.03	63	43
Colchicine 5 × 10⁻⁵ M	30 min. pretreatment 20 min. observation	7	+0.83 ± 0.04	59	37
Colchicine 5 × 10⁻⁴ M	30 min. pretreatment 20 min. observation	3[b]	+0.63 ± 0.07	33	30

[a] Chemotactic ratio = $\dfrac{\text{Net displacement toward gradient source}}{\text{Total distance traveled by the cell}}$. The plus sign indicates displacement *toward* the source.

[b] The reason for the small number of cells in some samples is because, for valid comparison, the table only includes observations made on a single day using one cell batch; however other experiments with other cells showed the same pattern of results.

[c] The mean starting distance of the cells from the source was about 50 μm and did not vary significantly among the different groups.

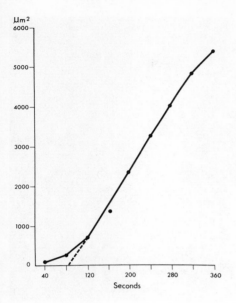

FIG. 2. Mean square displacement against time for human blood neutrophils migrating in the presence of casein (1 mg/ml: no gradient). The *dashed line* shows linear extrapolation to the time intercept.

some of the most interesting chemotactic factors which are soluble and not generated at a solid source. We have attempted to overcome this problem by allowing soluble chemotactic factors of known molecular weight to permeate into beads of Sephadex (Pharmacia, Uppsala, Sweden) of appropriate pore size such that the chemotactic factor enters the gel. We then place the Sephadex bead containing the chemotactic factor under a coverslip in a suspension of cells and study the locomotion of leukocytes in relation to it. If the experiment goes well, the chemotactic factor will diffuse out from the bead, and leukocytes will migrate toward it in response and accumulate under it. Neutrophil leukocytes can be shown to move toward such beads (Figs. 3 and 4). The gradient source is much larger than in the Candida assay, and, until now, results have proved to be somewhat more unpredictable. One reason is apparent from Fig. 4. In some sectors, cells were migrating in fairly direct paths toward the bead, whereas in other sectors their migration was random. This is probably because in those sectors the gradient was disturbed by local currents. The mean McCutcheon ratio for two experiments in which leukocytes were migrating toward casein diffusing from a Sephadex bead was +0.44 and +0.31, i.e., substantially lower than in the Candida assay, although many individual cells gave ratios higher than +0.7. Colchicine-treated cells gave a ratio near to zero, showing no mean net migration either toward the bead or away from it. This is an interesting result because it shows that the demonstration of chemotaxis and its abolition by drugs such as colchicine are very dependent on assay conditions. In the sharp, short-range gradients in the Candida assay, but not in the Sephadex bead assay, colchicine-treated cells still moved up the gradient chemotactically.

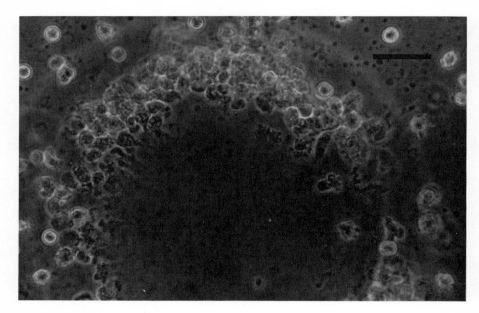

FIG. 3. Human blood neutrophils accumulating around a bead of Sephadex G200 which has been soaked in casein (1 mg/ml), rinsed, and added to a slide-and-coverslip preparation of leukocytes. Photograph was taken 30 min later. The bar represents 40 μm.

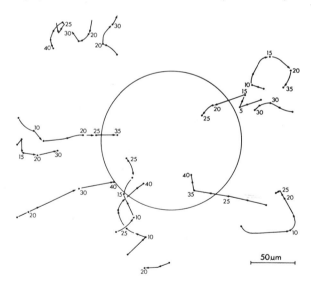

FIG. 4. Paths of human blood neutrophils migrating toward a bead of Sephadex G 200 containing casein (1 mg/ml). Observation was over a 45-minute period. The figures represent the position of individual cells at given times after starting the experiment. Note that in certain sectors cells are showing locomotion in fairly straight paths toward the bead, but that cells in other sectors (e.g., *upper left*) show little evidence that they are detecting a gradient.

At present, the Sephadex bead assay in our hands gives rather imprecise results possibly because the gradients obtained are easily disturbed. The method is promising but obviously requires further refinement.

From this brief account, it is apparent that visual assays of the movement of individual cells give much useful information. They provide an unequivocal demonstration of chemotaxis or chemokinesis and allow a detailed analysis of the locomotor behavior of cells. The changes that drugs and other chemical substances effect in this behavior can be equally studied in detail. None of this information can be obtained so clearly using the filter assay.

MICROPORE FILTER ASSAYS

The second group of assays of chemotaxis to be considered comprises those in which the effect of chemoattractants on locomotion of a whole population of cells, or of a sample of a population, is measured. In these assays, no attempt is made to follow the paths traveled by individual cells. Indeed, measurement is usually made after stopping cell migration, e.g., by fixation in alcohol. The micropore filter assay is the most widely used in this group, but other assays, e.g., the agarose assay, are essentially of the same type. There is no doubt that Boyden opened a new era in the study of leukocyte locomotion when he introduced the micropore filter assay (6). This assay was easy to use, gave a reasonably accurate and quantitative measurement of the movement of the cell population under study, and, in a period of a few years, allowed the study of numerous attractants and the documentation of their action. It became possible to make comparisons between the responses to chemoattractants of cells from patients and cells from control subjects. Many researchers were attracted to use the technique. As mentioned above, during this time it was assumed and seldom questioned that what was measured was chemotaxis when an attractant was placed below a filter and cells moved through the filter toward it. The paper of Zigmond and Hirsch (41) represented a watershed, since this was the first publication to examine this assumption in detail. This paper also introduced the "leading-front" measurement into filter studies. Briefly, in using the leading-front technique, cells are allowed to migrate into a filter but not to traverse its complete width. The experiment is stopped before the cells reach the lower surface, and the distance migrated by the leading front of cells (two or more cells per high-power field) is measured using the micrometer fine adjustment on the microscope. Previously, most workers had quantified cell migration by counting the number of cells reaching the lower surface of the filter. We do not want to embark upon a detailed comparison of different filter techniques here, since these have been discussed extensively elsewhere (32), but we may be permitted to reiterate our belief that the leading-front technique is much the best of those presently in use. The reasons are these: It allows discrimination of very small increases in migration above background. In our hands, increases in distance of 10 μm above the negative control reached by the leading front of cells moving toward a weak attractant are usually of statistical significance, increases which would not be detected by counting cells on the lower surface of the filter because the cells would only arrive there after a very prolonged interval. Those who have used both methods agree that leading-front method gives a lower scatter in single experiments and better reproducibility between experiments than lower surface counts. Some reasons for inaccuracy in the lower surface count have been reported elsewhere (16,32), particularly the tendency of cells to drop off the lower surface of filters. This inaccuracy is improved by double-filter techniques, but such techniques call for considerable migration on the part of the cells before any response is detected and do not pick up the small increases above background which the leading-front method picks up. Finally, the leading-front method is the only one that allows a detailed analysis of the influence of both the absolute concentration of the attractant and the concentration gradient of the attractant on cell locomotion, and it therefore allows the distinction to be made between chemotaxis and chemokinesis. Demonstration of this distinction is made by checkerboard assay and has now been achieved successfully by workers in a number of laboratories (1,24,25,34,41). Examples of its use are discussed later in this chapter (see Tables 2 and 3).

Analysis of the checkerboard does, however, depend on a number of assumptions, e.g., that the gradient in a filter is linear between two points, is stable, and has been accurately set up. It must be admitted that the visual assay gives a much clearer demonstration of the influence of attractants on the rate and direction of leukocyte locomotion than the checkerboard filter assay. Checkerboard assays can only be done using filters much wider than a cell diameter, e.g., the cellulose ester filters of 100 to 150 μm thickness which most workers use. They are unsuitable for use with the much thinner polycarbonate filters. The leading-front method has been criticized on the grounds that it might give misleading results if two cell populations migrating at different speeds were present (27). Since we are now interested in lymphocyte chemotaxis (24,38), this will present a problem if different lymphocyte subsets have different locomotor properties, as seems likely to be the case. An easy way to check this should be to make counts at intervals of 10 μm depth within the filter. Biphasic distribution curves should be detected in cases in which there are indeed two migrating populations. It remains to be seen how useful this will be.

Colchicine-treated leukocytes studied by the checkerboard assay lose the ability to detect gradients of chemotactic factors. We have published such a study of lymphoblasts (24) and have similar unpublished data on neutrophils and monocytes. Nevertheless, in the visual assay with Candida, the same cells orient toward the yeasts and reach toward them. Almost certainly, in filters, the nature of the substrate on which the cells move, which is a tortuous matrix, means that the cells have to take very indirect paths to reach the lower surface. Thus, it may only require a slight decrease in the efficiency of cellular orientation, as seen in colchicine-treated cells, for the chemotactic effect to be lost altogether. It might be said that the nature of the filter assay loads the dice against the cells, and it is perhaps remarkable that their chemotactic reactions are clearly demonstrable in filters.

ADVANTAGES AND DISADVANTAGES OF THE TWO METHODS

To summarize, both types of assay have advantages and disadvantages, some of which are listed below.

Visual assays allow detailed examination of the morphological events in moving cells and the influence on these of attractants, inhibitors, and drugs. By analysis of the paths taken by cells, a detailed description of the influence of these agents on cell velocity, direction of movement, turning behavior, etc., can be obtained. This provides essential information for interpreting the mechanism of locomotion at the cellular and molecular level. The disadvantages of the assay are that it is fairly difficult at present to quantify cell response to a given agent, i.e., to obtain dose-response curves. This is partly because such agents may affect many variables. Once there is a solid body of work showing which variables give useful information, it may be possible to study, e.g., turning angles or chemotactic ratios and the factors that influence them. The visual assay is relatively sophisticated and requires care, time, and patience to get good results. Dependence on a solid gradient source is a drawback, and there is at present no way of predictably obtaining a gradient of known steepness from a source of known strength.

Without the filter assay, it is certain that the rapid progress achieved in the chemotaxis field during the past decade could never have been made. It is technically simple and, in its better variants, fairly sensitive and reproducible. Dose-response curves are easily obtained, and the method has proved ideal for the assay of unknown factors for attractant or inhibitory activity; however it gives no information about the morphology, direction of path, or turning behavior of moving cells. It does not distinguish chemotaxis from chemokinesis except when the checkerboard assay is used, and even that is very indirect compared to the visual assay.

Since the two assays give different types of information and neither gives a complete picture of the locomotor behavior of leukocytes, it would seem sensible to use both techniques in parallel.

IMPORTANCE OF THE MEDIUM IN WHICH CELLS MOVE: ROLES OF SERUM ALBUMIN

In the remainder of this chapter, we shall discuss the influence of the medium in which cells are suspended on their locomotion and on their interaction with chemoattractants. There are a number of discussions in the literature of the effects of temperature and pH (8,32) and of composition of ions (3,8,26,29,33) in the medium on leukocyte locomotion, but here we shall consider a variable which has not been studied for a number of years, namely, the influence of protein added to the medium. It is well known that cells that are not otherwise under the influence of an attractant migrate better in an albumin-containing medium than in one without protein (15). Here we shall consider three aspects of the importance of albumin for leukocyte locomotion: (a) the chemokinetic effect of serum albumin: (b) the effect of albumin on the response of leukocytes to chemotactic factors, and (c) the effect of albumin on the modulation of chemotactic responses by drugs. All these studies were carried out using the micropore filter technique and quantified with the leading-front method.

The Chemokinetic Effect of Albumin

Table 2 shows a checkerboard assay for human blood neutrophils migrating into filters in the presence of different concentrations of bovine serum albumin (BSA) above and below the filter. No other attractant was present. The migration observed came very close to that expected (figures in parentheses) if the cells had been responding, not to the concentration gradient of the BSA but to the absolute BSA concentration in the cell's environment, and this may therefore be taken as evidence that the influence of BSA on leukocyte locomotion was chemokinetic and not chemotactic. Thus, the presence of BSA in the medium caused the cells to move faster at random. Leukocytes in HSA behaved in exactly the same way; however serum albumin could not be replaced by other proteins. Nonalbumin proteins such as IgG or gelatin did not have a chemokinetic effect on leukocyte locomotion in filters, and cells in media containing these proteins migrated like cells moving in the absence of protein.

Note that denaturation of HSA (or BSA) causes it to become chemotactic for leukocytes. It is necessary to demonstrate by a checkerboard assay that

TABLE 2. *Migration of human blood neutrophils in various absolute concentrations and concentration gradients of bovine serum albumin (BSA : Sigma)*

		Distance traveled in μm in a 3-μm pore-size filter in 75 min BSA concentration (μg, ml^{-1}) below filter				
		0	50	200	350	500
BSA	0	19				
Concentration	50		20	20(20)	21(21)	23(21)
Above	200		23(24)	24	27(25)	27(26)
Filter	350		33(31)	33(32)	33	35(34)
	500		41(37)	38(37)	38(38)	39

The figures on the diagonal from upper left to lower right represent migration in various absolute BSA concentrations but no gradient. Above the diagonal there is a positive gradient, below it a negative gradient. Figures without parentheses represent experimental observations. Those in parentheses represent theoretical migration expected if cells only detected the absolute concentration and not the gradient. They are based on the calculations described by Zigmond and Hirsch (41). Note that the observed migration is extremely close to migration expected on the basis of a response to the absolute concentration but not the gradient of BSA. In other words, BSA is acting as a chemokinetic not a chemotactic factor in this assay.

TABLE 3. *Migration of human blood neutrophils in various absolute concentrations and concentration gradients of alkali-denatured human serum albumin (HSA Behringwerke)*

		Distance traveled in μm in a 3-μm pore-size filter in 75 min Denatured HSA concentration ($\mu g \cdot ml^{-1}$) below filter				
		0	50	200	350	500
Denatured	0	50				
HSA	50		58	75(60)	76(61)	76(63)
Concentration	200		60(63)	65	77(67)	79(69)
Above	350		69(69)	66(71)	73	76(71)
Filter	500		63(70)	60(69)	67(67)	65

For explanation of experimental conditions, see footnote to Table 2, above. Since HSA is itself chemokinetic (cf. BSA, Table 2), the total HSA concentration in each chamber has been made up to 1 mg per milliliter. For example, in the chamber shown at the upper right, the cells were in 50 μg per milliliter denatured HSA + 950 μg per milliliter native HSA, and below the filter, the medium contained 500 μg per milliliter denatured HSA + 500 μg per milliliter native HSA. Thus any chemokinetic effect of the HSA should be the same throughout the test. Note in contrast to Table 2 that cells migrating in positive gradients of denatured HSA are traveling further into the filter than would be expected on the basis of a response to absolute concentration alone, and that cells migrating in negative gradients are traveling a shorter distance than would be expected. In other words, denatured HSA is acting as a chemotactic factor.

this effect of denaturation really is chemotactic and does not just represent a chemokinetic effect. Table 3 shows a checkerboard assay for human blood leukocytes migrating in various absolute concentrations and concentration gradients of HSA which had been denatured at pH 12 for 24 hours at 20°C in H_2O followed by return to physiological conditions. Since native HSA itself is chemokinetic, the total HSA concentration in all chambers both above and below the filter was made up to 1 mg per milliliter by adding sufficient native HSA to give this overall HSA (native + denatured) concentration throughout and thus to remove bias resulting from varying absolute protein concentrations. Table 3 shows that cells migrating in denatured HSA were responsive to the gradient, since the distance migrated in positive gradients was higher and in negative gradients was lower than that expected on the basis of random migration alone. We have suggested elsewhere that this chemotactic effect of denaturation of HSA (31,35) and of other proteins (30) is caused by exposure of hydrophobic groups that penetrate the phospholipid bilayer of the cell membrane. Since denatured proteins may be chemotactic, it is very important to use only good quality native albumin preparations for chemotaxis studies.

Effect of Serum Albumin on the Response of Leukocytes to Chemotactic Factors

Serum albumin is well known to bind a wide range of molecules. For example, it carries binding sites with fairly high association constants for fatty acids

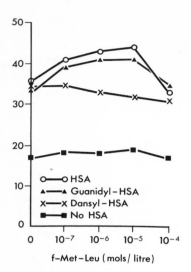

FIG. 5. Neutrophil migration. The response of human blood neutrophils in filters of 3-μm pore size to formyl-methionyl-leucine in the absence of serum albumin and in the presence of untreated serum albumin and of serum albumin conjugated to dansyl chloride or guanidylated with O-methyl isourea. Note that a response to the peptide is seen in the presence of HSA or guanidyl-HSA but not in the absence of HSA, or the presence of dansyl-HSA. Note also that background chemokinesis in the presence of all HSA preparations, including dansyl-HSA, is higher than in the absence of protein.

$[K = 10^6 - 10^8 \ (14)]$, for detergents (K *circa* 10^6), for indole, tryptophan, and many other small molecules [reviewed in (28)]. Many of the substances bound by albumin are anionic and partially hydrophobic in character. Since albumin is such a protean carrier of other molecules, it is possible and worth exploring that chemotactic factors in an albumin medium may become bound by the albumin and presented to the cell surface as an albumin-chemotactic factor complex.

We have studied the effects of serum albumin on the responses of leukocytes to a number of chemotactic factors, and a preliminary report has been published elsewhere (36). It was found (Fig. 5) that leukocytes which, when suspended in serum albumin, responded well to low-molecular-weight chemotactic factors such as formylmethionyl peptides, failed to respond to the same peptides when suspended in albumin-free media. Table 4 shows an extension of these findings. Human blood neutrophils and monocytes in albumin-free media did not respond to several low-molecular-weight chemotactic factors including formylmethionyl peptides, fatty acids, and dibutyryl cyclic AMP, but did respond to protein chemotactic factors such as casein and denatured HSA. When albumin was added, the cells responded normally to both low- and high-molecular-weight attractants. Albumin could not be replaced by other proteins in these experiments. Leukocytes in IgG, myoglobin, or gelatin did not respond to low-molecular-weight attractants.

To test the possibility that the low-molecular-weight factors were binding to albumin (a possibility for which there is firm evidence in the case of fatty acids) the chemoattractants were incubated with HSA, passed through a column of Sephadex G25, and the protein peak fraction and the low-molecular-weight peak fraction were separated and tested for activity (Table 5). Chemoattractant

TABLE 4. The effect of HSA and other proteins on migration of human blood leukocytes toward chemotactic factors

Attractant below filter	Neutrophil migration (μm in 75 min, 3-μm filter pore size)					Monocyte migration (μm in 2 hr, 12 μm filter pore size)	
	No added protein	HSA (1 mg/ml)	IgG (1 mg/ml)	Gelatin (1 mg/ml)	Myoglobin (1 mg/ml)	No added protein	HSA (1 mg/ml)
Negative control (Gey's only)	14 ± 0.6	24 ± 2.9	27 ± 1.6	23 ± 2.5	26 ± 1.0	36 ± 2.4	35 ± 3.0
fMet-Leu 10^{-5} M	16 ± 1.5	57 ± 2.0	24 ± 2.3	26 ± 2.5	21 ± 1.0	35 ± 1.9	46 ± 2.0
Linolenic acid 3×10^{-6} M (approx)	13 ± 0.7	41 ± 2.6	29 ± 2.5	19 ± 1.4	20 ± 1.3	36 ± 2.7	48 ± 2.8
Dibutyryl cAMP 10^{-5} M	11 ± 1.4	43 ± 1.4		15 ± 1.4			
CAT-CCT peptides (10 μg/ml approx)	16 ± 0.7	41 ± 3.3	15 ± 0.8	22 ± 1.0	18 ± 1.1		
Alkali-denatured HSA (1 mg/ml)	72 ± 5.4	60 ± 1.9	56 ± 2.1	68 ± 4.7	83 ± 3.9	84 ± 2.9	62 ± 4.2
Casein (1 mg/ml)	72 ± 3.7	71 ± 2.4	65 ± 2.1	82 ± 3.3		79 ± 3.2	54 ± 5.2
Succinyl-melittin (500 μg/ml)	50 ± 3.3	86 ± 2.2	59 ± 2.4	61 ± 2.4			

Note: Figures are means of 10 measurements in duplicate filters ±SEM PHA-transformed human lymphocytes, not shown, gave an identical pattern of results.

CAT-CCT peptides are anaphylatoxic peptides purified from dextran-activated serum by Dr. J. H. Wissler. From Wilkinson (36) with permission.

TABLE 5. *Chemoattractant activity of fractions from Sephadex columns for blood neutrophils*

Material placed on column (20 × 1 cm)	Migration (mean ± SEM) of neutrophils in Gey's solution toward	
	Protein fraction (tested at 1 mg/ml)	Low mol. weight fraction (tested at approx 10^{-5} M)
G25 column no.		
HSA alone 10 mg	32 ± 1.1	
HSA 10 mg + fMet-Phe 10^{-4} M	42 ± 1.5	21 ± 1.5 [a]
HSA 10 mg + fMet-Met 10^{-4} M	51 ± 1.8	31 ± 1.7
HSA 10 mg + linolenic acid 10^{-4} M	44 ± 2.0	23 ± 1.2
G100 column no.		
HSA 20 mg alone	32 ± 0.9	
HSA 20 mg + CAT-CCT peptides 2 mg	40 ± 1.2	26 ± 1.3 [b]

[a] Monitored by OD_{257} (λmax. fMet-Phe)
[b] Monitored by OD_{278}.
From Wilkinson (36), with permission.

activity appeared in the protein fraction rather than in the low-molecular-weight fraction, suggesting that it was albumin-bound chemotactic factor rather than free chemotactic factor which was attracting the cells.

The possibility exists that the chemokinetic effect of serum albumin is necessary for leukocytes to respond chemotactically to small molecular attractants, but not required for a response to large proteins. In other words, albumin somehow "turns on" locomotion, and this is necessary for a response to small molecules, but protein attractants can themselves replace albumin in this role. Recent experiments, however, suggested that the chemokinetic effects of albumin could be dissociated from its effects on chemotaxis of leukocytes to fMet peptides. Binding sites on albumin for many small molecules can be blocked by covalently bonding appropriate groups to the albumin molecule, one of which, the dansyl group, has been shown to block the albumin binding site for indole (12). This is apparently a fairly flexible site that binds a number of ligands with a wide range of affinities (13). Figure 5 shows a comparison of the effects of adding native HSA or dansylated HSA to a suspension of human blood neutrophils on their ability to migrate toward fMet-Leu. It was apparent that dansylated HSA did not support cell migration to fMet-Leu, whereas native HSA (and HSA conjugated to a different group, the guanidyl group) did allow such migration; however dansylated HSA still did act as a chemokinetic agent for leukocytes in the same way as native HSA, i.e., the migration in the absence of any chemotactic factor was the same in the presence of either protein.

In summary, these findings suggest that the presence of serum albumin is obligatory for the chemotactic activity of low-molecular-weight attractants such as peptides and lipids. (We have similar unpublished findings with ECFs-A

Val-Gly-Ser-Glu and Ala-Gly-Ser-Glu as attractants for neutrophils and monocytes.) Two explanations suggest themselves: first, that since albumin is demonstrably chemokinetic for leukocytes, this effect is necessary as a "support" for cell locomotion to other factors but that this support does not depend on binding of the chemotactic factor to albumin; second, that albumin binds to the chemotactic factors and presents them to the cell. We favor the second alternative (a) because chemoattractant activity appears in the albumin fraction when albumin-peptide mixtures are put through Sephadex, suggesting binding of peptides to albumin, and (b) because blocking-defined binding sites on albumin abolishes the ability of albumin to act as a support medium for migration to these factors, suggesting that the factors may bind to albumin at these sites. If this view is correct, it must be taken into account in interpreting the interactions of low-molecular-weight chemotactic factors with cells.

The Effects of the Presence of Albumin on Drug-induced Changes in Leukocyte Locomotion

Albumin binds to many small molecules used as pharmacological and therapeutic agents. We have recently carried out a survey of the effects of anesthetic drugs on leukocyte locomotion in filters (19). This study, which was largely based on measuring the locomotion of cells to protein attractants in albumin-free media, showed that anesthetics of all three major classes—local, intravenous (inductional), and inhalational—had varied but often profound inhibitory effects on leukocyte locomotion. These effects, however, could be partially protected against by addition of serum albumin to the medium. Figure 6 shows the effect of different doses of the intravenous anesthetic thiopentone on the response of blood neutrophils to casein in the presence and absence of HSA, and it is clear that the drug was less effective in the presence of HSA than in its absence. Thiopentone is a drug of the barbiturate group; it is known to bind to albumin, and it is possible that albumin-bound thiopentone is less able to enter cells and paralyze the locomotor mechanism than free drug. Since serum albumin

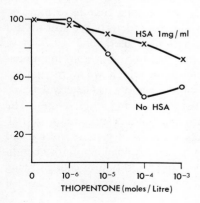

FIG. 6. Neutrophil migration. The inhibitory effect of thiopentone on human blood neutrophil migration toward casein (800 μg/ml) in filters in the presence and absence of HSA. The failure of thiopentone (no HSA) at 10^{-3}M to inhibit more than at 10^{-4}M is a result of the insolubility of this drug at high concentrations.

is a constituent of the normal environment of leukocytes, such protective actions need to be considered in evaluating the effects of many drugs on these cells.

These observations demonstrate clearly that albumin added to media used for chemotaxis assays, the presence of which is often taken for granted, has a variety of effects which can influence the results obtained. It is chemokinetic in its own right, it may bind chemotactic factors and act as a carrier to present them at cell membranes, and its presence will influence the actions of drugs on cells.

CONCLUSIONS

In closing this survey of some aspects of methodology in leukocyte chemotaxis, we have to come back to the questions posed in the first paragraph. To what extent are our techniques likely to help, and to what extent to impede, our search for the truth. Overall, it is the personal feeling of the authors that we are reasonably fortunate in the methods available. The best filter methods give a reproducibility that is a good deal superior to that of many other techniques used for the study of cells in immunology *in vitro.* Perhaps the main failing evident in the use of filter methods in recent years has been the confusion and lack of curiosity about the nature of the cellular response that was actually being measured. A wider appreciation of the nature of the chemokinetic and chemotactic reactions of leukocytes should remove this confusion. In any case, the use of time-lapse cinematographic studies of moving cells, and the development of improved methods for analyzing tactic and kinetic reactions, should supply a corrective and a control on data obtained using filters. It is this availability of two complementary, reasonably reproducible methods, which use different approaches but which optimally should be used side by side, that gives grounds for feeling progress can and will be made in the next few years.

On the other hand, there are areas in which progress has been slower. The comparison of two cell populations, e.g., blood leukocytes from a patient and a control subject, is still risky, and this makes progress in clinical studies difficult. Cells from blood samples taken and treated in as nearly an identical way as possible can still differ in locomotor capacity for reasons that have more to do with their treatment *in vitro* than with any intrinsic defect. We still do not understand the importance of factors like adhesion or metabolic behavior in regulating locomotion of leukocytes, or to what extent our laboratory manipulations upset these functions. Finally, the criticism to which we were perhaps most of all vulnerable is that we have not shown that chemotaxis (strictly defined) occurs *in vivo* or that it plays a role in inflammation in living tissues. The circumstantial evidence that it does is now enormous, but it is still circumstantial. It would seen extravagant for cells to possess such an elegant orienting and direction-finding mechanism if they only used it under artificial laboratory conditions. Nevertheless, the demonstration of directional migration of cells in living tissues is difficult and is not a goal which attracts many investigators. Even if it could be demonstrated, and there are reports that it can be (9), the experiment would still be open to the criticism that directional migration in tissues can as well be a result of contact guidance as of chemotaxis, and the two cannot be distinguished *in vivo*. At present, there seems little prospect of progress, from studies in living animals, in understanding the role of chemotaxis in inflammation. This is ironic, since many who are working on inflammation are convinced that it is only *in vivo* models of inflammation that give realistic information of possible use in developing therapeutic agents. The conditions of assay of chemotaxis *in vitro* are much too simplified for them to serve as models for inflammation; however, these assays are at present yielding a spate of information that is certainly increasing our understanding of the role of leukocytes in clearance, inflammation, and immune reactions, in maintaining the *status quo* of healthy tissues, and in removing destructive agents from foci of disease. They should also be of considerable use in unraveling the basic cellular and molecular biology of cell locomotion, a field in which it seems that striking advances will probably be made during the next few years.

ACKNOWLEDGMENT

R.B.A. is supported by a HERT grant to the Department of Anaesthesia, Royal Infirmary, Glasgow, Scotland.

REFERENCES

1. Anderson, R., Glover, A., Koornhof, H. J., and Rabson, A. R. (1976): *In vitro* stimulation of neutrophil motility by levamisole: Maintenance of cGMP levels in chemotactically stimulated levamisole-treated neutrophils. *J. Immunol.*, 117:428–432.
2. Armstrong, P. B., and Lackie, J. M. (1975): Studies on intercellular invasion *in vitro* using rabbit peritoneal neutrophil granulocytes (PMNs): I. Role of contact inhibition in locomotion. *J. Cell. Biol.*, 65:439–462.
3. Becker, E. L., and Showell, H. J. (1972): The effect of Ca^{2+} and Mg^{2+} on the chemotactic responsiveness and spontaneous motility of rabbit polymorphonuclear leukocytes. *Z. Immunitaetsforsch*, 143:466–476.
4. Bessis, M. (1974): Necrotaxis: Chemotaxis towards an injured cell. *Antibiot. Chemother.*, 19:369–381.
5. Black, J. (1803): *Lectures on the Elements of Chemistry,* Vol. I, p. 193. University of Edinburgh, Edinburgh, Scotland.
6. Boyden, S. V. (1962): The chemotactic effect of mixtures of antibody and antigen on polymorphonuclear leucocytes. *J. Exp. Med.*, 115:453–466.
7. de Bruyn, P. P. H. (1944): Locomotion of blood cells in tissue cultures. *Anat. Rec.*, 89:43–63.
8. Bryant, R. E., de Prez, R. M., Van Way, M. H., and Rogers, D. E. (1966): Studies on leukocyte motility: I. Effects of alterations of pH electrolyte concentration and phagocytosis on leukocyte migration, adhesiveness and aggregation. *J. Exp. Med.*, 124:483–499.
9. Buckley, I. K. (1963): Delayed secondary damage and leucocyte chemotaxis following focal aseptic heat injury in vivo. *Exp. Mol. Pathol.*, 2:402–417.
10. Gail, M. (1973): Time lapse studies on the motility of fibroblasts in tissue culture. In: *Locomotion of Tissue Cells,* Ciba Foundation Symposium *14,* edited by G. E. Wolstenholme and J. Knight, pp. 287–310. ASP, Amsterdam.
11. Gail, M. H., and Boone, C. W. (1970): The locomotion of mouse fibroblasts in tissue culture. *Biophys. J.,* 10:980–993.

12. Gambhir, K. K., and McMenamy, R. H. (1973): Location of the indole binding site in human serum albumin. *J. Biol. Chem.,* 248:1956–1960.
13. Gambhir, K. K., McMenamy, R. H., and Watson, F. (1975): Positions in human serum albumin which involve the indole binding site. *J. Biol. Chem.,* 250:6711–6719.
14. Goodman, D. S. (1958): The interaction of human serum albumin with long-chain fatty acid anions. *J. Am. Chem. Soc.,* 80:3892–3898.
15. Keller, H. U. (1966): Studies on chemotaxis: III. Modification of Boyden's technique for the evaluation of chemotactic agents. *Immunology,* 10:225–230.
16. Keller, H. U., Borel, J. F., Wilkinson, P. C., Hess, M., and Cottier, H. (1972): Reassessment of Boyden's technique for measuring chemotaxis. *J. Immunol. Methods,* 1:165–168.
17. Keller, H. U., Wilkinson, P. C., Abercrombie, M., Becker, E. L., Hirsch, J. G., Miller, M. E., Ramsey, W. S., and Zigmond, S. H. (1977): A proposal for the definition of terms related to locomotion of leucocytes and other cells. *Clin. Exp. Immunol.,* 27:377–380.
18. McCutcheon, M. (1946): Chemotaxis in leukocytes. *Physiol. Rev.,* 26:319–336.
19. Moudgil, G. C., Allan, R. B., Russell, R. J., and Wilkinson, P. C. (1977): Inhibitions by anaesthetic agents of human leucocyte locomotion towards chemical attractants. *Br. J. Anaesth.,* 49:97–105.
20. Popper, K. R. (1959): *The Logic of Scientific Discovery.* Hutchinson, London.
21. Ramsey, W. S. (1972): Analysis of individual leucocyte behaviour during chemotaxis. *Exp. Cell. Res.,* 70:129–139.
22. Ramsey, W. S. (1972): Locomotion of human polymorphonuclear leukocytes. *Exp. Cell. Res.,* 72:489–501.
23. Robineaux, R. L. (1964): Movements of cells involved in inflammation and immunity. In: *Primitive Motile Systems in Cell Biology,* edited by R. D. Allen and N. Kamiya, pp. 351–364. Academic Press, New York.
24. Russell, R. J., Wilkinson, P. C., Sless, F., and Parrott, D. M. V. (1975): Chemotaxis of lymphoblasts. *Nature,* 256:646–648.
25. Showell, H. J., Freer, R. J., Zigmond, S. H., Schiffmann, E., Aswanikumar, S., Corcoran, B., and Becker, E. (1976): The structure-activity relations of synthetic peptides as chemotactic factors and inducers of lysosomal enzyme secretion for neutrophils. *J. Exp. Med.,* 143:1154–1169.
26. Showell, H. J., and Becker, E. L. (1976): The effects of external K^+ and Na^+ on the chemotaxis of rabbit peritoneal neutrophils. *J. Immunol.,* 116:99–105.
27. Snyderman, R., and Mergenhagen, S. E. (1976): Chemotaxis of macrophages. In: *Immunobiology of the Macrophage,* edited by D. S. Nelson, pp. 323–348. Academic Press, New York.
28. Steinhardt, J., and Reynolds, J. A. (1969): *Multiple Equilibria in Proteins.* Academic Press, New York.
29. Ward, P. A., and Becker, E. L. (1970): Potassium reversible inhibition of chemotaxis by ouabain. *Life Sci.,* Part 2, 9:355–360.
30. Wilkinson, P. C. (1973): Recognition of protein structure in leukocyte chemotaxis. *Nature,* 244:512–513.
31. Wilkinson, P. C. (1974): Surface and cell membrane activities of leukocyte chemotactic factors. *Nature,* 251:58–60.
32. Wilkinson, P. C. (1974): *Chemotaxis and Inflammation.* Churchill-Livingstone, Edinburgh, Scotland.
33. Wilkinson, P. C. (1975): Leucocyte locomotion and chemotaxis: The influence of divalent cations and cation ionophores. *Exp. Cell Res.,* 93:420–426.
34. Wilkinson, P. C. (1975): Chemotaxis of leucocytes. In: *Primitive Sensory and Communication Systems: The Taxes and Tropisms of Microorganisms and Cells,* edited by M. J. Carlile, pp. 205–243. Academic Press, New York.
35. Wilkinson, P. C. (1976): Recognition and response in mononuclear and granular phagocytes. *Clin. Exp. Immunol.,* 25:355–356.
36. Wilkinson, P. C. (1976): A requirement for albumin as carrier for low molecular weight leucocyte chemotactic factors. *Exp. Cell. Res.,* 103:415–418.
37. Wilkinson, P. C., and McKay, I. C. (1972): The molecular requirements for chemotactic attraction of leucocytes by proteins: Studies of proteins with synthetic side groups. *Eur. J. Immunol.,* 2:570–577.
38. Wilkinson, P. C., Roberts, J. A., Russell, R. J., and McLoughlin, M. (1976): Chemotaxis of mitogen-activated human lymphocytes and the effects of membrane-active enzymes. *Clin. Exp. Immunol.,* 25:280–287.

39. Wilkinson, P. C., Russell, R. J., and Allan, R. B. (1977): *Leucocytes and Chemotaxis. Agents and Actions (suppl. in press).*
40. Zigmond, S. H. (1974): Mechanisms of sensing chemical gradients by polymorphonuclear leukocytes. *Nature,* 249:450–452.
41. Zigmond, S. H., and Hirsch, J. G. (1973): Leukocyte locomotion and chemotaxis: New methods for evaluation and demonstration of cell-derived chemotactic factor. *J. Exp. Med.,* 137:387–410.

DISCUSSION

Dr. Becker: We find, as you do, Dr. Wilkinson, that protein is needed for any sort of chemotactic response with the synthetic peptides. On the other hand, protein in the medium is not needed for synthetic peptide release of lysosomal enzymes. Evidence has accumulated that the lysosomal enzyme release and the chemotaxis response result from stimulation of the same receptor. I do not know what serum albumin is doing in the chemotactic response, but I suggest that it is not essential for binding but rather something that occurs after binding.

Dr. Schiffmann: With respect to the radio-labeled ligand binding, we do that in the absence of added protein, and it binds perfectly well; in fact, if we add protein, there seems to be slight inhibition of binding. The binding would not appear to depend upon added protein.

Dr. Wilkinson: The explanation usually put forward for the effect of protein has been that protein is "good" for moving cells, which is not very helpful. The whole thing obviously badly needs reexamination.

Dr. Goetzl: I am interested in the effect of high-molecular-weight serum albumin on chemotactic activity, as shown in Table 5. Serum albumin is not homogeneous and there is generally a varying percentage of polymers which are considerably more hydrophobic and more disordered than monomeric albumin. Thus, it would be critical to study the separate effects of denatured monomer albumin and polymeric albumin, both of which molecular species are more hydrophobic than native monomer.

Dr. Wilkinson: The albumin we use (Behringwerke, Marburg, Germany) is a pretty homogeneous product which, judged by its viscosity, surface activity, etc., is completely in native form and is lipid-free. On Sephadex G200 chromatography, there is little or no material forward of the monomer peak.

Dr. Snyderman: From my point of view, the requirement for protein with the formylated peptides is an artifact of the nitrocellulose system, and not really reflective of what is necessary for chemotaxis. We do our binding studies using radio-labeled fMet-Leu-Phe in the absence of any added protein using washed cells, and the binding is perfectly good. The equilibrium dissociation constants for binding have very similar ranges to the KD for chemotaxis.

We have found that with the 5 μ polycarbonate filter assay system, in monocytes that have migrated through the pores, the distance from the top to the bottom of the chamber is only about 15 μ, so that the cells have to go only a short distance.

To show that this assay is indeed measuring chemotaxis, we used lymphocyte-derived chemotactic factor with the checkerboard of doses above and below the filter. The chemokinesis was evident, as well as chemotaxis, when this system was used. This is in the absence of any added protein.

We found the same thing when we used activated human serum as the chemoattractant. When we used the leading-front method and a nitrocellulose filter with the same chemoattractant, we did not really see a chemotactic effect until there was a very high percentage of protein in the medium. With the formulated peptide, chemotaxis can be seen in the complete absence of protein, using the polycarbonate system. But in the nitrocellulose system, protein is needed. I think the protein requirement is an artifact of the nitrocellulose filter assay and does not reflect the effect of protein on the chemotactic response of cells.

Dr. Ward: In the early data that you presented, were the measurements representative of the entire cell population or were you selecting a small part of the total cell population?

Dr. Wilkinson: Not every cell is moving and only the moving cells were analyzed; however, the immobile cells are usually a minority in a carefully prepared neutrophil population.

Dr. Jenson: The protein effect depends very much on the cells. For human cells, for instance, we do not use any protein for chemotactic responses. If guinea pig cells are used, they will not migrate to C5a without any protein, so they have a very strong need for protein. It does not have to be albumin.

Leukocyte Chemotaxis, edited by John I. Gallin
and Paul G. Quie. Raven Press, New York
© 1978.

Chemotaxis of Human Leukocytes Under Agarose

*Robert D. Nelson,**Robert T. McCormack, and
*†Vance D. Fiegel

*Departments of Surgery and Laboratory Medicine-Pathology, and **Department
of Pediatrics, University of Minnesota Medical School, Minneapolis, Minnesota 55455;
*† Department of Surgery, University of Minnesota Medical School,
Minneapolis, Minnesota 55455*

We have recently described a new method for the study of spontaneous migration and chemotaxis of human leukocytes (13). Our method is based upon migration of cells under agarose gel, as described by Carpenter (5) for explanted tissue fragments and used by others (1,2,6,18) to study lymphokine-mediated inhibition of leukocyte migration. A similar assay for measurement of chemotaxis of guinea pig neutrophils has been described by Cutler (7). Our technique has application to both polymorphonuclear neutrophils and monocytes and quantitation of both spontaneous migration and chemotaxis of these cells.

This report describes our experience with the chemotaxis under agarose technique over the year since its original description. Included is an up-to-date summary of responses measured for spontaneous migration and chemotaxis of polymorphonuclear neutrophils and monocytes isolated from healthy volunteers. The correlation of these cell functions is discussed in addition to alternative approaches to assessing chemotactic responses to various cytotaxins. The contribution of anticoagulant, the presence of cells of other types, and medium components to variation in measurement of these cell functions are also discussed. Finally, we consider application of this technique to the study of other aspects of leukocyte migration.

THE AGAROSE METHOD

Isolation of Leukocytes

Blood is drawn using 5 to 10 units of sodium heparin (Upjohn, Kalamazoo, Michigan) per milliliter volume collected. The blood is then transferred to tubes and centrifuged at $200 \times g$ for 15 min to obtain a buffy coat layer. The plasma is transferred to another tube and the buffy coat leukocytes, together with the upper 5 mm of erythrocytes, are resuspended in this plasma. The majority of contaminating erythrocytes are removed by gravity sedimentation at 37° C. The leukocyte-rich plasma is decanted, diluted with an equal volume of minimal essential medium (MEM, supplemented to contain 2mM L-glutamine, 100 units/ ml penicillin and 100 μg/ml streptomycin; all from Grand Island Biologicals Co., Grand Island, N.Y.), layered over lymphocyte separation medium (LSM, Bionetics Laboratory Products, Kensington, Maryland), and leukocyte subpopulations fractionated as described by Boyum (4). Erythrocytes sedimenting with the PMN are eliminated by hypotonic lysis (12). Both PMN and mononuclear cells are washed 3 times in MEM before concentration for culture. The relative numbers of monocytes and lymphocytes in the mononuclear cell populations are determined using a stain for myeloperoxidase enzyme activity (11).

Use of a centrifugation step to sediment erythrocytes eliminates the requirement for addition of dextran, which may inhibit subsequent leukocyte migration (13). Removal of the majority of erythrocytes by centrifugation also reduces the time requirement for the subsequent gravity sedimentation step and thereby allows use of gravity sedimentation without dextran to obtain leukocyte-rich plasma from virtually all donors. Final elimination of erythrocytes contaminating PMN populations is achieved most effectively by brief exposure to water (12). We have observed that neither this lysis step itself nor exposure of the leukocytes to the erythrocyte components released is inhibitory for leukocyte migration.

Preparation of Agarose Plates

Agarose as Litex (type HSA, Accurate Chemical and Scientific Corp., Hicksville, N.Y.) is dissolved in sterile, distilled water at a concentration of 0.024 g/ml by heating in a boiling water bath for 10 to 15 min. After cooling in a 48° C water bath, the agarose is mixed with an equal volume of prewarmed (48°C) MEM diluted and supplemented as described below, and 5-ml volumes of the agarose medium are delivered to each 60 X 15 mm tissue culture plate (No. 3002, Falcon Plastics, Oxnard, California). In our experience, culture plates prepared for tissue culture are superior to nontissue culture types for leukocyte migration studies. To prepare 20 ml of agarose medium, the formula becomes:

Agarose: 0.24 g agarose in 10 ml sterile, distilled water
Medium: 2.0 ml 10 X MEM, 2.0 ml heat-inactivated, pooled human
serum, 0.2 ml 7.5% sodium bicarbonate, and 5.8 ml sterile, distilled water

Six series of three wells, 3 mm (11-gauge) in diameter and spaced 3 mm apart are cut in each plate using the punch and template described in Fig. 1. The plugs can be plucked out using a hypodermic needle or drawn out using a Pasteur pipette attached to a vacuum. Care must be taken not to score the plastic surface with the punch, since scratches become a barrier to cell migration. In order to prevent excessive bleeding of fluid into the prepared wells and to reestablish an appropriate pH, the plates are stored inverted in the incubator until used. Fluid accumulating in the wells can be removed using a microliter pipette or wicked out using a piece of tissue.

The center well of each three-well series receives a 10 μl aliquot of cell suspension (Fig. 2). We routinely use 2.5×10^5 PMN or monocytes per well. This

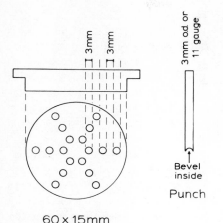

FIG. 1. Dimensions of tissue culture plate and the Plexiglas template and punch used to align and form wells in the agarose gel.

number of PMN requires a stock cell concentration of 2.5×10^7 PMN per milliliter. Because monocytes isolated with lymphocytes are used in these studies, the number of mononuclear cells transferred to the central well will vary from donor to donor. Monocyte numbers in such populations can be determined by application of a stain for myeloperoxidase activity (10). Since mononuclear cell populations usually contain approximately 25% monocytes, stock cell concentrations of approximately 1×10^8 mononuclear cells per milliliter will usually be required. The outer well receives 10 μl of chemotactic factor and the inner well 10 μl of the appropriate nonchemotactic control medium.

When volume of chemotactic factor is limited, the wells can be cut in an alternative pattern (Fig. 2) such that a single central well provides the gradient source for up to five replicate chemotaxis assays.

Quantitation of Migration

The culture plates are incubated at 37° C in a humidified atmosphere containing 5% CO_2 in air. After incubation for 2 hr for PMN or 10 to 18 hr for

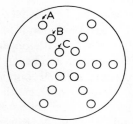
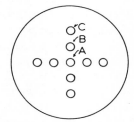

FIG. 2. Alternative patterns for arrangement of triplicate well series. **A,** cytotoxin; **B,** cells; **C,** control medium.

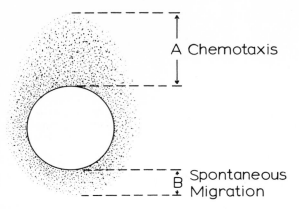

FIG. 3. Pattern of differential migration of leukocytes under agarose in response to chemotactic factor. Quantitation is accomplished by projection or observations by light microscopy of the migration pattern and measurement of the linear distances A (chemotaxis) and B (spontaneous migration). Alternative approaches to quantitation of migration are discussed in the text.

monocytes, the plates are flooded with 3 to 5 ml of methanol for 30 min, then with formalin for 30 min, the agarose is removed, and the cells stained with Wright's stain. When time is not available to complete fixation and staining, the plates can be stored with 3 ml methanol overnight or for the weekend at 4°C.

For quantitation of chemotaxis, the migration patterns are projected onto a white background at a magnification producing a well diameter of 5 cm using a microprojector (Tri-Ximplex, Bausch and Lomb, Rochester, N.Y.). Quantitation of chemotaxis is done, as shown in Fig. 3, by measuring in centimeters the linear distance the cells have migrated from the margin of the well toward the chemotactic factor (distance A). Spontaneous migration is represented by the distance the cells have migrated from the well margin toward the control medium (distance B). A "chemotactic index," A/B, and "chemotactic differential," A-B, can also be derived from these values.

Use of opposite sides of a single migration pattern to measure both spontaneous migration and chemotaxis now appears to have certain limitations. When incubation is limited to 2 hr and activated complement or microbial culture supernatants are used as chemotactic factors, the migration distance, B, is equal to the migration distance obtained when both wells receive control medium (13). Such short incubation periods in our experience apply only to PMN. With longer incubation times, these chemotactic factors appear to diffuse through and beyond the central well to influence migration of the cells moving toward the well containing control medium. Development of a cytotaxin gradient of sufficient strength in this area causes the cells migrating spontaneously to reverse their direction of movement such that the distance of spontaneous migration, B, is falsely reduced. We have also recently observed that a similar phenomenon occurs when the chemotactic dipeptide, N-formylmethionylphenylalanine, is used as the cytotaxin. Such low-molecular-weight chemotactic species appear to diffuse so rapidly that spontaneous migration, B, values are reduced even when the incubation period is limited to 2 hours.

In order to circumvent this problem under the conditions described and to eliminate all possibility of falsely reduced B values, we now routinely measure spontaneous migration of both PMN and monocytes using separate migration patterns obtained with control medium in both wells. Still another alternative to measurement of spontaneous migration is to measure migration from a well without use of adjacent wells containing control medium. We have observed, however, that values obtained for migration from single wells are somewhat less than those from control triplicate wells. This may be caused by diffusion of fluid into the space below the agarose, which can also affect leukocyte migration under agarose.

ALTERNATIVE APPROACHES TO QUANTITATION

Linear Distance of Migration

All our studies of leukocyte migration under agarose to date have employed this method of quantitation. Standard deviations of replicate measurements for tests quantitated by this means are consistently within 10% of the mean. Measurements of spontaneous migration of PMN isolated from more than 50 healthy volunteers over the past year average 2.1 ± 0.7 cm, with a range of 1.2 to 3.9 cm. Measurements of chemotaxis toward undiluted zymosan-activated serum (ZAS) average 4.6 ± 1.1 cm, with a range of 2.8 to 7.5 cm, and toward undiluted *Escherichia coli* culture supernatant average 3.7 ± 0.8 cm, with a range of 2.6 to 5.6 cm. The frequency distributions of the values obtained for these PMN functions are presented in Fig. 4A. Consideration of these distributions is interesting in that in no case is the distribution normal. The distribution of values for spontaneous migration, in fact, appears to be at least bimodal in nature. The distributions of values obtained for chemotactic responses to ZAS or *E. coli* culture supernatant (SEc) may be similarly multimodal in nature. The correlation coefficient for spontaneous migration and a chemotactic response to ZAS is $+0.61$, demonstrating a significant relationship between these functions. Whether the modality of the chemotactic responses is separate or related to that of spontaneous migration remains to be determined.

Measurements of spontaneous migration of monocytes isolated from more than 20 healthy volunteers in these studies average 3.7 ± 1.4 cm, with a range of 1.5 to 6.8 cm. Measurements of chemotaxis toward undiluted ZAS, with an incubation period of 18 hr average 5.8 ± 1.4 cm with a range of 3.0 to 8.7 cm. Frequency distributions of the values obtained for these monocyte functions are similar to those described for the respective PMN functions (Fig. 4 B). Not enough values have been accumulated to date to permit assessment

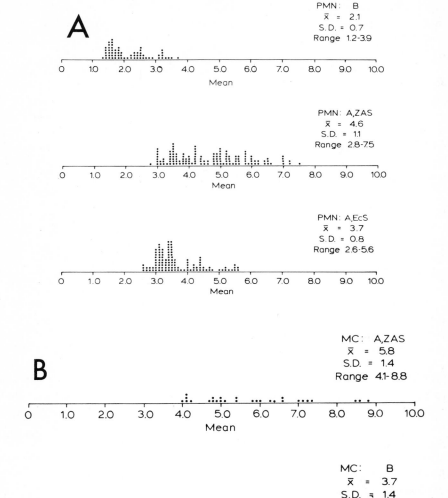

FIG. 4. A: Frequency distributions of the values obtained for spontaneous migration of PMN and their chemotactic responses to zymosan-activated serum (ZAS) and *Escherichia coli* culture supernatant (EcS). **B:** Frequency distributions of values obtained for spontaneous migration of monocytes and their chemotactic response to zymosan-activated serum (ZAS).

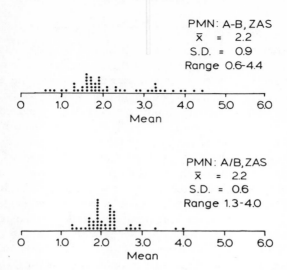

FIG. 5. Frequency distributions of values obtained for chemotactic index (A/B) and chemotactic differential (A-B) of PMN in response to zymosan-activated serum (ZAS).

of the modalities of these distributions, although subjectively they appear to be developing in a manner similar to those for the respective PMN functions. The correlation coefficient for spontaneous migration and chemotaxis in response to ZAS for monocytes is +0.88.

The possible bimodalities or trimodalities of the distributions of values for spontaneous migration and chemotaxis render use of mean and standard deviation values derived from these data less useful than anticipated. A more appropriate summary statistic in this situation might be the median, but the decision on how to consider patient data correctly must first await accumulation of additional normal data to describe these distributions accurately.

We have also begun to assess two alternative indices of the chemotactic response, the "chemotactic index," A/B, and "chemotactic differential," A-B. The distributions of these values for PMN in response to undiluted ZAS are presented in Fig. 5. The values for the chemotactic index appear to be more normalized in distribution. Whether these indices will be more useful in discriminating normal from defective leukocyte chemotaxis can be determined only after more patient data have been accumulated.

The values we have reported here for spontaneous migration and chemotaxis of PMN and monocytes are greater than the respective values reported in our original paper (13). We believe that this difference is the result of a change in agarose (Litex®, type HSA in place of indubiose A37) together with our identification and control of a number of factors which can have an inhibitory influence on these leukocyte functions.

Rate of Migration

The linear distance of migration values which have been discussed also provide a measure of migration rate, since the time of incubation is controlled. We have reported that an average migration rate for PMN in the agarose system is in the range of 0.2 to 0.4 mm per hr and for monocytes is approximately 0.04 mm per hr (13). Under the conditions currently employed, these values for PMN are nearly double those originally reported. Since migration rates determined by this method do not account for the nonlinear movement of cells as they migrate radially from the well margin and because the cells migrate as a population, without freedom from influences of proximal cells, the values noted must only approximate actual rates of migration of individual leukocytes.

Rates of migration of leukocyte populations under agarose can be assessed most easily by monitoring distance of migration of cells *in situ* over time, without fixation and staining, using a light microscope with an appropriate ocular micrometer (7) or grid (8). An inverted microscope is not essential for these observations, since the plates can be inverted without loss of the well contents.

Cell Density

The linear distance measurements described correspond to the leading-front method for quantitation of migration using membrane filters (19). We are currently assessing the use of an ocular grid for measurement of cell density within the migration pattern. This technique should provide data corresponding to the methods for measurement of migration through membrane filters which are based in some way on cell number (3,8,11).

In our preliminary studies of cell density, we have used a 1-cm square ocular grid divided into 2-mm squares. With this dimension, one can count approximately 30 cells per 4-mm^2 area using a 16 X objective. Although cells migrating radially from the round well must become diluted to some degree as a consequence of the increasing area covered, this dilution factor will be constant in comparisons of cell densities at similar distances from the well margins. Since identification of the peripheral limit of migration in measurements of linear distance is somewhat arbitrary, use of such a grid may also aid in definition of this limit; i.e., the limit might become the last 4-mm^2 area to contain a minimum of two cells.

CHEMOTACTIC RESPONSES TO VARIOUS CYTOTAXINS

Cellular Specificity of Cytotaxins

Over the past year, we have used five cytotaxins in studies of chemotaxis of human PMN and monocytes. These include the chemotactic dipeptide, *N*-formyl methionyl phenylalanine (15) (FMP, Sigma Chemical Co., St. Louis), activated complement as zymosan-activated serum (16), and filtered supernatants

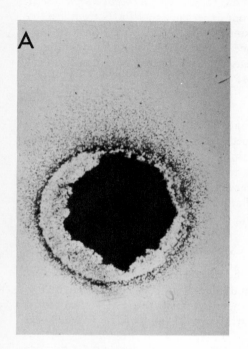

FIG. 6. **A:** Migration pattern of PMN in response to *Escherichia coli* culture supernatant. **B:** Migration pattern of PMN in response to zymosan-activated serum. **C:** Migration pattern of monocytes in response to zymosan-activated serum.

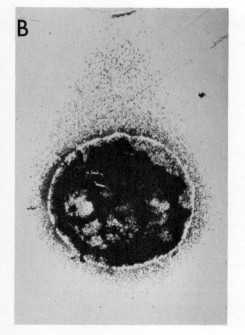

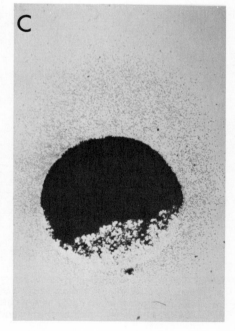

from 24-hr cultures of *Escherichia coli* (EcS) (17), *Staphylococcus aureus* (SaS), and *Candida albicans* (CaS). It has been our experience that PMN from healthy volunteers respond to all of these cytotaxins, although their strengths as attractants for PMN differ. When FMP at a concentration of 0.05 mg/ml and undiluted ZAS or microbial culture supernatant are used, their relative strengths as cytotaxins for human PMN are in the order FMP > ZAS > EcS > SaS > CaS. Monocytes isolated from healthy individuals, in contrast, respond chemotactically only to ZAS.

Another observation we have made is that migration patterns of PMN responding to ZAS are consistently rocket-shaped, whereas those obtained using any of the other cytotaxins are most often blunt in shape (Fig. 6). This difference is apparent throughout the migration period and remains at all concentrations of ZAS and may therefore reflect differences in the way in which PMN interact with and respond to these cytotaxins. Patterns of migration of monocytes responding to ZAS are blunt in shape (Fig. 6).

Titration of Cytotaxins

With the agarose method, ZAS and the microbial culture supernatants are all maximally active as cytotaxins in undiluted form. Data presented in Fig. 7 A illustrate the effect of dilution of these cytotaxins on PMN chemotaxis. For all factors, the relationship of concentration to chemotactic activity is linear

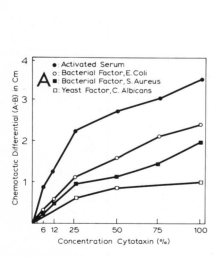
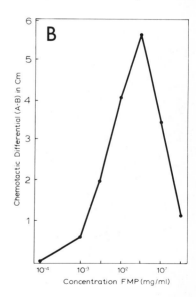

FIG. 7. A: Effect of dilution of chemotactic factors, zymosan-activated serum (ZAS), *Escherichia coli* culture supernatant (EcS), *Staphylococcus aureus* culture supernatant (SaS), and *Candida albicans* culture supernatant (CaS) on the chemotactic response of PMN. **B:** Relationship of concentration of *N*-formylmethionylphenylalanine to the chemotactic response of PMN.

to a concentration of 25%, at which there appears to be an inflection point. At dilutions greater than 3%, chemotactic activity is lost. Although the undiluted cytotaxins differ significantly in activity, serial dilution results in approximately parallel diminution of their respective activities.

Data presented in Fig. 7B illustrate the relationship of the chemotactic response of PMN to the concentration of FMP. In the agarose system, a concentration of 0.05 mg/ml produces the optimal response. Greater concentrations of this cytotaxin are inhibitory for PMN migration.

SOURCES OF VARIATION

In studies of leukocyte function *in vitro*, attention must be paid to the time at which blood specimens are drawn and the time taken and reagents used in isolation of the cell population(s) to be tested. We have recently identified several additional factors that are stimulatory or inhibitory for leukocyte spontaneous migration and chemotaxis under agarose. Failure to control these factors reduces the ability of this assay to differentiate between normal and defective cellular function, renders results obtained in different laboratories less comparable, and may also provide a basis for difficulties some individuals have reported in setting up this agarose technique. We have observed that heparin, and contamination of leukocyte subpopulations by erythrocytes and platelets, can inhibit leukocyte spontaneous migration and chemotaxis under agarose and that increasing cell number and supplementation of the medium with L-glutamine can enhance these cell functions.

Influence of Anticoagulant

In these experiments, we have compared spontaneous migration and chemotaxis of PMN and monocytes isolated from blood collected with heparin (sodium heparin, Upjohn, Kalamazoo, 10 units per ml blood), acid-citrate-dextrose (ACD, 0.07 mg per ml blood) or ethylenediamine tetraacetic acid (EDTA, 1.4 μg per ml blood). Data presented in Fig. 8 illustrate that neither spontaneous migration nor chemotaxis of PMN is influenced by anticoagulant at the concentrations used; however, collection of blood with heparin reduces both monocyte functions by approximately 30%. Monocytes, therefore, appear to be more sensitive in this respect to exposure of heparin.

Since clinical blood specimens may be drawn with variable amounts of heparin, we have also assessed the influence of a greater concentration of heparin on these leukocyte functions. For these experiments, blood was collected using either 10 or 50 units of heparin per milliliter of blood and the syringes allowed to stand at room temperature for 30 min to simulate the usual delay receiving clinical specimens. Data presented in Fig. 9 demonstrate that spontaneous migration of PMN and monocytes is not further reduced when blood is collected with a fivefold excess of heparin. In contrast, the chemotactic responses of

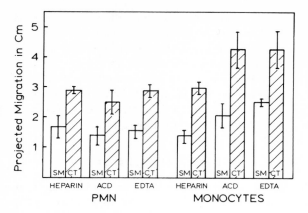

FIG. 8. Effect of anticoagulant on PMN and monocyte spontaneous migration and chemotaxis. Blood was collected with heparin (10 U/ml), ACD (0.07 mg/ml), or EDTA (1.4 mg/ml), and PMN and monocytes as mononuclear cells isolated as described. Leukocyte migration was measured, without re-addition of anticoagulant to the cell suspension medium. Cytotaxin: undiluted zymosan-activated serum.

cells of both types are inhibited by approximately 20% with the larger heparin dose. It remains to be determined whether heparin itself or the preservative, benzyl alcohol, is responsible for the effects observed.

Influence of Cells of Other Types

Because elimination of erythrocytes cosedimenting with PMN is not always complete with a single lysis step, we have assessed the influence of erythrocyte contamination on PMN migration. Data presented in Fig. 10 illustrate that the presence of erythrocytes with PMN at a ratio greater than 1 : 1 is inhibitory for both spontaneous migration and chemotaxis of PMN. The mechanism of

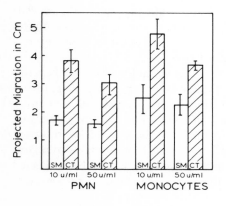

FIG. 9. Effect of excess heparin on PMN and monocyte spontaneous migration and chemotaxis. Blood was collected with heparin at concentrations of 10 U or 50 U/ml and the samples allowed to stand at room temperature for 30 min. PMN and mononuclear cells were isolated as described and migration measured without re-addition of heparin to the cell suspension medium. Cytotaxin: undiluted zymosan-activated serum.

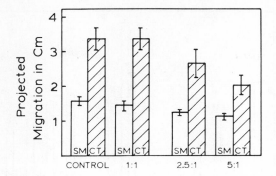

FIG. 10. Effect of erythrocytes on PMN spontaneous migration and chemotaxis. Leukocyte-free autologous erythrocytes were added to 2.5×10^5 erythrocyte-free PMN in ratios of 1 : 1, 2.5 : 1, and 5 : 1 RBC to PMN. Cytotaxin: undiluted zymosan-activated serum.

inhibition may not involve physical interference with movement, since chemotaxis is inhibited more than spontaneous migration.

In our experience, populations of mononuclear cells isolated from healthy volunteers contain 70 to 80% lymphocytes on the average, although values as low as 50% or as high as 95% may occur. Lymphocyte numbers therefore also represent a significant variable in using mononuclear cells as a source of monocytes for these studies. Since lymphocyte-free monocytes are difficult to prepare, we have assessed the influence of lymphocytes on monocyte migration by extrapolation from their effect on PMN migration. We have observed that addition of lymphocytes to PMN to provide a ratio as great as 2 : 1 has no significant influence on either PMN function (data not shown).

In routine studies of leukocyte function, little attention seems to be paid to the presence and possible influence of platelets. The presence of potent pharmacological agents in these cells makes their contamination of leukocyte subpopulations a very important consideration. Data demonstrating the inhibitory influence of platelets on leukocyte function are presented in Fig. 11. The presence of one platelet per 10^3 PMN inhibits chemotaxis by approximately 20%, but has no effect on spontaneous migration when the incubation perid is limited to 2 hr. Increasing the platelet to PMN ratio to 1 : 1 eliminates the chemotactic response. By increasing the incubation period to 18 hr, inhibition of PMN spontaneous migration and chemotaxis by one platelet per 10^2 PMN is reduced from 30 and 45%, respectively, to less than 10% of the respective control values. This effect of extending the incubation period on the inhibitory influence of platelets on PMN function suggests that pharmacological agents may be involved. This may also explain why these monocyte functions are not affected in the same way or to the same degree by platelet contamination.

In our experience, mononuclear cell populations are occasionally contaminated with PMN. We also find that nonsegmented (band) forms of PMN sediment with the mononuclear cells in Ficoll-Hypaque gradients. Since PMN migrate

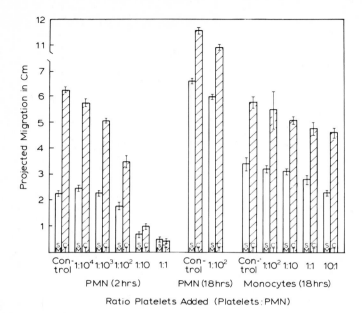

FIG. 11. Effect of platelets on PMN and monocyte spontaneous migration and chemotaxis. Autologous platelets were added to 2.5 X 10⁵ PMN and 2.5 X 10⁵ monocytes in ratios of 1 : 10⁴ to 1 : 1 and 1 : 10² to 10 : 1 platelets to leukocytes, respectively. Cytotaxin: undiluted zymosan-activated serum.

at a greater rate than monocytes, such contamination of mononuclear cells will result in falsely increased migration distances. We therefore recommend that all monocyte migration patterns be routinely checked by light microscopy for the presence of PMN.

Influence of Cell Number

We have reported that migration of PMN is positively related to the number of cells used in the migration assay (13). Data presented in Fig. 12 demonstrate that the same phenomenon occurs with monocytes. Doubling monocyte numbers produces an average increase in migration distance for both spontaneous migration and chemotaxis by approximately 40%. This effect of cell number on monocyte migration is similar to that observed on doubling PMN numbers.

Influence of L-Glutamine

The role of L-glutamine as a source of amide nitrogen in the biosynthesis of mucopolysaccharides in addition to purines suggested to us that L-glutamine supplementation of the medium in this assay may also be critical. To test this possibility, we isolated PMN and mononuclear cells in medium free of L-gluta-

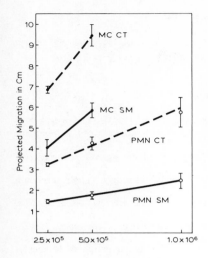

FIG. 12. Effect of cell number on PMN and monocyte spontaneous migration and chemotaxis. Number of PMN per well was 2.5×10^5, 5×10^5, or 1×10^6; number of monocytes per well was 2.5×10^5 or 5×10^5. Cytotaxin: undiluted zymosan-activated serum.

mine. Then, for measurement of migration, the leukocyte subpopulations were suspended in medium either free of or supplemented to contain 2 mM L-glutamine. Supplementation of the suspension with L-glutamine increased PMN spontaneous migration and chemotaxis by 15 and 20% on the average (data not shown). These monocyte functions were not significantly affected by addition of L-glutamine. This differential effect of L-glutamine on PMN and monocytes may be caused by the difference in incubation periods for these cells or by a difference in the requirements of cells of these types for exogenous amino acid. Loss of L-glutamine from stored medium may therefore provide an additional source of variation in this assay.

In spite of our current efforts to control these factors in our studies, a significant amount of variation remains in comparing results obtained with leukocytes from either different individuals or the same individual tested repeatedly. The relative contributions of the donor's dynamic physiological status and still other factors acting *in vitro* to this variation remain to be determined.

OTHER APPLICATIONS

The monolayer of PMN or monocytes formed on migration of these leukocytes under agarose also provides cells which can be easily prepared for examination by electron microscopy. Such studies are obviously useful in identification of morphological changes associated with a chemotactic response (14).

Leukocytes migrating under agarose can also be stained to reveal intracellular enzyme activities, i.e., myeloperoxidase (10). Since PMN are known to secrete lysosomal enzymes on exposure to certain cytotaxins (9), comparison of leukocytes migrating spontaneously and in response to cytotaxins by application of such cytochemical techniques might provide evidence of cell-cytotaxin interaction in the absence of a chemotactic response.

ACKNOWLEDGMENTS

Supported in part by United States Public Health Service Grants AI 12402 and CA 11605 and National Cancer Institute Contract NO1-CB 43948.

REFERENCES

1. Astor, S. H., Spitler, L. E., Frick, O. L., and Fudenberg, H. H. (1973): Human leukocyte migration inhibition in agarose using four antigens: Correlation with skin reactivity. *J. Immunol.,* 110:1174–1179.
2. Ax, W., and Tautz, C. (1974): Assay of leukocyte migration under agarose. *Behring Inst. Mitt.,* 54:72–80.
3. Boyden, S. (1962): The chemotactic effect of mixtures of antibody and antigen on polymorphonuclear leukocytes. *J. Exp. Med.,* 115:453–466.
4. Boyum, A. (1968): Separation of leukocytes from blood and bone marrow. *Scand. J. Clin. Lab. Invest.,* 21(Suppl. 97):77–89.
5. Carpenter, R. R. (1963): In vitro studies of cellular hypersensitivity. *J. Immunol.,* 91:803–818.
6. Clausen, J. E. (1971): Tuberculin-induced migration inhibition of human peripheral leukocytes in agarose medium. *Acta Allergol.* (Kbh), 26:56–80.
7. Cutler, J. (1974): A simple in vitro method for studies on chemotaxis. *Proc. Soc. Exp. Biol. Med.,* 147:471–474.
8. Gallin, J. I., Clark, R. A., and Kimball, H. R. (1973): Granulocyte chemotaxis: An improved in vitro assay employing ^{51}Cr-labeled granulocytes. *J. Immunol.,* 110:233–240.
9. Goldstein, I., Hoffstein, S., Gallin, J., Weismann, G. (1973): Mechanisms of lysosomal enzyme release from human leukocytes: Microtubule assembly and membrane fusion induced by a component of complement. *Proc. Natl. Acad. Sci. USA,* 70:2916–2920.
10. Kaplow, L. S. (1965): Simplified myeloperoxidase stain using benzidine dehydrochloride. *Blood,* 26:215–219.
11. Keller, H. U., Borel, J. F., Wilkinson, P. C., Hess, M. W., and Cottier, J. (1972): Re-assessment of Boyden's technique for measuring chemotaxis. *J. Immunol. Meth.,* 1:165–168.
12. Nelken, D., Gibboa-Garber, N., and Gurevitch, J. (1960): A method for simultaneous separation of human thrombocytes and leukocytes. *J. Clin. Pathol.,* 13:266.
13. Nelson, R. D., Quie, P. G., and Simmons, R. L. (1975): Chemotaxis under agarose: A new and simple method for measuring chemotaxis and spontaneous migration of human polymorphonuclear leukocytes and monocytes. *J. Immunol.,* 115:1650–1656.
14. Nelson, R. D., Fiegel, V. D., and Simmons, R. L. (1976): Chemotaxis of human polymorphonuclear neutrophils under agarose: Morphologic changes associated with the chemotactic response. *J. Immunol.,* 117:1676–1683.
15. Schiffmann, E., Corcoran, B. A., and Wahl, S. M. (1975): N-formyl methionyl peptides as chemoattractants for leukocytes. *Proc. Natl. Acad. Sci. U.S.A.,* 72:1059–1062.
16. Ward, P. A. (1968): Chemotaxis of mononuclear cells. *J. Exp. Med.,* 128:1201–1221.
17. Ward, P. A., Lepow, I. H., and Neuman, L. H. (1968): Bacterial factors chemotactic for polymorphonuclear leukocytes. *Am. J. Pathol.,* 52:725–736.
18. Weisbart, R. H., Cunningham, J. E., Bluestone, R., and Goldberg, L. S. (1973): A modified agarose method for detection of migration inhibitory factor and delineation of its antigen dependency. *Int. Arch. Allergy Appl. Immunol.,* 45:612–619.
19. Zigmond, S. H., and Hirsch, J. G. (1973): Leukocyte locomotion and chemotaxis: New methods for evaluation, and demonstration of a cell-derived chemotactic factor. *J. Exp. Med.,* 137:387–410.

DISCUSSION

Dr. Gallin: I have two comments and one small question. Dr. Mark Klempner, working in my laboratory, has recently been using the agarose assay for a variety of situations, and we have been impressed by its usefulness in distinguishing migration of different populations of polymorphonuclear leukocytes, for example, the eosinophils and neutrophils.

We have also been struck, however, by its property of being rather insensitive to certain stimuli. I think our data show that very high concentrations of the chemoattractant are needed to see the response. More importantly, we have had some difficulty demonstrating abnormal chemotaxis in some of our patients with abnormal chemotaxis using the filter method (i.e., Chediak-Higashi syndrome). Have you used this technique to assess clinical patients or clinical abnormalities?

The effects of heparin were apparently irreversible in your system. Several years ago, we published a paper on the effects of heparin on human polymorph chemotaxis using the micropore filter system, and found that heparin effects were 80% reversible. Perhaps all this is evidence that the two techniques measure different aspects of cell locomotion.

Dr. Nelson: I do not agree that the agarose method is less sensitive than the membrane filter method. The requirement for higher concentrations of attractants in the agarose method may be a consequence of the geometry of this system. For example, with the agarose method we use 10 μl of undiluted activated serum per replicate, whereas approximately 1.0 ml of 10% activated serum is optimal in the standard Boyden chamber. The agarose method actually requires *10 X less* complement, not more. This reduced requirement for complement in the agarose method applies in spite of the much greater sink size and the greater physical distance over which the gradient is established. This distance is at least 3×10^3 to 3×10^4 greater than that existing in the membrane filter method using cellulose or Nucleopore filters, respectively. Using the chemotactic dipeptide, N-formylmethionylphenylalanine, however, 10 times more attractant is required to achieve the minimum effective dose in the agarose system. Since this attractant may be molecularly much smaller than activated complement components, it will diffuse much more rapidly. In this case, the increased sink size and greater physical distance over which the gradient is established in the agarose system may contribute to increased dose requirements.

Concerning the clinical application of this technique, my experience has been somewhat limited as yet. Your experience with Chediak-Higashi patients suggests to me that there is some fundamental difference between the agarose and membrane filter methods. My feeling is that less deformation of the cell is required for movement under agarose. Thus, you may find normal chemotaxis of Chediak-Higashi neutrophils under agarose. Parallel application of the agarose and membrane filter methods may permit one to distinguish between defects in the basic locomotory apparatus (results concordantly depressed) and defects in deformability because of membrane changes or the presence of large inclusions (results discordantly depressed in the membrane filter system).

With respect to the effect of heparin on neutrophil chemotaxis, our results are in agreement with yours. When we isolated neutrophils from blood using

50 U heparin per milliliter blood, we observed depression of neutrophil chemotactic function on the order of 20%.

Dr. Lynn: I would like to comment on the data on the platelets. They, of course, are really a source of chemotactic factors.

Dr. Nelson: Yes, I agree with you that the "inhibitory" effect of platelets on neutrophil chemotaxis could be a result of their release of chemotactic factors. If the platelet factor gradient were to overwhelm that of the activated complement, the cells would be drawn back toward the central well. Migration will appear to have been inhibited; however, when we put platelets in the well which would otherwise receive attractant, no chemotaxis is observed. Our results, therefore, do not support your hypothesis.

Dr. Ward: This method seems to be another version of the leading-front, and I think one runs into difficulties in being able to detect abnormalities of chemotactic function if the leading-front is the only method used. The question I am asking is does the agarose method detect perturbations in leukocyte function that are detected by other methods?

Dr. Nelson: I do not know. We have had limited opportunity to compare patient leukocyte chemotaxis using the agarose and other methods. I agree with you that quantitating the way I do is analogous to the leading-front method used with the membrane filter system. We do, however, see variation in the number of cells which form the migration pattern, even though we are very careful to apply a constant number of leukocytes to the well. Determination of cell density, as I have described in the text, would therefore complement the distance measurement. Both pieces of information are needed and both can be obtained from a single migration pattern.

Leukocyte Chemotaxis, edited by John I. Gal
and Paul G. Quie. Raven Press, New Y
© 1978.

A Modified Micropore Filter Assay of Human Granulocyte Leukotaxis

Eufronio G. Maderazo and Charles L. Woronick

Medical Research Laboratory, Division of Infectious Diseases, Department of Medicine, Hartford Hospital, Hartford, Connecticut 06115

Clinical studies showing the association between abnormalities of leukotaxis and serious or recurrent infections has lead to a commonly accepted concept that leukocyte mobilization is an important part of the host defense against microbial invasion; however, progress in the understanding of the mechanism of leukotaxis has been slow, and some clinical studies have given conflicting results (3,7), perhaps in part because of the inherent difficulty with the assay system (the Boyden's micropore filter technique) which may be unreliable in detecting subtle leukotactic abnormalities owing to the detachment of migrated cells from the distal surface of the micropore filter (4) and the lack of standardization of these filters. An important additional problem with cell surface counting is that cells reaching the distal surface of the filter are counted, and given a grade of 100% migration, while cells that do not reach the surface, regardless of how far or near the distal surface they have reached, are not counted and given a grade of 0% migration. This has often led to a clinical-laboratory discrepancy in which a relatively well patient has a 90 to 100% leukotaxis inhibition. This magnification of defects would have been occasionally an asset were it not for the fact that errors are magnified as well. Furthermore, as a result of our continuing clinical studies and studies of the humoral regulators of leukotaxis, we have uncovered evidence of the importance of measuring both the *number* of migrating cells and the *distance* (depth) of migration in the calculation of the leukotactic index. Consequently, Boyden's method was modified to correct, if not reduce to a minimum, most of the above-mentioned problems.

The following report is a description of this modified method and includes some discussion of the kinetics of leukotaxis *in vitro* (in micropore filter), to illustrate some of the less well-known pitfalls encountered in leukotaxis assessment with Boyden's technique.

METHOD

Description

Leukotactic assays were performed as described in detail elsewhere (5). Modified transparent acrylic Boyden chambers (Ahlco Corp., Southington, Connecti-

43

TABLE 1. *Sample calculation of leukotactic index*

(A) Distance from origin (μm)	(B) Number of cells per level	A $\times$ B
0	26	0
10	54	540
20	52	1,040
30	47	1,410
40	30	1,200
50	32	1,600
60	22	1,320
70	16	1,120
80	9	720
90	5	450
100	3	300

Total (including monolayer): 296   9700
Total (excluding monolayer): 270
Leukotactic Index (LI) = 9700 ÷ 270 = 35.9 μm
LI (monolayer included)[a] = 9700 ÷ 296 = 32.8 μm

[a] This is used in all nonstimulated migration (experiments in the absence of chemotactic factor in the lower compartment, or plasma or serum in the upper compartment).

cut 06489) and 13-mm diameter 5-μm pore size filters (Millipore Corp., Bedford, Massachusetts 01730) were used. The chemotactic attractant or medium 199 was used in the lower compartment and the cell suspension (5×10^5 cells per chamber) was introduced into the upper compartment. The prepared chambers were incubated at 37°C for 60 or 90 min. After incubation, the filters were removed, stained, and mounted on slides. This short incubation period prevented complete migration of cells to the opposite surface of the filter, removing the variability introduced by cell detachment from the distal filter surface.

The cells were then counted at every 10-μm interval from the original monolayer to the distal surface. The number of cells counted per level was multiplied by the distance of that level from the starting surface. Then the products were added and the sum was divided by the total[1] number of cells counted per field. The number obtained was then called the leukotactic index (LI), which was the average distance migrated by the cells in 60 or 90 min of incubation. (See Table 1 for sample calculation.) Three or more fields were counted per filter and the mean LI calculated from duplicate filters.

---

[1] When a majority of the cells have responded and have moved distal to the original monolayer, such as when cells are preincubated with serum or plasma, the monolayer cell count is not included in the calculation; however, when a majority of the cells do not respond and remain at the origin, the monolayer cell count significantly affects the index and therefore is included in the calculation.

Day-to-Day Stability of Leukotactic Indices

To test for stability of the leukotactic index, cells and serums were obtained and tested from 5 normal volunteers in 2 to 5 separate days. Cells incubated in 7% autologous serum were tested for chemotactic response to 10% bacterial chemotactic factor. Micropore filters from the same lot number were used in all experiments to minimize filter variability in the study. Indices obtained from experiments done on separate days were then compared. As shown in Table 2, the coefficient of variation ranged between 8 to 12%. These results indicate

TABLE 2. *Stability of leukotactic index for individual leukocyte donors*

Subjects	No. of days	No. of filters	No. of fields	Index (mean ± SD)	Coefficient of variation
IS	5	10	30	45 ± 3	8
DL	4	8	24	44 ± 5	12
RP	3	6	18	44 ± 4	9
NW	2	4	12	48 ± 4	8
MT	2	4	11	39 ± 4	11

Cells were incubated in 7% autologous serum, and chemotactic response to 10% bacterial chemotactic factor was determined.

the day-to-day stability of the leukotactic indices of individuals as calculated by this method.

Reader Variability of Leukotactic Index Determination

A study was made to compare reader variability of counting different fields on the same filter at two different times. Filters in the same lot number were again used in all studies. Two readers were used, of whom one (B) was inexperienced in cell-counting (this was introduced in the experiment to determine if experience is necessary for accuracy in cell-counting). Three fields were counted for each filter and reader A counted 16 filters while reader B counted 14 filters. Analysis of the results showed no significant difference between the first and second counts made by both readers (reader A, $p > 0.2$ and reader B, $p > 0.5$ by Student's t test).

Another experiment compared counts on different fields of the same filter performed at different times by the same two readers. Thirty-two filters were counted, and the significance of the differences of the leukotactic indices obtained was analyzed. The results again showed no significant differences between counts of the two readers ($p > 0.05$).

A third experiment compared counts performed on the same field by two readers. The difference of the two counts was also found to be insignificant

($p > 0.1$). These studies demonstrate that despite the seeming complexity of the counting and calculations of this method, reader variability is minor and counting and leukotaxis index calculations are in fact sufficiently simple that even inexperienced technicians can perform them accurately.

Nonhomogeneity of Migrating Cell Population

The relationship between the log of the number of cells counted at a given depth in the filter and the square of that depth was examined. As shown in Fig. 1, at least two different populations of migrating cells were observed. One

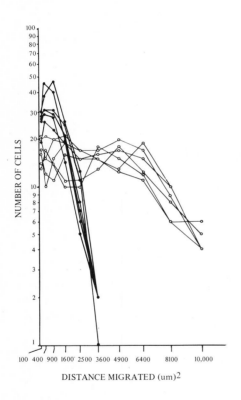

FIG. 1. Relationship between log of the number of cells and the square of the distance migrated, showing nonhomogeneity of migrating cell population: one population being rapidly moving with the characteristics of randomly moving particles, and another a slowly moving population with a more horizontal slope. Data plotted in closed circles (●) were results from cell migration in the absence of plasma, serum, or chemotactic factor in the upper or lower compartment; data in open circles (○) illustrate results of cells incubated with 7% serum in the upper compartment. A point represents a field in duplicate experiments.

population was rapidly moving and consisted of cells that migrated first or the only cells seen in the filters in nonstimulated experiments (cells incubated in the absence of plasma or serum). The distribution of the cells in the filter resembled the characteristics of randomly moving particles (9). The other population of cells was slowly responding. The peak concentration of these cells remained in the monolayer in nonstimulated experiments. Their presence and their distinct behavior, however, became quite obvious in experiments using cells preincubated with serum.

STUDIES ON SERUM AND PLASMA

Thirty-five different serum samples collected from normal laboratory personnel of both sexes and of various age groups were tested simultaneously. Various aliquots of cells (5×10^5) from a single normal donor were incubated with 7% concentration of the various serum samples, and the responses of the treated cells were tested without chemotactic factor in the lower compartment. Using the new method of calculation, the mean LI was 41.3 ± 5.8 SD μm/90 min with a coefficient of variation of 13.99% and standard error of the mean of 0.34. When compared with the mean index in the absence of serum (20.8 ± 5.9), this was a 98.6% increase.

To determine if plasma and serum have the same effects on polymorphonuclear leukotaxis, the responses of cells pretreated with plasma (obtained from heparinized blood) or serum were compared and analyzed as to the depth of migration and the number of cells responding. As depicted in Fig. 2, the fastest of the plasma-treated cells reached a distance slightly farther than those of the serum-treated cells (in some experiments, the depth of migration was similar). Of greater interest, however, is that more of the plasma-treated cells were nonresponsive and remained in the original monolayer. These results have been a consistent finding on numerous subsequent studies. The differences between the effects of normal plasma and serum became more apparent when the monolayer cell count was included in the calculation of the leukotactic index but was not detectable when the leading-front technique of Zigmond and Hirsch (9) was used.

The effects of abnormal serum were likewise studied. Serums were collected

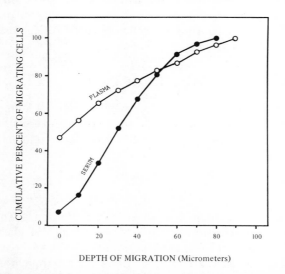

DEPTH OF MIGRATION (Micrometers)

FIG. 2. Comparison of migration characteristics of plasma- and serum-treated cells using 7% plasma or serum. Each point represents the mean of six fields in duplicate experiments.

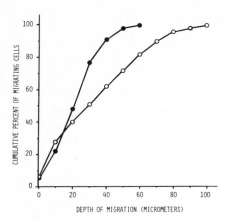

FIG. 3. Effect of serum from a patient with liver cirrhosis (●) as compared to that of normal serum (○) on migration characteristics of normal cells. Cells were incubated in the presence of 7% normal or abnormal serum in the upper compartment. Each point represents the mean of six fields in duplicate experiments.

from patients with liver cirrhosis, and their direct effects on polymorphonuclear leukotaxis were tested. In the presence of serum from cirrhotic patients, normal cells still migrate en masse, but unlike cells treated with normal serum, the depth of migration is shallow (Fig. 3). In this instance, the Zigmond and Hirsch technique (9) will be valuable and accurate; however, since the cells treated with the abnormal serum would not have reached the distal surface of the filter at the time when a majority of the cells treated with normal serum would have, the use of Boyden's original method of leukotaxis evaluation would lead to a magnification of defect and would result in a clinical-laboratory discrepancy of a relatively well patient with a 90 to 100% reduction of leukotaxis. Moreover, no defect will be apparent when sufficient time is allowed for the slow cells (treated with abnormal serum) to reach the surface. This error is common to all micropore filter methods using the cell population reaching a predetermined distance as the index of leukotactic response.

STUDIES OF CELLS

The method was also used to study migration of normal human polymorphonuclear leukocytes, including nonstimulated migration (in the absence of chemotactic factor and plasma or serum) and the effects of chemotactic factor.

Nonstimulated Migration

The response of various washed cells obtained from 19 normal donors of both sexes of various age groups was studied at different times. To test nonstimulated migration, experiments were done in the absence of chemotactic factor and plasma or serum. (In these early experiments monolayer counts were not included in LI calculations.) The mean LI of 28 determinations in duplicate experiments was 20.8 ± 5.9 SD μm/90 min (range : 15.1 to 35.8). Cell variability, therefore, is greater than variability among serums. This is similar to Gallin's findings using a radioassay technique (2).

Effect of Chemotactic Factor

Chemotactic response of cells from 7 normal donors was tested simultaneously in the presence of 10% bacterial chemotactic factor in the lower compartment. The mean index was 28.6 ± 5.3 SD μm/90 min. The effect of chemotactic factor was then further examined in terms of distance migrated and the number of cells migrating. Figure 4 illustrates the results of experiments performed on

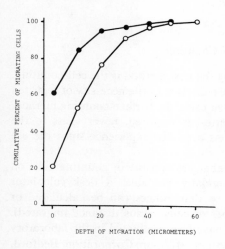

FIG. 4. Comparison of leukotactic responses of normal cells in the presence (○) or absence (●) of 10% bacterial chemotactic factor in the lower compartment. A point represents the mean of six fields in duplicate experiments.

cells with and without chemotactic factor in the lower compartment, which shows that the more consistent and obvious effect of chemotactic factor is its ability to increase the number of responding cells rather than its effect on the depth of migration. Experience in our laboratory has shown that measurement of the depth of migration is not a sensitive measure of chemotactic factor effect, and as a corollary, not sensitive in detecting serum chemotactic factor inactivator (CFI) activity (Maderazo, *unpublished observation*). [CFI has been discussed in detail elsewhere (6,8)]. Consequently, to maximize the sensitivity of the assay, we have included monolayer counts in the index calculations of experiments in which the nonmigrating cells account for the majority of the total cell population, such as those done on washed cells when not reincubated in serum.

PROBLEMS OF THE MICROPORE FILTER ASSAY

Filters

Despite the many modifications and refinements of the original Boyden's method, many problems have defied solution and continue to exist. The most serious persistent problem is the lack of well-standardized cellulose micropore filters. We have tested various filters from different companies (Millipore, Gelman, and Schleicher and Schuell), but none provided us with filters of 3-, 5-, and 8-μm pore size giving consistent results on simultaneous duplicate or triplicate experiments. Previously, pretesting of samples from various uncut sheets or lot numbers before ordering has helped in the selection of better filters from one company. Recently, however, none of the samples sent has been satisfactory. It is claimed by one company that their filters with small pore sizes are better standardized. This possibility, in addition to the continued search for better filters from other sources, is worth pursuing, since no solution for this problem is in sight.

Tediousness of Counting

The other problem that is made worse by the new method is the cell-counting. This disadvantage is, however, offset by the reduction of the necessity of repeated testing, which has often been necessary when using the surface-counting method. In clinical studies where patient cooperation is required, fewer visits to the laboratory is a distinct advantage. This has been our experience since the use of the new method.

Moreover, automatic particle counters that are capable of counting cells on and in micropore filters are now commercially available. A desk calculator can also be interfaced with the counter so that indices can be calculated or results even instantly plotted (e.g., number of cells versus distance migrated). Automatic counters from two companies have been evaluated in the laboratory (ΠMC Particle Measurement Computer System, Millipore Corporation, Bedford, Massachusetts 01730, and the Omnicon Alpha Image Analysis System, Bausch & Lomb, Rochester, New York, 14625). The two systems performed similarly, but the latter is less bulky and less expensive.

SUMMARY

A method of leukotaxis assay is described in which the index of migration takes into account both the number of migrating cells and their depth of migration. The advantages of this method include: (a) all cells in a field (not merely representative cells) are counted; (b) cells are graded according to their speed of migration, and thus the magnification or minifying of defects is avoided; (c) calculation corrects for nonuniformity of cell distribution between fields; (d) bias is reduced because the index is not known until calculated; (e) incubation period is shorter; (f) precision and accuracy are greater; and (g) the relative number of the rapidly and slowly migrating cell populations can be estimated by plotting the log of the number of cells against the square of their depths of migration. The disadvantages include: (a) it is more tedious; (b) reproducibility is limited by the micropore filters used which are usually poorly standardized; and (c) although more precise, it is less sensitive in detecting chemotactic factor effect (counting the number of migrating cells is more sensitive but less precise).

APPENDIX: MODIFIED MICROPORE FILTER ASSAY

Materials

1. Patient's and normal leukocytes and serums: Venous blood is drawn into a plastic syringe containing 50 units of heparin (sodium) per milliliter of blood. Standing the syringe on its plunger allows the erythrocytes to sediment at room temperature. After 30 to 60 min, the leukocyte-rich plasma is delivered into a plastic 40 ml test tube; a bent needle or a polyethylene catheter attached to the tip of the needle is used. The cell pellet is removed by centrifugation at $500 \times g$ for 10 min, and the cells are resuspended and adjusted to a concentration of 5×10^6 cells per milliliter medium 199, pH 7.4. Serum is prepared from freshly clotted blood.
2. Leukotactic chambers (Ahlco Corp., Southington, Connecticut 06489) (Fig. 5).

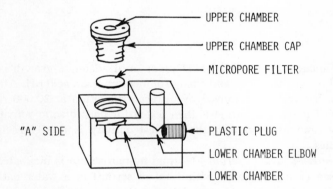

UPPER CHAMBER

UPPER CHAMBER CAP

MICROPORE FILTER

"A" SIDE

PLASTIC PLUG

LOWER CHAMBER ELBOW

LOWER CHAMBER

FIG. 5. Modified clear acrylic leukotactic chamber.

3. Micropore filter 13-mm diameter, 5-μm pore size (Millipore).
4. Sodium heparin without preservative.
5. TC medium 199, pH 7.4 (Difco).
6. Staining materials:
   a. Staining cassettes for micropore filters (Ahlco Corp., Southington, Connecticut 06489) (Fig. 6).
   b. Isopropyl alcohol, 70%, 90%, and 100%.
   c. Hematoxylin, with 4 ml concentrated acetic acid per 100 ml.
   d. Acid-alcohol (3 drops of HCl per 200 ml 70% isopropyl alcohol).
   e. Bluing agent (20 gm $MgSO_4$ + 2 gm $NaHCO_3$ in 1 liter of water).
   f. Xylene.
7. Preparation of chemotactic factors:
   a. *Bacterial chemotactic factor*—A loop of *Escherichia coli* in broth culture or 1 to 2 colonies in agar are inoculated into 1,000 ml medium 199

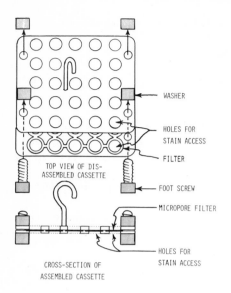

WASHER

HOLES FOR
STAIN ACCESS

FILTER

TOP VIEW OF DIS-
ASSEMBLED CASSETTE

FOOT SCREW

MICROPORE FILTER

HOLES FOR
STAIN ACCESS

CROSS-SECTION OF
ASSEMBLED CASSETTE

FIG. 6. Staining cassettes for 13-mm diameter micropore filters (Ahlco Corporation, Southington, Conn.)

and incubated at 37°C for 24 hr or until adequate growth is observed as shown by turbidity and change of medium to an acid pH. After incubation, bacteria are removed by ultracentrifugation at 20,000 rpm for 20 min. The culture filtrate is then tested for chemotactic activity and the least amount producing the greatest activity is used for chemotactic studies.

b. *Zymosan-activated serum*—Normal human serum is incubated with zymosan (5 mg zymosan with 1 ml of serum) in a water bath at 37°C for 30 min. (This treatment will trigger the alternate or properdin pathway of complement to produce the complement-derived chemotactic factors.) A 1:10 dilution of this preparation in medium 199 is used as the attractant in the lower compartment of the chemotactic chamber.

Method

1. *Preparation of chambers*—The upper chamber cap is unscrewed, and a micropore filter is placed on the floor of the upper compartment. The upper chamber cap is replaced and tightened slightly. (Excessive tightening may produce corrugations of the filter and irregular deposition of cells.) With the leukotactic chamber tilted so that its A-side is facing downward, the properly diluted chemotactic factor is injected into the lower chamber with the use of a Pasteur pipette. (This maneuver will prevent air bubbles under the micropore filter.) With the lower chamber filled only up to the elbow, 0.1 ml of the cell suspension containing 5×10^6 cells/ml is added into the upper compartment which is then filled completely with medium 199. Following this, the lower compart-

TABLE 3. *Sample protocol*

Upper compartment (cells + serum)	Lower compartment (factor)	To test for
Normal + No	No	Nonstimulated migration
Patient's + No	No	
Normal + No	Chemotactic factor	Chemotaxis
Patient's + No	Chemotactic factor	
Normal + Normal	No	Cell-directed inhibitor of leukotaxis, or leukotaxis-enhancing factor
Normal + Patient's	No	
Patient's + Normal	No	
Patient's + Patient's	No	
Normal + No	Chemotactic factor + normal serum	Chemotactic factor inactivator
Normal + No	Chemotactic factor + patient's serum	
Normal + No	Activated normal serum	Complement-derived chemotactic factors
Normal + No	Activated patient's serum	

ment is similarly filled with medium 199. (Filling the lower compartment completely before the upper compartment is filled will lead to seepage of the chemotactic factor through the filter into the upper compartment.) The prepared chambers are then incubated in air at 37°C for 90 min. This short incubation period prevents polymorphonuclear leukocytes from reaching the lower surface of the filter, thus avoiding the variable of cell detachment from that surface into the attractant fluid of the lower compartment. Table 3 shows the usual protocol for leukotaxis workup.

2. *Staining of filters*—After incubation, the filters are removed, placed in specially made staining cassettes (Fig. 6), and quickly fixed in 100% isopropyl alcohol for 30 sec. (Drying of the filter resulting from delayed fixing will lead to cell disruption and loss of cell outline.) Then the filters are stained in hematoxylin for 2 min, quickly rinsed in water, decolorized in acid alcohol for 30 sec, rinsed in water again, immersed in the bluing agent for 30 sec, rinsed in water, dehydrated successively in 75%, 95%, and absolute isopropyl alcohol for 30 sec each, and finally cleared in xylene for 5 min. The stained filters are mounted on slides with Permount and covered with a thin cover slip.

3. *Calculation of the leukotactic index*—Under 400 × magnification, the cells are counted at every 10-μm interval from the original monolayer to the distal surface. The number of cells counted per level are multiplied by the distance of that level to the starting surface. Then the products obtained are added, and the sum is divided by the total number of migrated cells counted. The number obtained is the *leukotactic index* (LI), which is the

average distance migrated by the cells in 90 minutes of chamber incubation. (Table 3 gives a sample calculation.) Three or more fields are counted and the mean LI is calculated for each duplicate or triplicate filter.

4. *Evaluation of results*—The mean LI of control cells or serum is arbitrarily 0% leukotactic inhibition. Changes from this value can be calculated using the following equation.

$$\% \text{ leukotactic inhibition} = \frac{\text{control LI} - \text{patient LI}}{\text{control LI}} \times 100$$

Leukotactic inhibition exceeding 14% is considered significantly abnormal.

This method can also be used to measure monocyte chemotaxis, by using peripheral blood monocytes isolated by density gradient centrifugation (1), 8-μm pore size filters, and incubation period for prepared chambers of 2-1/2 to 3 hr.

ACKNOWLEDGMENTS

I would like to thank Dr. Richard Quintiliani and Dr. Peter A. Ward for their suggestions in the preparation of this manuscript. These studies were supported in part by The Hartford Hospital Research Free Funds and NIH grant A1–12225.

REFERENCES

1. Boyum, A. (1968): Isolation of mononuclear cells and granulocytes from human blood. *Scand. J. Clin. Lab. Invest.,* 21 (Suppl. 97):77–89.
2. Gallin, J. I. (1974): Radioassay of granulocyte chemotaxis: Studies of human granulocytes and chemotactic factors. In: *Antibiotics and Chemotherapy, Vol. 19: Chemotaxis: Its Biology and Biochemistry,* edited by E. Sorkin, pp. 146–160. S. Karger, Basel.
3. Hill, H. R., Gerrard, J. M., Hogan, N. A., and Quie, P. G. (1974): Hyperactivity of neutrophil leukotactic responses during active bacterial infection. *J. Clin. Invest.,* 53:996–1002.
4. Keller, H. U., Hess, M. W., and Cottier, H. (1974): The in vitro assessment of leukocyte chemotaxis. In: *Antibiotics and Chemotherapy, Vol. 19: Chemotaxis: Its Biology and Biochemistry,* edited by E. Sorkin, pp. 112–125. S. Karger, Basel.
5. Maderazo, E. G., and Ward P. A. (1977): Leukocyte function tests. In: *Methods in Immunodiagnosis,* edited by N. R. Rose and P. E. Biggazi. John Wiley and Sons, New York.
6. Maderazo, E. G., Ward, P. A., Woronick, C. L., Kubik, J., and DeGraff, A. C., Jr. (1976): Leukotactic dysfunction in sarcoidosis. *Ann. Intern. Med.,* 84:414–419.
7. Mowat, A. G., and Baum, J. (1971): Polymorphonuclear leukocyte chemotaxis in patients with bacterial infections. *Br. Med. J.,* 3:617–619.
8. Ward, P. A. (1974): The regulation of leukotactic mediators. In: *Antibiotics and Chemotherapy, Vol. 19: Chemotaxis: Its Biology and Biochemistry,* edited by E. Sorkin, pp. 333–337. S. Karger, Basel.
9. Zigmond, S. H., and Hirsch, J. G. (1973): Leucocyte locomotion and chemotaxis: New methods for evaluation and demonstration of a cell-derived chemotactic factor. *J. Exp. Med.,* 137:387–410.

DISCUSSION

Dr. Clark: I would like to reemphasize the comment made concerning the assumption in the Zigmond-Hirsch article (9) that here is homogeneity of the migrating cell population. We ran into this as a problem a couple years ago when we were looking at eosinophils, since eosinophils are not homogeneous in their response. A plot of log eosinophils versus distance squared does not give a straight line; moreover, there is a great difference among eosinophil populations from patient to patient.

Dr. Wilkinson: Heterogeneity of leukocyte populations can provide a problem with our micropore filter assays.

Dr. Gallin: Not only are eosinophils a heterogeneous population but as Dr. Maderazo implied there is evidence that neutrophils also are a heterogeneous population of cells. Dr. Wilkinson's photographs suggest that some cells do not eat *Candida albicans.* Moreover, Dr. Klempner in our laboratory has just completed a project and submitted an abstract to the American Federation of Clinical Research (1977) demonstrating two populations of neutrophils. We have found that about 80% of neutrophils rosette with human erythrocytes coated with rabbit antihuman IgG (7SEA). We can separate the rosetting and nonrosetting neutrophils. The cells which rosette migrate much better than cells which do not.

Dr. Ward: I wonder if in the method of isolating your two neutrophil populations you are doing something to the cells by the rosetting technique to turn something on, thereby, causing them to be more hyperresponsive. One would have to be very careful to determine if this were a turn-on mechanism in the process of isolating cells, rather than actually defining intrinsic cell differences in functional reactivity, of two cell populations.

Dr. Gallin: We do not have the answer to that now.

Leukocyte Chemotaxis, edited by John I. Gallin
and Paul G. Quie. Raven Press, New York
© 1978.

A New Visual Assay of Leukocyte Chemotaxis

Sally H. Zigmond

Department of Biology, University of Pennsylvania, Philadelphia, Pennsylvania 19104

Most recent studies of leukocyte chemotaxis have utilized one of a number of variations of a millipore filter system introduced by Boyden in 1962 (3). In these assay systems, the cells are allowed to migrate into the pores, usually 3 μm in diameter, of the filter which is placed between two chambers. By varying the solutions placed in the chambers, a gradient is established across the filter. Studies using such a system have been useful in identifying a number of chemotactic agents (13). They have also demonstrated that most chemotactic factors stimulate locomotion (chemokinesis) as well as directed locomotion (chemotaxis) and that high concentrations of the factors inhibit these cell responses (12,13,15).

In spite of these impressive advances, the millipore techniques have several shortcomings. They are relatively slow (often incubation times greater than 2 hr are used), thus making it difficult to study initial or short-term effects. The techniques depend on active locomotion by the cells and allow one to investigate locomotion and directed locomotion but not orientation in the absence of locomotion. The sensitivity of the assays appears to be greatest with rapidly locomoting cells. Finally, the opaque filter prevents observation of the cell behavior during the response. It is difficult or impossible, for example, to differentiate between an enhanced chemotactic response brought about by alterations in (a) the percentage of responding cells, (b) the accuracy of orientation, (c) the frequency or magnitude of turns, or (d) the rate of movement by cells with a certain orientation. Behavioral studies complementing and extending the information obtainable in the millipore system would thus be useful.

Cell behavior can be observed directly by phase microscopy and can be altered with drugs and physical parameters such as temperature and pressure. Microscopic studies of cells under conditions that alter their behavior can be correlated with biochemical information on the effects of the drugs or physical conditions on *in vitro* variables such as the amount of actin polymerized or the sol-gel equilibrium of a cell extract. In addition, as the interaction of chemotactic factors with the cell membrane is studied, it is important to examine carefully the effects on cell behavior of agents which compete for chemotactic factor binding sites or agents which inhibit digestion of the chemotactic factors by the cells.

Most of the studies in which the behavior of cells was visualized have used immobilized agents which generate chemotactic factors (2,6,7,9,14,15). In these studies, the amounts of chemotactic factor formed can only be roughly known. The few studies using soluble material have only been semiquantitative with regard to the concentration and concentration gradient to which the cell was exposed (10) or have reported cell responses so insensitive to the concentration of stimulant that the results must be questioned (5).

I felt that it would be useful to have a system in which one could examine the behavior of individual cells in known concentrations and concentration gradients of chemoattractants. It is possible to establish a linear gradient of a chemical in a solution across a bridge or semipermeable membrane if two concentrations of the chemical are present in large stirred volumes on each side of the bridge (4). These conditions are approximated for creating a gradient in the Boyden millipore systems. For a visual assay in which cells exposed to a gradient can be observed, a Plexiglas chamber was designed which allows evaluation of orientation of cells on a bridge that connects two wells containing chemotactic agents. Cells can be continuously observed, and orientation can be scored in less than 15 min, thus permitting investigation of early responses to chemical stimuli. I have used the chamber to investigate the optimal concentration and minimal concentration gradient required for cell orientation, and to provide evidence on the reversibility of the response and on the inactivation of chemotactic factors by the cells.

VISUAL SYSTEM

A Plexiglas microscope slide 3-mm thick was cut to have two wells across the width of the slide 1-mm deep and 4-mm wide, separated by a 1-mm bridge. A 22- X 40-mm coverslip placed over the wells and across the 1-mm bridge. was held firmly in place by clips on the top of both ends of the slide (Fig. 1).

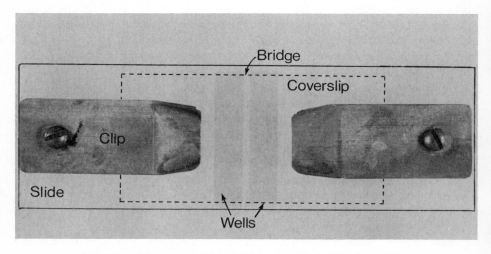

FIG. 1. Plexiglas chamber for visual assay of leukocyte chemotaxis.

Fluid then placed in one well is drawn by capillary action over the bridge, but the resistance to flow is sufficiently great that the fluid does not flow into the second well. The second well can then be filled with another solution. With two different concentrations of fluorescein isothiocyanate in the wells, the development of a gradient across the 1-mm bridge was examined using a fluorescence microscope. A gradient across the bridge was apparent in one min; it increased in steepness over the first 15 to 30 min. It was then reasonably stable for about 60 min before it began to decline.

For assays of cell orientation, human peripheral blood leukocytes were allowed to settle and stick to the central region of a 22- X 40-mm coverslip. The coverslip was then inverted onto the Plexiglas slide such that the cells were over the bridge where they could be observed by phase microscopy. In order to make preparations that had a very thin fluid layer over the bridge (about 5 μm thickness of fluid was optimal for establishing a good gradient and for observing the cells), the two ends of the coverslip in contact with the ends of the Plexiglas slide had to be dry and clean as the preparation was assembled. When the wells were filled, fluid flowed to the ends of the coverslip as well as onto the bridge. Different concentrations of chemotactic peptides, either *N*-formylmethionylmethionylmethionine (FMMM) or *N*-formylmethionylleucylphenylanine (FMLP), the generous gifts of Drs. E. L. Becker and E. Schiffmann, were placed in the wells. For most tests, the peptides were dissolved in Hanks' medium containing 1% gelatin. The cells over the center of the bridge were observed with a 40X objective (field diameter about 0.4 mm) and either photographed or scored as moving into the 180°-sector toward one or the other well. The direction of locomotion of a polymorphonuclear leukocyte (PMN) can be judged morphologically since the front of a cell is marked by a granule-free pseudopod and the rear by a knob-like tail. The results are expressed as the percentage of scorable cells moving toward the well containing the higher concentration of peptide.[11]

RESULTS

Orientation Toward N-Formylmethionyl Peptides

The PMNs showed marked orientation toward both FMMM and FMLP with often greater than 90% of the cells responding (Fig. 2). The orientation was apparent 10 to 15 min after making the preparation, and reached maximal levels between 20 and 30 min; it then remained nearly constant until 90 min. Orientation was routinely scored between 20 and 60 min. The cell response was reversible by reversing the gradient. Whereas 87% of the PMNs had oriented toward the right well which contained 3×10^{-6} M FMMM and 13% toward the well containing 3×10^{-7} M FMMM, 15 min after the solutions in the wells were removed and replaced with the opposite polarity, 71% of the cells were oriented toward the 3×10^{-6} M FMMM, which was now in the left well.

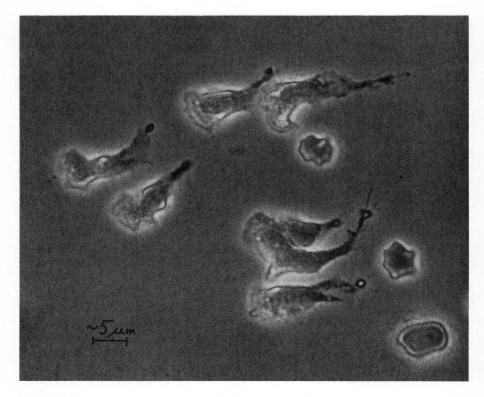

FIG. 2. Phase micrograph of cells over the Plexiglas bridge oriented in gradient of 3×10^{-7} to 3×10^{-6} M FMMM.

Concentration Dependence of the Orientation Response

The magnitude of the cell response, as measured by the percentage of scorable cells oriented toward the well containing the higher concentration of peptide, depended upon the mean concentration of peptide present over the bridge. In a constant gradient, e.g., a 10-fold increase in concentration across the bridge, the cells responded best between 10^{-6} and 10^{-5} M FMMM with $91 \pm 2\%$ (mean $\pm$ SEM, N = 8) of the scorable cells oriented toward the higher concentration. The percentages of oriented cells in nonoptimal gradients of FMMM were: 10^{-8} to 10^{-7} M, $66 \pm 2\%$ (N = 11); 10^{-7} to 10^{-6} M, $77 \pm 2\%$ (N = 10); 10^{-5} to 10^{-4} M, $65 \pm 10\%$ (N = 2). The optimal concentration range for FMLP was between 10^{-8} and 10^{-9} M. Evidence of an optimal concentration range for the chemotactic response has been demonstrated by studies using a millipore filter system (12), although in these studies the optimal concentration for chemotaxis was lower, between 10^{-7} and 10^{-6} M FMMM. The chemotactic response thus differs from that predicted by the Weber-Fechner law of sensory physiology according to which the response would be solely a function of the gradient. The concentration-dependent orientation is consistent with a response mechanism that depends upon the interaction of the peptide with a cell receptor having a particular binding constant, K_d. A cell that senses a gradient by detecting a different proportion of receptors bound on its two sides would be able to do this best in the concentration range of the K_d. In this range, the slope of a plot of the percentage of receptors bound versus the log of peptide concentration is steepest. Optimal orientation should occur at that concentration of chemotactic factor that corresponds to the functional interaction of the factor with the cell, the K_d. A similar dose-response relationship can be seen in bacterial systems in which the concentration of the optimal response and that of the binding constant correspond closely. The optimal concentration for leukocyte chemotaxis remains in some doubt, since cell inactivation of the factor may alter the concentration present. This complication will be discussed below.

Sensitivity of the Sensory Mechanism

The ability of a cell to sense a shallow gradient should also be optimal in the region of the binding constant. There was significant cell orientation, $69 \pm 4\%$ (mean $\pm$ SEM, $N = 4$) to a twofold gradient across the 1-mm bridge between 5×10^{-6} and 10^{-5} M FMMM. Under these conditions, the concentration difference across the dimensions of a given cell would be about 1%. As the steepness of the gradient was increased to 10-fold in the same concentration range, approximately a 10% difference in concentration across a cell's dimensions, the orientation response increased to greater than 90%.

As the steepness of the gradient was increased, the accuracy with which cells oriented toward the well containing the higher concentration increased along with the percentage of the population oriented into the correct 180° sector. Photographs of microscope fields with different percentages of the cells oriented were analyzed to determine the exact direction of movement, measured as degrees deviation from the direct path to the well. In optimal gradients where 90% of the cells oriented toward the well containing the high concentration of peptide, greater than 60% were oriented less than or equal to 30° from the direct path to the well.

Inactivation of the Peptides by the Cells

When high cell concentrations were present over the bridge (approximately 500 cells per mm^2), the cells tended to orient toward the closer side of the bridge. With 10^{-6} M FMMM present in both wells (i.e., no gradient), the cells in the 40X fields adjacent to the edge of the bridge were not randomly oriented; 86% of the cells on each side were oriented toward the edge near them. The orientation toward the near edge was dependent on high cell concentrations;

only 62% oriented toward the edge when the cell population was reduced to 10 cells per mm². This orientation, termed *the edge effect,* appears to be a result of inactivation of the peptides by cells over the bridge. As fresh peptide diffuses in from both sides, a gradient is established from each edge to the center, causing the orientation observed. No such gradient could be formed unless active peptide was present in the wells. Thus, even at high cell concentrations, edge orientation was not observed toward a well containing buffer rather than active peptide.

Aswanikumar et al. (1) have reported chemical evidence that PMNs can cleave and inactivate N-formylmethionyl dipeptides. This digestion can be inhibited by 0.1 mM tosyl-L-phenylalanyl chloromethyl ketone, TPCK, and by 0.1 mM N-benzoyltyrosine ethyl ester, BTEE. In behavioral tests in the visual chamber, I have found that the two inhibitors used at the concentration mentioned above prevent cell locomotion. At lower concentrations (0.01 mM), both locomotion and the edge effect can be observed. Both cell locomotion and the edge effect can be observed in the presence of other proteolytic inhibitors including 1 mg/ml lima bean trypsin inhibitor, soybean trypsin inhibitor, or human alpha 1 antitrypsin or of 1 mM either ethylenediaminetetraacetic acid (EDTA) or ethylene bis (oxyethylenenitro) tetraacetic acid (EGTA) in the absence of divalent cations.

Below about 50 cells per mm², the cell concentration did not significantly alter either the percentage of cells in the center of the bridge oriented toward the well containing the higher concentration of peptide or the optimal concentration range for chemotaxis. At higher cell concentrations, the presence of the edge effect did reduce the percentage of cells oriented toward the well containing the higher concentration of peptide. As mentioned above, cells responded to a twofold concentration difference across the 1-mm bridge. To ensure that the estimate of a 1% difference in concentration across the cell's dimensions was not in error because of digestion of the chemotactic factors, which would cause a steeper gradient, preparations with about 100 cells per square millimeter were reexamined in a twofold gradient. Cells adjacent to the well with the low concentration of factor were scored, and more than 65% oriented toward the well with the high concentration of peptide. Cell inactivation of peptide over the bridge would lead to a shallower rather than a steeper gradient in this region of the bridge.

DISCUSSION

The visual assay allows a rapid evaluation of cell orientation in specified concentrations and concentration gradients of chemotactic factors. The assay is sensitive; cell responses to shallow gradients can be detected. The estimate of the cell's ability to detect a 1% difference in concentration across its dimensions is in keeping with estimates by Ramsey (10) and by Grimes and Barnes (5).

The optimal concentration of chemotactic peptide for orientation in the visual assay was higher than that which was optimal for chemotaxis in the millipore system. Experiments were carried out to determine if this difference was because of the length of the assay, the cell concentrations present, or the species of PMNs used. None of these factors on their own accounted for the difference, nonetheless some combination of these factors may contribute to the difference. Even at low cell concentrations, there may be inactivation of the factors by cells in the small volume over the bridge decreasing the concentration of peptide present. The discrepancy could also be caused by the different parameters measured by the two techniques: the visual system measures exclusively cell orientation and requires only enough motility for a cell to develop a polarized morphology; the millipore assay measures oriented movement and requires active cell locomotion.

The orientation of cells toward the edge of the bridge nearest them (the edge effect) was particularly prominent when high concentrations of cells were present over the bridge. It did not occur toward an edge adjacent to a well that did not contain active peptide. These observations suggest that the effect is a result of inactivation of the peptide by the cells, presumably through absorption, ingestion, or digestion. Behavioral evidence for inactivation of chemotactic factors has not been previously reported, although Oldfield described cells which avoided regions between two centers of high cell density through what was believed to be a repulsive interaction between the cell populations (8). This "no-man's-land" might be a result of cell inactivation or depletion of stimulatory agents in the medium. Cell inactivation of chemotactic factors *in vivo* may play a role in limiting the inflammatory response.

It would be useful to inhibit digestion of the chemotactic factors while allowing cell locomotion. So far, an inhibitor has not been found that will inhibit digestion and yet allow locomotion; presumably, this is because of a general toxicity of the inhibitors at the doses that must be used; however, the possibility remains that the actions of the inhibitors on locomotion are specific and that proteolysis is a necessary part of cell locomotion.

The visual assay system is being used to analyze further the cell behavior by filming cells under varying conditions. In addition, the method may prove useful as a clinical tool, since it is relatively rapid and requires only the amount of blood available from a finger prick.

ACKNOWLEDGMENTS

I would like to thank Dr. George Palade for space and equipment used for these studies; Dr. Frank Ruddle for the use of the fluorescence microscope; and Dr. Nigel Godson for the use of a Joyce Loble densitometer. The author was supported by the American Cancer Society and as a Special Fellow of the Leukemia Society of America.

REFERENCES

1. Aswanikumar, S., Schiffmann, E., Corcoran, B. A., and Wahl, S. M. (1976): Role of a peptidase in phagocyte chemotaxis. *Proc. Natl. Acad. Sci. U.S.A.,* 73:2439–2442.
2. Besis, M. (1974): Necrotaxis: Chemotaxis towards injured cell. *Antiobiotics and Chemotherapy, Vol. 19: Chemotaxis: Its Biology and Biochemistry,* edited by E. Sorkin, pp. 369–381. S. Karger, Basel.
3. Boyden, S. (1962): Chemotactic effect of mixtures of antibody and antigen on polymorphonuclear leukocytes. *J. Exp. Med.,* 115:453–466.
4. Finkelstein, A., and Mauro, A. (1963): Equivalent circuits as related to ionic systems. *Biophys. J.,* 3:215–237.
5. Grimes, G. J., and Barnes, F. S. (1973): A technique for studying chemotaxis of leukocytes in well-defined chemotactic fields. *Exp. Cell Res.,* 29:375–385.
6. Harris, H. (1953): Chemotaxis of granulocytes. *J. Pathol. Bacteriol.,* 66:135–146.
7. Lotz, M., and Harris, H. (1956): Factors influencing chemotaxis of the polymorphonuclear leucocyte. *Br. J. Exp. Pathol.,* 37:477–480.
8. Oldfield, F. E. (1963): Orientation behavior of chick leukocytes in tissue culture and their interactions with fibroblasts. *Exp. Cell Res.,* 30:125–138.
9. Ramsey, W. S. (1972): Analysis of individual leukocyte behavior during chemotaxis. *Exp. Cell Res.,* 70:129–139.
10. Ramsey, W. S. (1974): Retraction fibers and leukocyte chemotaxis. *Exp. Cell Res.,* 86:184–187.
11. Schiffman, E., Corcoran, B. A., and Wahl, S. M. (1975): N-formylmethionyl peptides are chemotactic for leukocytes. *Proc. Natl. Acad. Sci. U.S.A.,* 72:1059–1062.
12. Showell, H. J., Freer, R. J., Zigmond, S. H., Schiffmann, E., Srivinivesaldratt, A., Corcoran, B., and Becker, E. L. (1976): The structure activity relations of synthetic peptides as chemotactic factors and inducers of lysosomal enzyme secretion for neutrophils. *J. Exp. Med.,* 143:1154–1169.
13. Wilkinson, P. C. (1974): *Chemotaxis and Inflammation.* Churchill Livingston, Edinburgh, pp. 150–157.
14. Zigmond, S. H. (1974): Mechanisms of sensing chemical gradients by polymorphonuclear leukocytes. *Nature,* 249:450–452.
15. Zigmond, S. H., and Hirsch, J. G. (1973): Leukocyte locomotion and chemotaxis: New methods for evaluation and demonstration of a cell-derived chemotactic factor. *J. Exp. Med.,* 137:387–410.

DISCUSSION

Dr. Gallin: Dr. Wilkinson's studies of cells migrating under conditions of chemokinesis demonstrated that such cells travel in straight paths rather than a random-walk pattern. He showed cells in a uniform concentration of stimulus with no gradient; individual cells were oriented about an axis, but the population of cells were not oriented uniformly. Do you conclude that the machinery for locomotion, whether it be random or directed, is likely to be the same? The difference is the uniformity of orientation of the entire cell population.

Dr. Zigmond: Yes.

Dr. Quie: Dr. Zigmond, have you had a chance to use this method for evaluation of activated serum, or bacterial chemotactic factors? Would it be a good idea to use synthetic peptides for evaluation of chemotaxis in clinical situations?

Dr. Zigmond: No, I really have not done a survey on other factors and I am uncertain about the clinical relevance of lack of response to peptides.

Dr. Becker: This is an answer to Dr. Quie's question. As Dr. Schiffmann demonstrates (in Chapter 9), there is some limited evidence suggesting that the receptor for the C5 fragment is different from the peptide receptor. This suggests that in the clinical studies one would not want to depend upon a single chemoattractant; however, I would make a plea that in doing clinical studies, except in the preliminary exploratory stages, one does not use activated serum, which is a mess.

Dr. Wilkinson: But the mess is what the cells see *in vivo.*

Dr. Becker: Yes, but if one is attempting to define the mechanisms involved, it is desirable to have a little more control than is possible with whole activated serum. In fact, this is why the cells are taken out of the body to study.

Dr. Ward: Have you ever looked for the effects of any of these peptides on lymphocyte orientation?

Dr. Zigmond: No, in fact, most of the preparations that I use in this assay are with an adherent cell population. I do not have any lymphocytes there. It is, in fact, possible that I am selecting for an adherent population among the neutrophils.

Dr. Quie: There may be little inconsistency in your observation—that all cells orient in a gradient—and the observation of Dr. Klempner that Dr. Gallin told us about—two populations of granulocytes in terms of locomotion and behavior. You have selected those cells which stick to the glass and have probably made a preselection of one population.

Dr. Snyderman: I would like to get back to whether protein is necessary for the f-Met peptides to cause orientation change. You said you had gelatin in your study. What are your data concerning the requirement for protein to get orientation changes?

Dr. Zigmond: Most of my studies were done in the presence of 1% gelatin. I did other studies in 0.9% sodium chloride, first washing cells with 1 millimolar EGTA or EDTA. The cells do not look good for very long, but it is possible to get an orientation response under those conditions.

Dr. Wilkinson: The trouble is your assay shows only orientation and not the whole chemotactic response.

Dr. Zigmond: Quite true, unless you also film the response.

Dr. Wilkinson: Chemotaxis is a sustained locomotion.

Dr. Zigmond: I think that chemotaxis is a complicated phenomenon, including orientation and locomotion. I am quite sure that cations are required for cell adherence. Cells have a difficult time translocating in the absence of calcium or magnesium because they are not sticking to the glass. A real question is how much external cation one needs for a motile process to occur.

Dr. Becker: It also is important, in terms of the analysis, to consider the possibility that for orientation, per se, one does not need cations, but for the locomotion, one does.

Dr. Zigmond: There is motility involved in developing that locomotive orientation, however, I think that cations are required for adhesion, which is necessary for locomotion.

Dr. Snyderman: I think it is very dangerous to make assumptions about the effects of extracellular calcium by using calcium-free medium, or even medium treated with EDTA. This is because we have recently shown that when such medium is used, where one can, perhaps, get cellular migration, the addition of lanthanum chloride, which essentially washes all calcium off the cells, results in inhibition of directed cell movement. In other words, unless one gets the calcium off the extracellular matrix of the cell one really does not know how much extracellular calcium is functionally present for the cells to utilize.

Dr. Zigmond: Operationally, I can tell you that I had 1 millimolar EDTA.

Dr. Stossel: There is no way that there can be calcium on the outside of the cell under those conditions. There is also no way there can be calcium in flux.

Dr. Snyderman: That is not true. EDTA will only chelate Ca^{+2} within the binding limits ($K_D \simeq 10^{-8}$ for Ca^{+2}) and then only freely ionizable Ca^{+2}.

Dr. Williams: Are you not curious as to what these peptides do? It would be fascinating to label them to see if the degree of orientation were directly correlated with the number of cell receptors.

Dr. Zigmond: This is an important question. There is a good correlation between the optimal concentration of fMet peptides for chemotaxis and orientation. I also think there are going to be a number of interesting studies showing the distribution of these receptors during orientation. Clearly, these questions need further investigation.

Dr. Schiffmann: Dr. Zigmond, you mentioned the effect of colchicine. Have you studied the effect of ouabain on orientation?

Dr. Zigmond: No, I have not looked at ouabain.

Leukocyte Chemotaxis, edited by John I. Gallin
and Paul G. Quie. Raven Press, New York
© 1978.

Modified Boyden Chamber Method Of Measuring Polymorphonuclear Leukocyte Chemotaxis

K. Lynn Cates, Casann E. Ray, and Paul G. Quie

*Department of Pediatrics, University of Minnesota School of Medicine,
Minneapolis, Minnesota 55455*

The method used for evaluation of human neutrophil chemotaxis in the authors' laboratory at the University of Minnesota is a modification of methods originally described by Boyden. Most of the modifications of the Boyden method used in our laboratory were developed by Peter Ward and, indeed, the earliest evaluations of human neutrophil chemotaxis at the University of Minnesota School of Medicine were done by A Todd Davis after observing the method in Dr. Ward's laboratory. Further evolution of the method occurred during the Harry Hill years at Minnesota, and details of those methods are described by Hill et al. (2). The Boyden method has been modified even further during the past several months, and the present method used for the evaluation of neutrophil chemotactic activity in patients suspected of having abnormal neutrophil function and for investigation of chemotaxis is described.

The procedures are detailed in step-by-step fashion with the expectation that investigators will be able to set up their laboratories and begin experiments.

MATERIALS

1. Chemotaxis Modified Boyden Chambers, #B-312, Neuroprobe, Inc., 7621 Cabin Road, Bethesda, Maryland 20034.
2. Hanks' Balanced Salt Solution (10x), #406, Gibco, 3175 Staley Road, Grand Island, New York 14072.
3. Hepes Buffer, #H3375, Sigma Chemical Company, P.O. Box 14508, St. Louis, Missouri 63178.
4. Millipore Filters, #SMWP 013 00 5μ-pore size, 13-mm diameter, Millipore Corporation, Bedford, Massachusetts 01730.
5. Hematoxylin-Harris' Alum Hematoxylin, #638, Harleco, Gibbstown, New Jersey 08027.
6. Staining Tank and filter holder template, University of Minnesota Scientific Apparatus Shop, Minneapolis, Minnesota 55455.
7. Sorvall GLC-1 centrifuge.

8. Tissue Culture Medium 199, #12–109, Microbiological Associates, 5221 River Road, Bethesda, Maryland 20016.
9. Zymosan A (from *S. cerevisiae* yeast), #Z-4250, Sigma Chemical Company, P.O. Box 14508, St. Louis, Missouri 63178.
10. Dextran, 6% Gentran 75 (Dextran 75) and 0.9% Sodium Chloride Injection, Travenol Laboratories, Inc., Deerfield, Illinois 60015.

PREPARATION OF REAGENTS

1 M Hepes buffer is obtained by dissolving 23.8 g Hepes buffer in 60.0 ml sterile distilled H_2O and then adding NaOH (50%) to the solution dropwise at 25°C until a pH of 7.85 is reached. This mixture is poured into a volumetric flask and diluted to the 100.0-ml mark with sterile distilled H_2O; 3.1-ml aliquots are stored at −70°C. Once thawed, the solution is not refrozen.

Buffered Hanks' Balanced Salt Solution (HBSS) (1X) 100 ml is made by combining 10.0 ml HBSS (10X), 87.0 ml sterile distilled H_2O, and 3.0 ml Hepes buffer.

The chemoattractant, *Escherichia coli* bacterial factor (BFE), is prepared by inoculating 100 ml of Tissue Culture Medium 199 with one loopful of *E. coli* (originally obtained from Peter Ward, Farmington, Conn.) and growing at 37°C for 24 hr. This suspension is then centrifuged for 20 min at 10,000 rpm in a Sorvall bottle and the supernate filtered (0.22-μ pore size) for sterility. It is divided into 1.1-ml aliquots for storage at −70°C. For use, it is thawed and resuspended in buffered HBSS (1X) for a final concentration of 50 μl BFE/ml HBSS.

In preparing activated serum (AS), 0.025 g of zymosan is needed to activate 1.0 ml of serum. The appropriate amount of zymosan is weighed out and washed with phosphate-buffered saline (about 1 ml PBS/0.025g zymosan), vortexed to mix, and then spun at 2,000 rpm for 10 min, and the supernate is decanted. Serum is added to the zymosan precipitate and vortexed vigorously. After 30 min incubation in a 37°C water bath, it is spun at 2,000 rpm for 10 min, and the supernate is removed and stored in aliquots at −70°C. For chemotaxis, the activated serum is diluted to a concentration of 100 μl AS/ml of buffered HBSS (1X).

20 g $MgSO_4 − 7H_2O$ plus 2 g $NaHCO_3$ is diluted up to 1,000 ml with sterile distilled H_2O to make the bluing agent used for staining filters.

Leukocyte diluting fluid is made by diluting 1% gentian violet 1:100 in 1.5% glacial acetic acid.

PREPARATION OF LEUKOCYTES

Heparinized blood (0.1 ml of 1,000 units per milliliter heparin per 10 ml whole blood) is drawn and gravity- or dextran-sedimented. For gravity sedimentation, the blood is left in an upright syringe for 1 hr at room temperature and then leukocyte-rich plasma (LRP) is expelled through a bent needle. Dextran sedimentation is performed by adding 2 ml dextran to 10 ml heparinized whole blood in a plastic tube. This is left to settle at a 45° angle for 45 to 60 min and then the LRP is removed with a Pasteur pipette. LRP is spun at 800 rpm for 10 min and then the plasma is removed and saved. The cells are washed twice with buffered HBSS (1X) by gently resuspending the cells in approximately 3 to 5 ml of HBSS, spinning at 800 rpm for 5 min, and then discarding the supernate. The wash is repeated.

The washed cells are resuspended in a convenient amount of buffered HBSS (1X) (2 to 5 ml) and a leukocyte (WBC) count and wet differential are performed. The WBC suspension is diluted in a WBC diluting pipette with WBC diluting fluid. The count is done with a hemacytometer, under high power (45X). The number of PMNs in 4 squares times 50×10^{-3} is equal to the number of PMNs $\times 10^6$ per milliliter of cell suspension.

The cell suspension is then diluted to the desired concentration of PMNs (usually 2×10^6 PMN/ml final suspension) using buffered HBSS (1X) and the desired concentration of plasma or serum (usually 10%) or other additives as required.

Cells suspended in homologous plasma or serum or heterologous substances are preincubated for 15 min at 37°C. No preincubation is necessary for cells suspended in autologous plasma or serum.

FILLING CHAMBERS

The bottom of a petri dish is covered with buffered HBSS (1X) and the filters are floated *rough side up* on the HBSS. Filters that do not absorb media *quickly* and *evenly* are discarded. One filter at a time is placed into the Boyden chambers, and the top of the chamber is screwed on. The chemoattractant is added to the lower compartment (up to the level of the bend) with a Pasteur pipette, tilting the chambers to avoid bubble accumulation under the filters. The final cell suspension 0.4 ml is then placed in the upper compartment. Enough additional chemoattractant is added to the lower compartment to fill it to the same level as the cell compartment. Filled chambers are placed in centrifuge carriers and spun in a Sorvall centrifuge for 3 min at 300 rpm. The cell compartment is then filled to the top with buffered HBSS (1X) and the attractant compartment to the top with the appropriate attractant. The chambers are covered to prevent evaporation and then incubated at 37°C for 120 min.[1]

STAINING OF FILTERS

Fluids on both sides of the filter are removed by shaking. The tops are removed from all chambers, and the filters are placed on edge to allow quick removal.

---

[1] Time curves should be performed in each laboratory to determine optimal incubation time. The usual range is 75 min to 3 hr.

Filters are not allowed to dry out. Just before loading the staining rack, each filter is dipped quickly in methanol to fix the cells. The filters are loaded, cell side down, into the filter holder and stained as follows, draining on gauze gently after each dunking:

- filtered hematoxylin for 2 min
- H_2O rinse
- 70% alcohol for 1/2 min
- H_2O rinse
- bluing agent for 2 min
- H_2O rinse
- 70% propanol for 1/2 min
- 95% propanol for 1/2 min
- 100% propanol for 2 min
- 100% propanol for 2 min
- 100% propanol for 3 min
- xylene for 2 min
- xylene for 2 min

To mount filters, one drop of Permount is put on a glass slide, the filter is placed, *cell side down,* on the Permount, one more drop of Permount is added and a coverslip is dropped onto the filter. All solutions are changed daily except the stain, which is reused after refiltering.

COUNTING FILTERS

The number of PMN adhering to the chemoattractant side of the filter (i.e., cells that have come completely through filter) inside a 5- X 5-mm grid in 10 randomly selected high-power fields (10X ocular and 45X objective) is counted. The mean number of cells migrating in response to buffered HBSS alone is subtracted from the mean number of cells migrating in response to the chemoattractant to determine the chemotactic activity. The result is usually a 2- to 3-digit number.

To correct for day-to-day variation in the absolute chemotactic activity, results are expressed as percent of the control chemotactic activity, 100% being normal.

$$\% \text{ control chemotactic activity} = \frac{\text{experimental chemotactic activity}}{\text{control chemotactic activity}} \times 100$$

A major problem in measuring chemotactic response by the Boyden method is lack of uniformity of the micropore filters. This problem continues to plague us and, for that reason, all assays must be run in triplicate. If an abnormality of chemotaxis is observed, the test must be repeated to document reproducibility. Ideally, neutrophil locomotion should be studied by different methods (i.e., leading-front or under-agarose) to confirm abnormal locomotion.

REFERENCES

1. Boyden, S. V. (1962): The chemotactic effect of mixtures of antibody and antigen on polymorpho-nuclear leucocytes. *J. Exp. Med.*, 115:453–466.
2. Hill, H. R., Hogan, N. A., Mitchell, T. G., and Quie, P. G. (1975): Evaluation of a cytocentrifuge method for measuring neutrophil granulocyte chemotaxis. *J. Lab. Clin. Med.*, 86:703–710.

Leukocyte Chemotaxis, edited by John I. Gallin
and Paul G. Quie. Raven Press, New York
© 1978.

Methodology for Monocyte and Macrophage Chemotaxis

Ralph Snyderman and Marilyn C. Pike

*Division of Rheumatic and Genetic Diseases, Duke University Medical Center,
Durham, North Carolina 27710*

MATERIALS

Chemotaxis Chambers and Filters

Several types of chambers are available for the quantification of chemotaxis *in vitro.* They generally contain an upper compartment into which a standardized cell suspension is placed and a lower compartment into which is placed the chemotactic or control stimulus (Figs. 1 and 2). The upper and lower compartments are separated by a porous filter. For studying macrophage chemotaxis, two types of filters are used in the authors' laboratory (3,5,6). The polycarbonate (Nuclepore) filters with a 5.0-μm pore size and 15-μm thickness can be purchased from Wallabs Inc., San Rafael, California; Neuroprobe Inc., Bethesda, Maryland 20014; or BioRad Inc., Richmond, California 94802. These filters have through-and-through round holes with a diameter of 5.0 μm. Cellulose nitrate filters with a pore size of 8 μm and a thickness of approximately 150 μm can be obtained from the Sartorious Division, Brinkman Instruments, Westbury, New York 11590. These filters have convoluted pores. Chemotaxis chambers can be purchased from Neuroprobe Inc. or can be made by any good instrument shop.

Cell Preparation

Human Mononuclear Leukocytes

Preparations of human peripheral blood mononuclear leukocytes are obtained from Ficoll-Hypaque gradients as follows (3,6): heparinized (10 μ/ml) venous blood is diluted 1 : 4 in physiological saline and approximately 35 ml placed in Falcon No. 2070 conical centrifuge tubes. Twelve milliliters of a mixture containing 2.4 parts of 9% Ficoll (Pharmacia Fine Chemicals, Piscataway, New Jersey 08854) and 1 part 33.9% hypaque (Winthrop Laboratories, Atlanta, Georgia 30304) is injected below the diluted blood using a 50-ml syringe and a 16-gauge, 4-inch spinal needle. Following centrifugation at 20°C for 40 min at

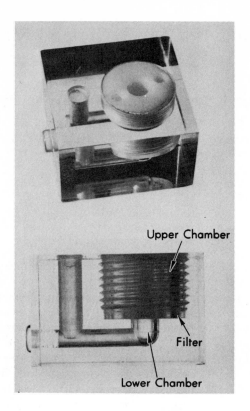

FIG. 1. Modified Boyden chemotaxis chamber. A standardized cell suspension (0.4 ml) is placed in the upper compartment of the chamber and is separated from the chemotactic stimulant or medium alone (0.85 ml) in the lower compartment by a polycarbonate or nitrocellulose filter. (From Snyderman et al., ref. 9, with permission.)

400 g, the diluted plasma is aspirated and the buffy coat removed, using a 9-inch Pasteur pipette. A maximum of 7.5 ml of the cell suspension is placed in 50-ml Falcon centrifuge tubes and to this is added 40 ml of phosphate buffered (pH 7.0) isotonic saline containing 0.1% gelatin (PBS). The tubes are centrifuged for 15 min at 300 g, 4°C. The cell pellets are washed once more with PBS and then are combined, resuspended in medium RPMI 1640, pH 7.0 (Grand Island Biological Co., Grand Island, New York 14072), and standardized to contain 1.5×10^6 monocytes per milliliter for use in the chemotaxis assay.

Guinea Pig Peritoneal Macrophages

Approximately 25 to 30 ml of 0.5% shellfish glycogen in isotonic saline is injected into the peritoneal cavities of guinea pigs (10). Four days later, the

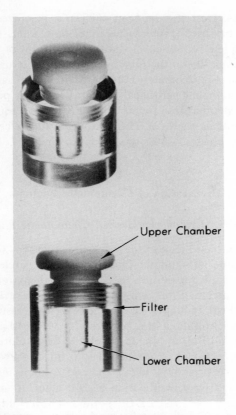

FIG. 2. Blind well chemotaxis chamber. A standardized cell suspension (0.2 ml) is placed in the upper compartment of the chamber and is separated from the chemotactic stimulant or medium alone (0.2 ml) in the lower compartment by a polycarbonate or nitrocellulose filter. (From Snyderman and Pike, ref. 6, with permission.)

guinea pigs are killed, and the peritoneal cavities lavaged vigorously with 150 ml Gey's balanced salt solution containing 0.01M Hepes buffer (Calbiochem, La Jolla, California 92037), pH 7.0 (Gey's BSS). Following one wash in Gey's BSS, the exudate cells, which contain approximately 75% macrophages and 25% lymphocytes, are standardized to contain 1.5×10^6 macrophages/ml in Gey's BSS for use in the chemotaxis assay (10).

Mouse Peritoneal Macrophages

Mice are injected intraperitoneally with 35 μg phytohemagglutinin (PHA, Burroughs Wellcome Co., Beckenham, England) or 50 μg concanavalin (Con A, Pharmacia Fine Chemicals Co., Piscataway, New Jersey 08854) contained in 2-ml sterile, isotonic saline or with 2 ml of a 9% solution of proteose peptone

(Difco Laboratories, Detroit, Michigan 48233) in deionized water (8,9). Two (PHA or Con A) or three (proteose peptone) days later, the abdominal wall is exposed by complete retraction of the skin, and 9 ml of Gey's BSS injected vigorously into the midline of the intact peritoneal cavity using a 10-ml syringe and 19-gauge needle. Approximately 8.0 ml are withdrawn using the same syringe and needle. The individual peritoneal exudates are then pooled, washed once in Gey's BSS, and standardized to contain 2.2×10^6 macrophages per milliliter for use in the chemotaxis assay (9). The peritoneal exudate cells contain approximately 70% macrophages, 28% lymphocytes, and 2% polymorphonuclear leukocytes.

Preparation of Chemotactic Factors

Human Lymphocyte-derived Chemotactic Factor

Human peripheral blood leukocytes are sedimented for 20 min at room temperature; equal volumes of undiluted blood and 3% (w/v) dextran (T500, Pharmacia, Piscataway, New Jersey) are used, contained in sterile isotonic saline. The supernatant is decanted following sedimentation, centrifuged, and washed twice with sterile RPMI 1640, pH 7.2. The cells are then resuspended to contain 2×10^6 total cells per milliliter in serum-free RPMI 1640, and 25-ml aliquots placed in sterile 250-ml Falcon No. 25100 plastic tissue culture flasks, to which is then added 250 μg of Con A contained in 5 ml of RPMI 1640. Following incubation for 24 to 48 hr at 37°C in 5% CO_2, 95% humidified air, the supernatant fluid is harvested by centrifugation at 500 g for 10 min, aliquoted, and stored at −70°C until use. The LDCF is diluted threefold to 20-fold for use as a positive control stimulant in the chemotaxis assay. Medium alone, culture supernatants from unstimulated leukocytes, or unstimulated supernatants to which Con A is added after culture can serve as negative controls (1,3).

Chemotactically Activated Serum

One milliliter of human, guinea pig, or mouse serum is incubated with 0.1 ml isotonic saline containing 1 mg of *Salmonella typhosa* 0901 endotoxin (Difco Laboratories, Detroit, Mich.) or zymosan for 60 min at 37°C, followed by 56°C for 30 min. The activated serum, the chemotactic activity of which is predominantly a result of the production of C5a, is diluted to approximately 0.5 to 3.0% in the appropriate medium for use as a positive chemotactic stimulus (3,9,10).

METHODOLOGY

Prior to the chemotaxis assay, the filters can be numbered along the edge using ball-point ink. Forceps should always be employed for handling the filters.

When the blind well chemotaxis chamber is used, 0.2 ml of the chemotactic or control stimulus is placed in the lower compartment of the chamber and the filter is placed above, just touching the liquid. When polycarbonate filters are used, the filter is placed *dull side* up. The cellulose nitrate filters have no readily apparent means for identifying either side. After the filter is placed in the chamber, the cap is secured in place and 0.2 ml of the appropriate cell suspension is placed in the upper well. Care must be taken to avoid air bubbles above or below the filter (6).

When the modified Boyden chambers are used, the filters are first placed in the chamber and the cap secured in place. The substance being tested for chemotactic activity is delivered into the lower compartment of the chamber using a 6-inch Pasteur pipette. Immediately after the liquid makes contact with the filter, the cells (about 0.4 ml) are introduced with a Pasteur pipette into the upper compartment and both sides of the chamber are filled simultaneously (6).

The chambers containing cells and stimulants are incubated at 37°C in humidified air for 90 min when human monocytes or guinea pig macrophages are used, or for 4 hours when mouse macrophages are used. Following incubation, the residual cells and stimulants are aspirated with pasteur pipettes and the filters placed into staining trays (Duke University Surgical Instrument Shop, Durham, North Carolina 27710). The filters are then fixed in ethanol for 15 sec, stained with Mayer's hematoxylin for 6 min, followed by 1 min each in acid alcohol and bluing solution, respectively (4). After staining, the filters are placed right side up on 22- X 50-mm glass cover slips, air-dried, and mounted upside down onto glass slides using immersion oil. Chemotaxis is quantified by counting and averaging the total number of macrophages that have migrated per oil immersion microscopic field (1000 to 1500 X). When the cellulose nitrate filters, which require a dehydrating step, are used, they are placed sequentially for 1 min each in 70%, 95%, and absolute alcohol following the staining procedure. The filters are then clarified in xylene and placed upside down directly onto glass slides under cover slips (10).

CRITICAL COMMENTS

The monocyte and macrophage chemotaxis assays described herein are quantitative, reproducible means of measuring unidirectional cell migration. It should be noted that these assays enable one to distinguish between chemotaxis, random migration, and chemokinesis (7). Use of the blind well chambers is preferable when small amounts of cells or chemotactic stimuli are available; however, the modified Boyden chambers are easier and faster to load. Using the polycarbonate filters permits shorter incubation times as well as easier determination of morphology of the migrated cells. This is important when heterogeneous cell populations are being tested. A disadvantage of the polycarbonate filter is its thinness, which allows only the scoring of cells on either side of, but not within, the filter (see below). Another is the danger of cells falling off the bottom of the filter; this may be greater with the polycarbonate filter than with the nitrocellulose filter, although it has not been a problem in our hands.

An alternative method for quantifying chemotaxis is to measure the distance into the cellulose nitrate filter to which the leading front of cells have migrated (11). This method can be tedious and requires a homogeneous cell population, but it is accurate, reproducible, and it alleviates the danger of cells falling off the bottom of the filter. Chemotaxis can also be quantified using a radioassay (2). Cells are labeled with ^{51}Cr and placed above two filters in the modified Boyden chambers. After incubation, the bottom filter is counted for gamma radiation. This method allows a more objective scoring of chemotaxis, but should be used only for homogeneous cell populations.

REFERENCES

1. Altman, L. C., Snyderman, R., Hausman, M. S., and Mergenhagen, S. E. (1973): A human mononuclear leukocyte chemotactic factor: Characterization, specificity, and kinetics of production by homologous leukocytes. *J. Immunol.,* 110:801–810.
2. Gallin, J. I., Clark, R. A., and Kimball, H. R. (1973): Granulocyte chemotaxis: An improved in vitro assay employing ^{51}Cr-labeled granulocytes. *J. Immunol.,* 110:233–240.
3. Snyderman, R., Altman, L. C., Hausman, M. S., and Mergenhagen, S. E. (1972): Human mononuclear leukocyte chemotaxis: A quantitative assay for humoral and cellular chemotactic factors. *J. Immunol.,* 108:857–860.
4. Snyderman, R., Gewurz, H., and Mergenhagen, S. E. (1968): Interactions of the complement system with endotaxic polysaccharides: Generation of a chemotactic factor for polymorphonuclear leukocytes. *J. Exp. Med.,* 128:259–275.
5. Snyderman, R., and Mergenhagen, S. E. (1976): Chemotaxis of macrophages. In: *Immunobiology of the Macrophage,* edited by D. S. Nelson, pp. 323–348. Academic Press, New York.
6. Snyderman, R., and Pike, M. C. (1976): Chemotaxis of mononuclear cells. In: *In Vitro Methods in Cell Mediated and Tumor Immunity,* edited by B. R. Bloom and J. R. David, pp. 651–661. Academic Press, New York.
7. Snyderman, R., and Pike, M. C. (1977): Pathophysiological aspects of leukocyte chemotaxis: Identification of a specific chemotactic factor binding site on human granulocytes and defects of macrophage function associated with neoplasia. *(This volume.)*
8. Snyderman, R., Pike, M. C., Blaylock, B. L. and Weinstein, P. (1976): Effects of neoplasms on inflammation: Depression of macrophage accumulation after tumor implantation. *J. Immunol.,* 116:585–589.
9. Snyderman, R., Pike, M. C., McCarley, D., and Lang, L. (1975): Quantification of mouse macrophage chemotaxis in vitro: Role of C5 for the production of chemotactic activity. *Infect. Immun.,* 11:488–492.
10. Snyderman, R., Shin, H. S., and Hausman, M. H. (1971): A chemotactic factor for mononuclear leukocytes. *Proc. Soc. Exp. Biol. Med.,* 138:387–390.
11. Zigmond, S. H., and Hirsch, J. G. (1973): Leukocyte locomotion and chemotaxis: New methods for evaluation and demonstration of cell derived chemotactic factor. *J. Exp. Med.,* 137:387–410.

Leukocyte Chemotaxis, edited by John I. Gallin
and Paul G. Quie. Raven Press, New York
© 1978.

Radioassay of Leukocyte Locomotion: A Sensitive Technique for Clinical Studies

*John I. Gallin, **Robert A. Clark, and †Edward J. Goetzl

*Laboratory of Clinical Investigation, National Institute of Allergy and Infectious Diseases, National Institutes of Health, Bethesda, Maryland 20014; **Department of Medicine, University of Washington, Seattle, Washington 98195; and †Laboratory for the Study of Immunological Diseases, Howard Hughes Medical Institutes, Harvard Medical School and Robert Bent Brigham Hospital, Boston, Massachusetts 02120*

Over four years have passed since the development of a radioassay of leukocyte locomotion. The assay, which utilizes 51-chromium (^{51}Cr)-labeled leukocytes and a double micropore filter system, was initially developed for assessment of polymorphonuclear leukocyte (PMN) locomotion (13,18), and has now also been adapted for measurement of monocyte locomotion (14,26). Working independently, we have accumulated considerable experience using this technique. We feel the method is a reliable, objective, and practical screening test of human leukocyte locomotion. The purpose of this chapter is to summarize the method, review our recent clinical experience with the technique, and suggest possible roles of this assay in an assessment of apparent aberrations in leukocyte locomotion.

MATERIALS AND METHODS

Acrylic chemotactic chambers (Neuroprobe, Bethesda and Ahlco Scientific, Granby, Conn.) were designed to hold two 13 mm-diameter cellulose nitrate micropore filters. The filters, which separate upper (cell) and lower (stimulus) compartments, were obtained from either Millipore Corp., Bedford, Mass. or Särtorius, Gottingen, West Germany (distributed by Beckman Instruments, Mountainside, N.J.). Medium 199 or Gey's Tissue Culture Medium pH 7.2 containing 2.0% bovine serum albumin, 2% penicillin and streptomycin (Microbiological Associates, Bethesda) were used for cell suspensions during chemotaxis, and Hanks' solution was used for cell labeling with chromium-51 (^{51}Cr), which was obtained from New England Nuclear (Boston) or Amersham-Searle Corp. (Arlington Heights, Illinois)

Leukocyte and Chemotactic Factor Preparation

For PMN chemotaxis, leukocytes were obtained from citrated or heparinized peripheral blood by dextran sedimentation. Residual erythrocytes were removed

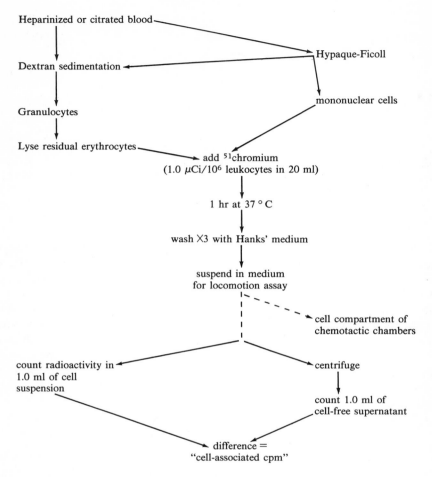

FIG. 1. Leukocyte preparation for radioassay.

by either ammonium chloride (18) or hypotonic saline lysis (5), and the leuko-cytes were then washed in Hanks' solution. For monocyte chemotaxis, mononu-clear cells were isolated from peripheral blood by the Hypaque-Ficoll technique (2). The mononuclear cells were washed twice in Hanks' solution.

Leukocytes free of erythrocytes were labeled with ^{51}Cr (Fig. 1) by either incubating 10^8 cells with 200 μCi of ^{51}Cr in 1.0 ml for 20 min at 25°C (E.G.) or incubating 10^6 cells with 1.0 μCi of ^{51}Cr for 1 hr at 37° (Gallin and Clark). The labeled cells were then washed two (Goetzl) or three times (Clark and Gallin) in Hanks' media and then suspended in the media used for chemotactic assay (medium 199 with 0.5% ovalbumin pH 7.4) (Goetzl) or Gey's tissue culture media with 2.0% bovine serum albumin and penicillin and streptomycin (Clark and Gallin). Such labeled cells contained 10,000 to 30,000 cpm/10^6

cells, depending on the specific activity of the ^{51}Cr used. Any chemotactic stimulus can be used for the assay. The standard stimuli we use include endotoxin-activated serum (2.5%) (5), sodium caseinate (Difco Laboratories, Detroit, Michigan, 5 mg per milliliter, 0.85% NaCl) (13), kallikrein (21), or C5a obtained by trypsinization of C5 (28) or partially purified from endotoxin-activated serum (16).

Assembly of Chemotactic Chambers

Two micropore filters are inserted into a recessed upper compartment in the acrylic chambers (see Fig. 5 of Chap. 2, by Maderazo and Woronick), and held in place by a threaded Teflon cylinder, which forms the side walls of the leukocyte well. The well can vary in diameter to hold 0.3 to 0.8 ml cells. For PMN locomotion, two 3.0-μm or two 5.0-μm pore micropore filters are used, and for mononuclear cells two 8.0-μm pore filters are used. The chemotactic factor is added to the bottom compartment first, with tilting as needed to allow air bubbles to escape. The ^{51}Cr-labeled leukocytes (2.3 × 10[6] for PMNs and 3.0 × 10[6] for mononuclear cells) are added to the upper compartment using a pipette gun to deliver a set volume of cells. After loading, chambers are incubated in high humidity at 37°C for varying times. For PMN migration, standard incubation is 3 hr, and for mononuclear cells, incubation is 4 hr. The chambers are then dismantled (Fig. 2), the bottom filters rinsed x3 in saline (the apparatus shown in Fig. 3 is convenient), and then the radioactivity counted. For each cell preparation, portions are incubated in the dilutions of stimuli studied and in buffer alone and then are centrifuged, and the cell-associated radioactivity is determined as the difference in radioactivity of the cell suspension before centrifugation and the corresponding supernatants after centrifugation. For quantitation of the results, the responses are either expressed as counts per 4 min in the lower filter, per 50,000 counts per 4 min in the

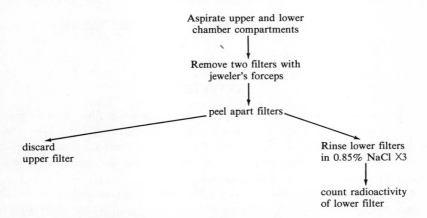

FIG. 2. Handling of filters after chemotaxis. (See Fig. 3 for basket used to rinse filters.)

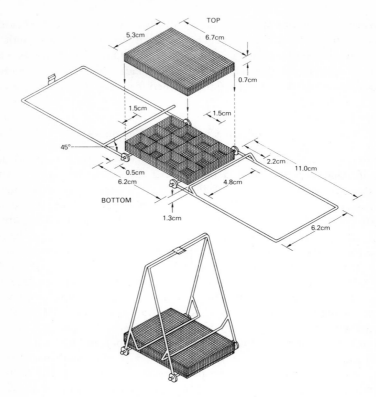

FIG. 3. Basket for rinsing filters.

initial 0.5 ml of cell suspension (18), or as cells in the lower filter as reflected by counts per min in the lower filter based on arbitrary standard uptake of 10,000 cpm/10^6 cells and computed according to the formula (13):

$$\begin{array}{l} \text{cells in lower} \\ \text{filter as} \\ \text{corrected cpm} \end{array} = \frac{\text{observed cpm lower filter} \times 10,000}{\text{cpm/}10^6 \text{ cells}}$$

RESULTS

Leukocytes migrate through the upper and into the lower filter with no apparent barrier to migration offered by the interface between the filters. With PMN migration through 3.0-μm filters, mixed leukocytes freed of erythrocytes by dextran sedimentation are acceptable, as the mononuclear cells do not cross the top filter during the incubation period.

The ^{51}Cr has no detectable effect on the leukocyte migration (13,18), and the isotope remains within the cells. With the ^{51}Cr technique, individual observer variability and subjectivity and observer-to-observer variability, which is considerable in the morphologic assay (13), are eliminated. The sources of variability in the assay include inherent differences among cells from different individuals; this variability exceeds day-to-day variability using a single cell source (9). This variability is comparable to that noted with the morphologic techniques (9,13).

CLINICAL APPLICATIONS

Humoral defects in the generation of chemotactic activity in serum or plasma have been found by the ^{51}Cr radioassay in patients with C1r deficiency (10), C4 deficiency (7, and Chap. 24), C2 deficiency (12, and Chap. 24), C3 deficiency (Chap. 24), and Fletcher factor deficiency (29). These abnormalities were clearly demonstrable by the ^{51}Cr assay, even though they were for the most part rather subtle, requiring a careful examination of serum concentration or kinetics of chemotactic factor generation.

Even more examples of cellular defects in leukocyte chemotaxis detected by the radioassay can be cited. In the Chediak-Higashi syndrome (CHS), the neutrophil chemotactic dysfunction was initially demonstrated with a conventional morphologic assay (5), but a subsequent study (13) showed virtually identical defects in two CHS patients studied in parallel with the conventional and ^{51}Cr assays. CHS mice were found to have a similar neutrophil defect by the radioassay (11). Monocyte chemotactic defects were detected in CHS humans and mink, when both morphologic and ^{51}Cr assays were used (14). A number of patients with the syndrome of hyperimmunoglobulinemia E and defective neutrophil chemotaxis have been studied by the radioassay. The defect in the initial patient was detected by both assays (8,10,13). Two Job's syndrome patients were studied in parallel with both assays showing similar chemotactic defects (20). When the morphologic and radioassay have been used, it has recently been shown that levamisole, *in vitro* and *in vivo,* corrects these abnormalities toward normal (30). A patient with icthyosis and elevated serum levels of IgE had defective neutrophil chemotaxis by the ^{51}Cr assay (24), and atopic dermatitis patients had defects by both morphologic and radioassays (25). Many patients in a large group of subjects receiving bone marrow transplants were found to have decreased neutrophil chemotaxis using the ^{51}Cr assay (4). Other examples of diseases characterized by defective PMN leukocyte migration, which has been detected by this assay, include α-mannosidosis (15), hypogammaglobulinemia (10), periodontosis (Chap. 24), and an isolated patient with recurrent infections (3).

More recently the ^{51}Cr assay has proven superior to the morphologic filter assay in revealing abnormalities in leukocyte motility in some conditions. Several studies of *in vitro* chemotaxis of polymorphonuclear (PMN) leukocytes from patients with rheumatic diseases have revealed intrinsic defects in the chemotactic response in rheumatoid arthritis, Felty's syndrome, and some subjects with systemic lupus erythematosus (6,17,23,32). Discrepancies among the results in individual reports have generally been attributed to differences in the characteristics of the patients in each series; however, the methods employed to quantitate PMN chemotaxis varied considerably with respect to leukocyte purification and concentration, filter type and pore size, and chemotactic stimuli. The concomitant application of both a modified single-filter Boyden assay and a double-filter radiomigration assay to study *in vitro* leukotaxis in 13 consecutive untreated subjects with rheumatic diseases revealed the greater sensitivity of the radiomigration assay of detecting intrinsic cell defects (17). PMN leukocytes from four patients with systemic lupus erythematosus showed both defective spontaneous migration ($p < 0.05$) and depressed chemotactic responsiveness to C5a and kallikrein ($p < 0.01$) compared to normal PMN leukocytes in a double-filter radiomigration assay, but not with a conventional single-filter Boyden technique (17). The latter assay did not uncover any defects in spontaneous migration or chemotaxis which were less prominent in the radioassay.

Numerous investigators have detected abnormalities in the *in vitro* mononuclear leukocyte chemotactic responses of patients with melanoma and other tumors (1,19,26,27). Differences among the chemotactic methods as well as the patient series have precluded a precise interpretation of the origin and evolution of the monocyte defect. The assessment of monocyte chemotactic responses to C5a utilizing both the single-filter Boyden method and a double-filter radiomigration technique with cells from nine subjects with stage III melanoma revealed a more significant depression of monocyte chemotaxis with the latter assay ($p < 0.01$) than with the conventional Boyden method ($p < 0.05$) (26). Serial studies in six of these patients utilizing both assays always showed that the defect in monocyte chemotactic responsiveness was more prominent with the double-filter radioassay.

COMMENT

The radioassay of leukocyte locomotion has proven the most reliable functional screening test for clinical studies. The method is easy to learn and eliminates the time-consuming task of microscopic enumeration of leukocytes in stained filters. The double-filter radioassay is in one sense a leading-front technique that measures the response of the leading population of cells which enter the lower filter and comprise 15 to 20% of the entire cell population. This renders the method preferable to the morphologic leading-front method, which measures only a small sample of the cell population (31). This increased population sampling renders the technique more sensitive in the clinical situations studied than the morphologic leading-front method. The radioassay does not, however, provide as much information about the entire population of responding cells as the time-consuming morphologic technique of counting cells at different depths into a single cellulose nitrate filter as described originally by Zigmond and Hirsch (31).

Some limitations of the technique need to be emphasized. A major limitation of the radioassay is the inability to distinguish cell types (i.e., eosinophils from neutrophils). When such morphologic distinction is required, either a standard single-filter Boyden assay (Chap. 5, by Cates, Ray, and Quie) or the agarose technique (Chap. 2, by Nelson, McCormack, and Fiegel) is particularly useful. The radioassay is suitable for distinguishing enhanced random migration from directed migration by testing different concentrations of chemotactic stimuli in both the cell and stimulus compartments of the chemotactic chambers (16); however, the technique does not yield direct information on cell orientation for which either the orientation assay of cells stuck to glass (see Chap. 4, by Zigmond) or to micropore filters (22) can be utilized. Cells must be labeled with ^{51}Cr, which adds 1 to 2 hr to cell preparation. Standard controls must be included, which rule out or quantitate loss of cellular ^{51}Cr with any unknown or new chemotactic stimulus. The potential hazards of using a chromium-51 radioisotope are minimal and easily controlled. After recognition of these limitations, we conclude that the ^{51}Cr assay has a unique function in laboratories studying leukocyte migration, and in particular it is critical to a complete evaluation when screening patients suspected of having abnormal leukocyte locomotion.

REFERENCES

1. Boetcher, D. A. (1974): Abnormal monocyte chemotactic response in cancer patients. *J. Natl. Cancer Inst.*, 52:1091–1099.
2. Boyum, A. (1968): Isolation of mononuclear cells and granulocytes from human blood. *Scand. J. Clin. Lab. Invest.*, 21(Suppl. 97): 77–89.
3. Chusid, M. J., Gallin, J. I., Dale, D. C., Fauci, A. S., and Wolff, S. M. (1976): Defective polymorphonuclear leukocyte chemotaxis and bactericidal capacity in a boy with recurrent pyogenic infections. *Pediatrics,* 58:513–520.
4. Clark, R. A., Johnson, F. L., Klebanoff, S. J., and Thomas E. D. (1976): Defective neutrophil chemotaxis in bone marrow transplant patients. *J. Clin, Invest.,* 58:22–31.
5. Clark, R. A., and Kimball, H. R. (1971): Defective granulocyte chemotaxis in the Chediak-Higashi syndrome. *J. Clin. Invest.,* 50:2645–2652.
6. Clark, R. A., Kimball, H. R., and Decker, J. L. (1974): Neutrophil chemotaxis in systemic lupus erythematosus. *Ann. Rheum. Dis.,* 33:167–172.
7. Clark, R., Klebanoff, S., Ochs, H., Gilliland, B., Schaller, J., and Wedgwood, R. (1975): C4 deficient human serum: Opsonic and chematactic activity. *Clin. Res.,* 23:410A.
8. Clark, R. A., Root, R. K., Kimball, H. R. and Kirkpatrick, C. H. (1973): Defective neutrophil chemotaxis and cellular immunity in a child with recurrent infections. *Ann. Intern. Med.,* 78:515–519.
9. Gallin, J. I. (1974). Radioassay of granulocyte chemotaxis: Studies of human granulocytes and chemotactic factors. In: *Chemotaxis: Its Biology and Biochemistry, Vol, 19: Antibiotic and Chemotherapy,* edited by E. Sorkin, pp. 146–160. S. Karger, Basel.
10. Gallin, J. I. (1975): Abnormal chemotaxis: Cellular and humoral components. In: *The Phagocytic Cell in Host Resistance,* edited by J. A. Bellanti and D. H. Dayton, pp. 227–248. Raven Press, New York.
11. Gallin, J. I., Bujak, J. S., Patten, E., and Wolff, S. M. (1974): Granulocyte function in the Chediak-Higashi syndrome of mice. *Blood,* 43:201–206.
12. Gallin, J. I., Clark, R. A., and Frank, M. M. (1975): Kinetic analysis of the generation of the chemotactic factor in human serum via activation of the classical and alternate complement pathways. *Clin. Immunol. Immunopathol.,* 3:334–346.
13. Gallin, J. I., Clark, R. A., and Kimball, H. R. (1973): Granulocyte chemotaxis: An improved *in vitro* assay employing ^{51}Cr-labelled granulocytes. *J. Immunol.,* 110:233–240.
14. Gallin, J. I., Klimerman, J. A., Padgett, G. A., and Wolff, S. M. (1975): Defective mononuclear leukocyte chemotaxis in the Chediak-Higashi syndrome of humans, mink, and cattle. *Blood,* 45:863–870.

15. Gallin, J. I., Wright, D. G., Fauci, A. S., Rosenwasser, L. J., Chusid, M. J., Taylor, H. A., Thomas, G., Libaers, I., Shapiro, L. J., and Neufeld, E. F. (1976): Defective leukocyte chemotaxis in mannosidosis. *Clin. Res.,* 24:344A.

16. Gallin, J. I. and Rosenthal, A. S. (1974): Regulatory role of divalent cations in human granulocyte chemotaxis: Evidence for an association between calcium exchanges and microtubule assembly. *J. Cell Biol.,* 62:594–609.

17. Goetzl, E. J. (1976): Defective responsiveness to ascorbic acid of neutrophil random and chemotactic migration in Felty's syndrome and systemic lupus erythematosus. *Ann. Rheum. Dis.,* 35:510–515.

18. Goetzl, E. J., and Austen, K. F. (1972): A method for assessing the *in vitro* chemotactic response of neutrophils utilizing ^{51}Cr-labeled human leukocytes. *Immunol. Commun.,* 1:421–430.

19. Hausmann, M., Brosman, S., Fahey, J. L., and Snyderman, R. (1973): Defective mononuclear cell chemotactic activity in patients with genitourinary carcinoma. *Clin. Res.,* 21:646.

20. Hill, H. R., Ochs, H. D., Quie, P. G., Clark, R. A., Pabst, H. F., Klebanoff, S. J., and Wedgwood, R. J. (1974): Defect in neutrophil granulocyte chemotaxis in Job's syndrome of recurrent "cold" staphylococcal abscesses. *Lancet,* 2:617–619.

21. Kaplan, A. K., Kaye, A. B., and Austen, K. F. (1972): A prealbumin activator of prekallikrein: III. Appearance of chemotactic activity for human neutrophils by the conversion of human prekallikrein to kallikrein. *J. Exp. Med.,* 135:81–97.

22. Malech, H. L., Root, R. K., and Gallin, J. I. (1977): Structural analysis of human neutrophil migration: centriole, microtubule, and microfilament orientation and function during chemotaxis. *J. Cell Biol.,* 75 (*in press*).

23. Mowat, A. G., and Baum, J. (1971): Chemotaxis of polymorphonuclear leukocytes from patients with rheumatoid arthritis. *J. Clin. Invest.,* 5:2541–2549.

24. Pincus, S. H., Thomas, I. T., Clark, R. A., and Ochs, H. D. (1975): Defective neutrophil chemotaxis with variant icthyosis, hyperimmunoglobulinemia E and recurrent infections. *J. Pediatr.,* 87:908–911.

25. Rogge, J. L., and Hanifin, J. M. (1976): Immunodeficiencies in severe atopic dermatitis: Depressed chemotaxis and lymphocyte transformation. *Arch. Dermatol.,* 112:1391–1396.

26. Rubin, R. H., Cosimi, A. B., and Goetzl, E. J. (1976): Defective human mononuclear leukocyte chemotaxis as an index of host resistance to malignant melanoma. *Clin. Immunol. Immunopathol.,* 6:376–388.

27. Snyderman, R., Dickson, J., Meadows, L., and Pike, M. (1974): Deficient monocyte chemotactic responsiveness in humans with cancer. *Clin. Res.,* 22:430A.

28. Ward, P. A., and Newman, L. J. (1969): A neutrophil chemotactic factor from human C'5 *J. Immunol.,* 102:93–99.

29. Weiss, A. S., Gallin, J. I., and Kaplan, A. P. (1974): Fletcher factor deficiency: A diminished rate of Hageman factor activation caused by absence of prekallikrein with abnormalities of coagulation, fibrinolysis, chemotactic activity, and kinin generation. *J. Clin. Invest.,* 53:622–633.

30. Wright, D. G., Kirkpatrick, C. H., and Gallin, J. I. (1977): Effects of levamisole on normal and abnormal leukocyte locomotion. *J. Clin. Invest.,* 59:941–950.

31. Zigmond, S., and Hirsch, J. (1973): Leukocyte locomotion and chemotaxis: New methods for evaluation and demonstration of a cell derived chemotactic factor. *J. Exp. Med.,* 137:387–410.

32. Zivkovic, M., and Baum, J. (1972): Chemotaxis of polymorphonuclear leukocytes from patients with systemic lupus erythematosus and Felty's syndrome. *Immunol. Commun.,* 1:39–49.

Leukocyte Chemotaxis, edited by John I. Gallin
and Paul G. Quie. Raven Press, New York
© 1978.

A Model for Understanding Millipore Filter Assay Systems

Sally H. Zigmond

Department of Biology, University of Pennsylvania, Philadelphia, Pennsylvania 19104

Millipore filter assay systems have been developed to study leukocyte locomotion and chemotaxis (1,3,4,6,7,9,11,12,13). There are two different parameters that these assays generally measure: either the *distance* from the origin that a criterion number of cells has moved, i.e., the distance into the filter that the front of the cell population has moved (12,13), or the *number* of cells that have moved some predetermined distance, e.g., to a certain depth in the filter, or completely through the filter (1,3,4,6,7,9). The new investigator may well be confused as to the relative advantages of one system over another. The assays can be compared with regard to the information they provide and the practical factors involved in using them. The assays differ in their ability to (a) measure stimulated locomotion reliably and sensitively; (b) measure the cell response at various times; (c) detect the number (or percentage) of cells responding; and (d) differentiate directional from nondirectional locomotion.

The assays also differ in their incubation times and in the time required for scoring the filters (3,10,11). In several cases, the scoring of the filters has been automated (3,7). These practical aspects must be judged on an individual basis depending upon the facilities available and the number of filters which must be processed.

In studying the locomotion of a population of cells, there are a number of interesting questions that can only be answered if one understands the locomotion assay. For example, if a given substance stimulates locomotion, does doubling the concentration of this substance cause the rate of locomotion to double? Or does addition of a second substance increase the locomotion in an additive manner? To answer these questions, one has to know whether doubling the rate of locomotion will double the distance to the front of the cell population, or double the number of cells which have moved through the filter. If the cells move at a constant rate over a certain time period, should one expect the distance to the front of the cell population or the number of cells through the filter to increase linearly over this time? What is involved in differentiating a factor that induces directed locomotion (chemotaxis) from one that merely stimulates locomotion (chemokinesis)?

By understanding a simple theoretical model of cell behavior in the millipore assays, an investigator can have a basis for choosing an assay appropriate to a particular question and for interpreting the results correctly. In this chapter, I will describe a model that allows one to determine which parameters a particular assay can measure effectively (12,13).

The model holds that in an ideal case cells move from the top of the filter into and through the filter in a pattern similar to that of particles of a gas or solute diffusing from a source. In a chemotactic gradient, the cells still move out from the source but, in addition, they are pulled toward the chemotactic agent, as charged particles would diffuse out from a source and move directionally toward the site of an opposite charge. By inspecting curves describing the diffusion process, one can get a picture of how the population of cells looks at various times as it moves through the filter. This diffusion or random-walk model does not imply that the cells move through the filter passively but only that the pattern of their distribution with time can be roughly described by diffusion equations. Experimental evidence has shown that this approximation is reasonable (12,13).

The model represents a simplified picture of leukocyte movement. In the figures that follow, I have assumed among other things (a) a uniform population of cells moving at constant rates of locomotion; (b) in the absence of a gradient, cells exhibit a random walk into the filter and are not able to swim off the top of the filter (the top of the filter is considered as a reflecting barrier); (c) if a chemotactic gradient is present, the force on the cells is constant over the distance of the filter and the duration of the assay; (d) if cells have completely traversed the filter, they are still able to reenter the filter (for example, return from a second filter). These assumptions are made to simplify the presentation but are not necessary; alternative curves could be drawn illustrating different basic assumptions. The figures included are solutions to diffusion equations and are intended to give the nonmathematical experimenter some idea of how an ideal population of cells might distribute itself with time.

Figure 1 represents the number of cells at increasing distances from the origin (top of the filter) after various incubation times in the absence of a chemotactic gradient. These curves represent the population distribution of cells moving at a constant level of locomotion, stopped and examined at various times. At time 0 (not shown), all the cells would be at the top of the filter. After the first incubation time, cells have begun to move into the filter, but the number of cells remaining at the top of the filter is too high to be included in Fig. 1. At later times, the population spreads progressively into the filter and the number remaining on the top declines. A measure of the distance to the cell front after the second incubation time would correspond to the distance along the x-axis to the point where the curve almost intersects the x-axis. If 0.2 were the bottom of the filter, a measure of the number of cells through the filter after the twelfth incubation time would correspond to the area under the portion of that curve beyond 0.2.

Although this series of curves was designed to examine the movement of cells after varying times, the same series of curves also describes the movement

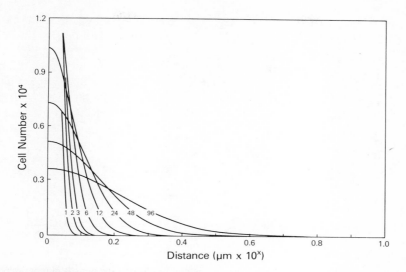

FIG. 1. Particle distribution for a random-walk process.

The particle (cell) number is plotted versus distance from the origin at various times (1,2,6 . . . 96). The curves are solutions of the diffusion equation: for particles starting at x = 0 (2) and with a reflecting barrier at x = 0:

$$\mu = \frac{\mu_0}{\sqrt{\pi DT}} \left[e^{\frac{-(x-AT)^2}{4DT}} + e^{\frac{-(x+AT)^2}{4DT}} + \frac{A}{D} e^{\frac{AX}{2D}} \left(1 - \Phi\left(\frac{X+A}{4DT}\right) \right) \right]$$

Where x = distance = μm D = diffusion coefficient = 8 μm/min; μ in total particle number = 10^6; A = flux = 0 μm/min; and T = time = 30 min X the curve number μ_0 and $(1 - \Phi)$ is the standard normal integral. The same curves can be obtained (while A = 0 X e) for a constant T and varying D. The diffusion coefficient and total cell number were chosen to be in a reasonable range, but long times and distances were included for illustrative purposes. Distance is plotted as μm X 10^3.

of cell populations moving at different rates and assayed at a constant time (i.e., one can get the same series of curves by keeping the diffusion coefficient, D, constant and varying the time, T, as by keeping T constant and varying D). Increasing the rate of locomotion would increase both the distance to the front of the cell population and the number of cells that have crossed the filter.

Figure 2 shows a similar series of curves, which represents the population distribution after various incubation times for cells moving in a positive chemotactic gradient. With time, the cell population spreads as in Fig. 1, but in addition, the whole population moves directionally into the filter. With time, the cell peak, the highest cell concentration at any one position, moves through the filter. This contrasts with the situation shown in Fig. 1, where the cell peak remains at the top of the filter. As in Fig. 1, the distance along the x-axis and the area under the curve past the *arrow* are comparable to measures of the distance to the population front and the number of cells through the filter, respectively.

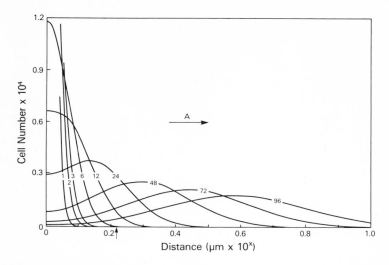

FIG. 2. Particle distribution for a random walk with a flux. The particle (cell) number is plotted versus the distance from the origin for conditions similar to those of Fig. 1 except A = a positive flux of 0.2 µm/min.

Figure 3 represents the change in the population distribution that would occur when the cell number, or the percentage of cells moving, is doubled. The distance to the cell front is only slightly affected by this change, while the number of cells at any point in the filter or the number of cells through

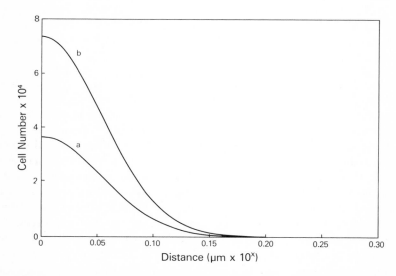

FIG. 3. Particle distribution for two population sizes. The particle (cell) distribution is plotted for a population moving in the absence of a flux but where population size of a ($\mu_0 = 2.5 \times 10^6$) is one half the size of population b ($\mu_0 = 5 \times 10^6$); other values are as in Fig. 1.

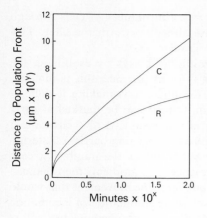

FIG. 4. Time course of distance to the population front of randomly (R) and directionally (C) moving populations. The distance along the x-axis to the point where each curve approached (= 2mm) the x-axis was measured for the curves in Figs. 1 (R) and 2 (C). The distance ($\times 10^3$) is plotted against the time of each curve.

the filter is doubled. Thus, a measure of cell number at any point below the top of the filter is sensitive to the cell number responding. In fact, the number at any position is proportional to the number of responding cells.

A time course of the distance to the cell front for an ideal population of cells moving in a homogeneous medium (R) or in a chemotactic gradient (C) is illustrated in Fig. 4. The curves are not linear with time but level off with longer incubations. This relative decrease in the progress of the cell front with time is inherent in the assay (or model of the assay) and would *not* indicate that the cells were moving more slowly. A similarly shaped curve would arise from measuring, at a constant time, populations of cells with increasing rates of locomotion. Thus, a given increase in the rate of movement of cells moving slowly would be expected to have a greater effect on the distance to the population front than the same increase of cells moving rapidly.

Figure 5 shows a time course of the number of cells expected to have crossed the filter if the cells were moving in a homogeneous medium (R) and in a chemotactic gradient (C). The number of cells through the filter rises more rapidly if the cells are incubated in the presence of a positive gradient than in

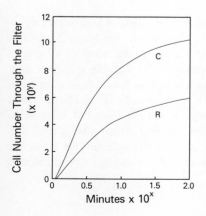

FIG. 5. Time course of the number of particles having moved beyond a certain distance for populations moving randomly (R) and with a flux (C). The area under the curves beyond 0.1 was measured by weighing for each of the curves in Figs. 1 and 2. The weight is plotted against the time ($\times 10^3$) of each curve.

the absence of a gradient. With time, the increase in number of cells through the filter levels off, since most of the cells are already beneath the filter. This is particularly obvious in the presence of the gradient (C).

Directed locomotion can be detected in millipore assays by examining the movement of the cell peak through the filter (13). In practice, this is difficult, since the peak spreads as it moves through the filter, thus making it difficult to define its location. In addition, the peak movement can be masked at early times by the fact that the cell distribution is not symmetrical (cells cannot move up off the filter: the top of the filter acts as a reflecting barrier). Alternatively, one can measure the distance to the cell front, or the number of cells through the filter, after incubating in the presence of a gradient, then one can correct this measure by an amount which accounts for the movement that would have occurred had the cells been exposed to the same stimulation of locomotion (chemokinesis) in the absence of a gradient. Since most chemotactic factors affect the rate of locomotion in a dose-dependent manner, cells part way through the filter in the presence of a positive gradient will be moving faster than cells still near the top of the filter. This fact must be taken into account when correcting the measure of cell movement in a gradient for the chemokinetic effects. A method has been described for correcting measures of the distance to the cell front for these chemokinetic effects (10,11,12,13). Thus far, no adaptation has been presented correcting a measure of cell numbers.

In conclusion, the choice of assay depends upon the questions being asked and the practical needs of each investigator (3,7,10,11,12). Measuring the distance to the cell front appears to be advantageous when one wants to differentiate directed locomotion, chemotaxis, from stimulated random locomotion (chemokinesis). This assay is also useful when short incubation times are required, since one does not have to wait for cells to cross the filter. Assays of the number of cells through (or into) the filter are sensitive to changes in the number of cells moving. Since at low concentrations, chemotactic factors may increase the number of cells moving, counting the cells which enter the filter may be particularly sensitive in detecting low concentrations of stimulants (7). Neither measure, distance, nor cell number, would be expected to show a linear time course or linear dose-response curve.

The model presented here is certainly an oversimplification of leukocyte migration through a millipore filter. Among other deviations, we know that cells do not exhibit a true random walk, since they do not make turns of all angles with equal probability (8). In addition, the presence of a suitable substrate may draw the cells directionally into the filter. The leukocytes may not be a uniform population of cells all responding equally (7); the chemotactic gradient would not be expected to remain constant over time; and cells may not be able to return to the filter from a second filter, etc. Nevertheless, the model is probably sufficiently correct to help interpret results, and, in fact, deviations from the ideal behavior may illuminate interesting features of leukocyte locomotion and chemotaxis.

ACKNOWLEDGMENTS

I would like to thank Drs. John Gillespie and Mitchell Baker for help with the mathematics of diffusion with a reflecting barrier, and Dr. Joann Otto for reading the manuscript.

REFERENCES

1. Boyden, S. (1962): Chemotactic effect of mixtures of antibody and antigen on polymorphonuclear leukocytes. *J. Exp. Med.,* 115:453–466.
2. Cox, D. R., and Miller, H. D. (1965): *The Theory of Stochastic Processes.* Spottiswoode, Ballantyne and Co., Ltd., London, p. 224.
3. Gallin, J. I., Clark, R. A., and Goetzl, E. J. (1977): Radioassay of Leukocyte Locomotion: A sensitive technique for clinical studies. *(This volume.)*
4. Goetzl, E. J., and Austen, K. F. (1972): A method for assessing the *in vitro* chemotactic response of neutrophils utilizing ^{51}Cr-labeled leukocytes. *Immunol. Commun.,* 1:421–430.
5. Jacobs, M. H. (1967): *Diffusion Processes.* Springer-Verlag, New York, pp. 61–65.
6. Keller, H. U., Borel, J. F., Wilkinson, P. C., Hess, M., and Cotlier, H. (1972): Reassessment of Boyden's technique for measuring chemotaxis. *J. Immunol. Methods,* 1:165–168.
7. Maderazo, E. G. (1977): A modified micropore filter assay of human granulocyte leukotaxis. *(This volume.)*
8. Nossal, R., and Zigmond, S. H. (1976): Chemotropism indices for polymorphonuclear leukocytes. *Biophys. J.,* 16:1171–1182.
9. Showell, H. J., Freer, R. J., Zigmond, S. H., Schiffmann, E., Srivinivesabhatt, A., Corcoran, B., Becker, E. L. (1976): The structure-activity relations of synthetic peptides as chemotactic factors and inducers of lysosomal enzyme secretion for neutrophils. *J. Exp. Med.,* 143:1154–1169.
10. Wilkinson, P. C. (1974): *Chemotaxis and Inflammation.* Churchill Livingstone, Edinburgh and London.
11. Wilkinson, P. C., and Allan, R. B. (1977): Assay systems for measuring leukocyte locomotion: An overview. *(This volume.)*
12. Zigmond, S. H. (1974): A modified millipore filter method for assaying polymorphonuclear leukocyte locomotion and chemotaxis. In *Chemotaxis: Its Biology and Biochemistry,* edited by E. Sorkin, pp. 126–145. S. Karger, Basel.
13. Zigmond, S. H., and Hirsch, J. G. (1973): Leukocyte locomotion and chemotaxis: New methods for evaluation and demonstration of a cell-derived chemotactic factor. *J. Exp. Med.,* 137:387–410.

APPENDIX: GENERAL DISCUSSION OF METHODS

Dr. Maderazo: Dr. Wilkinson, did you ever find a chemotactic response that was not chemokinetic?

Dr. Wilkinson: No, not with neutrophils.

Dr. Gallin: In regards to nomenclature, no one has used the term *stimulated random locomotion.* Should *chemokinesis* replace *stimulated random locomotion?* Are they equivalent terms?

Dr. Wilkinson: My own feeling is that they are the same; however, chemokinesis like chemotaxis describes a reaction of the cell to its environment; stimulated locomotion describes the results of that reaction, i.e., the locomotion. I think terms like *stimulated locomotion* should be used when we are not sure what reaction is occurring.

Dr. Becker: One does not use the placing of the same concentrations of agent above and below filters in chemotactic chambers with a resulting decreased locomotion as an indicator that the agent is, in fact, chemotactic.

Dr. Ward: But if one puts the factor in the bottom compartment and obtains a good response, whereas placing the factor in the cell compartment yields a response that is 10 to 15% the former, why do you object to this being a strong suggestion that one is in fact looking at the effects of a chemotactic agent? With purely chemokinetic agents, there is no such dramatic effect.

Dr. Becker: I object on the basis that if one does have chemokinesis, and one generally will, then what one is really showing is that the chemokinetic effect is being blotted out.

Dr. Jensen: But how can the chemokinetic effect be blotted out if you have the same concentrations on both sides?

Dr. Zigmond: The difficulty is if you put 100% serum below the filter, and then on top of the filter you may have a concentration of 10%, that stimulates locomotion. But with 100% of serum on the top, the high concentration could inhibit locomotion and you would see an inhibition and perhaps deactivation. That is the problem you want to avoid.

Dr. Jensen: Yes, but addition of different concentrations (a dose-response) to the cell compartment would eliminate that.

Dr. Gallin: I would like to comment on the chromium-51 radioassay for chemotaxis which is used by Goetzl, Clark, and me. the technique, which is outlined in the appendix section, uses a double-micropore filter system. Cells migrate through an upper filter and into a lower filter; 15 to 20% of the total cell population migrate into the lower filter. So in a sense the radioassay is a leading-front technique which measures a large sample of migrating cells. For this reason, we feel it is a much more valid measure of the population of cells than just the leading couple of cells measured by the single-filter morphologic leading-front technique; however, we feel that Zigmond's assay, where one counts through the entire filter, gives the most data about the entire population of cells. But it is also the most laborious. The chromium assay is very simple to quantitate (it is all done by machine), which means there is no observer subjectivity. We find it a sensitive test clinically.

Dr. Quie: I would like to follow up Gallin's remarks about methodology. When Nelson perfected the "under agarose" technique originally described by Cutler (1), there was a happy expectation that this, a simple method, would replace existing methods for measuring chemotaxis or locomotion in clinical situations. We have found some correlation between the micropore filter method and under agarose method, i.e., patients with a marked defect in chemotaxis using micropore filters show a defect in distance of migration under agarose. More subtle defects, however, such as those found in patients with burns, patients on chronic dialysis, and patients with the hyper-IgE syndrome, are not abnormal with the under agarose method. The two techniques may be measuring two different cellular functions, or the micropore filter may provide a greater challenge than under agarose migration. Nelson has evidence that assays with micropore filters of larger pore size correlate better with the under agarose assay. He was not able to show this because of time.

Dr. R. A. F. Clark: In Zigmond and Hirsch's paper (4), they derived a formula for migration of cells, assuming a homogeneous cell population. There is a correction to that formula and that correction bears immediately on Dr. Maderazo's work presented here. The formula, as presented in their paper, fails to predict the drift (*en masse* movement) of the cell population toward a chemotactic factor, as described in their experiments. What needs to be added to this equation is a time-dependent shift in the abscissa (−2CT) (2). The constant, "C", is the drift, but the product of the drift by the incubation time relates directly to Dr. Maderazo's patient index. We found that for normal subjects "C" was usually 0.5 and 2C therefore 1.0. This means that in 60 min the *en masse* movement of cells was about 60 mm into the filter; for 30 min, it was 30 mm; and so on. How long did you incubate?

Dr. Maderazo: Ninety min.

Dr. R. A. F. Clark: Ninety min? In our system, cells are moving faster.

Dr. Maderazo: It depends upon your filters. Our old lot of filters from 1975 required 90 min of incubation. The new lot of the same 5μm-pore size filters purchased in 1976 from the same source require only 60 min of incubation in order for the cells (neutrophils) to reach approximately the same distance. So filters can differ not only from one pore size to another, but also from lot to lot.

Dr. R. A. F. Clark: At 30 min we would get essentially the same patient index as you would get for 90 min.

Dr. Zigmond: The equation was for a homogeneous population undergoing a random walk. It was formulated for cells in the absence of flux. In addition, in the appendix that Knight added to my paper in *Antibiotics and Chemotherapy,* (3) these aspects of cell movement were considered. I think your formulation is probably an oversimplification of the situation. Knight's mathematics took into account the fact that the diffusion coefficient, D, was changing as the cells moved through the filter.

Dr. Clark: It seems to me it is really the "C" that is critical.

Dr. Zigmond: As soon as a gradient is through the filter, the rate of locomotion varies at different points in the filter. So your diffusion coefficients vary.

Dr. Clark: Yes, but all D is defining is the spread of the population; it has nothing to do with the *en masse* movement.

Dr. Zigmond: Yes, but are you not assuming that all these cells are exposed to the same concentration of material and therefore have one diffusion coefficient? I do not think you can assume that.

Dr. Clark: The formula does not take that into consideration; it is still greatly oversimplified.

Dr. Wilkinson: The whole question of how to measure leukocyte locomotion looked two or three years ago as if it would never change. Now everybody is thinking very hard about what they are measuring and what is the best way to measure it. This is very encouraging.

REFERENCES

1. Cutler, J. *Proc. Soc. Exp. Biol. Med.*
2. Feller, W. (1950): *Probability, Theory and Its Application.* John Wiley & Sons, New York, p. 295.
3. Zigmond, S. H. (1974): A modified millipore filter method of assaying polymorphonuclear leukocyte locomotion and chemotaxis. *Antibiotics and Chemotherapy*, Vol. 19. S. Karger, Basel.
4. Zigmond, S. H., and Hinsch, J. G. (1973): Leukocyte locomotion and chemotaxis: New methods for evaluation and demonstration of a cell-derived chemotactic factor. *J. Exp. Med.*, 137:387–410

Leukocyte Chemotaxis, edited by John I. Gallin
and Paul G. Quie. Raven Press, New York
© 1978.

Molecular Events in the Response of Neutrophils to Synthetic *N*-fMET Chemotactic Peptides: Demonstration of a Specific Receptor

Elliott Schiffmann, B. A. Corcoran, and S. Aswanikumar

Laboratory of Developmental Biology and Anomalies, National Institute of Dental Research, National Institutes of Health, Bethesda, Maryland 20014

Leukocytes respond to a variety of chemoattractants (15) most likely by way of specific receptors on the cell surface. Previous studies by others have established the role of receptors for chemoattractants in other systems. Binding proteins have been isolated for ribose, galactose, and serine, which are attractants for microorganisms (2,8). The absence of one of these proteins renders mutants unresponsive to the specific attractant. Chemotactic competence is restored when the missing part of the genome is recovered by a "revertant" mutation (1). The cellular slime mold has been shown (7) to have cyclic AMP receptors at the cell surface during the aggregation stage of its morphogenetic cycle. Since the leukocyte responds to levels of C5a, estimated to be in the nanomolar range (12), as well as to concentrations of bacterial factor which may be even lower (11), it seems likely that specific receptors of high affinity exist in this cell. Here we shall review some evidence on the nature of interaction between attractant and cell which has led to a direct demonstration of a chemotactic receptor on the neutrophil.

FORMYLMETHIONYL PEPTIDES AS LEUKOATTRACTANTS

We started by trying to isolate and characterize the chemoattractants produced by bacteria which induce leukotaxis. These studies were made in collaboration with Dr. Becker, Dr. Ward, and their associates at the University of Connecticut. Although the exceedingly low levels of this material in culture fluid have hampered this work, we established that the attractant consisted of heat-stable peptides of low molecular weight ($\leq$ 2,000 daltons), anionic at neutral pH, and perhaps with blocked *N*-termini (11). From considerations of these types of peptides that might be uniquely produced by prokaryotes, we decided to test the effects of formylmethionyl (fMet) peptides upon leukocytes, since for bacteria an fMet compound is obligatory in initiating protein synthesis, whereas in eukaryotes it is not. As Fig. 1 shows, these peptides are indeed attractants for neutrophils, with nonpolar residues in the C-terminal position enhancing potency (10). Similar results were found with macrophages. Based upon these findings, Drs. Becker, R. Freer, and their associates, along with us, undertook a systematic

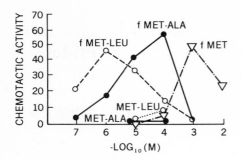

FIG. 1. Chemotactic activity of neutrophils in response to formylated and nonformylated peptides. Activity is expressed as the mean of triplicate samples in the Boyden chamber assay. Negative control activity was 3.2. Positive contol (C5a) activity was 46.4. The SEM did not exceed 10% for the values above 10. (From Schiffmann et al., ref. 10.)

study of the structure-activity relations of synthetic peptide attractants (12). As shown in Table 1, there are some exceedingly potent (10^{-11}M) attractants which also induce lysosomal enzyme release (not shown), an event contributing to inflammation. The correlation between chemotactic activity and enzyme release is very close. The presence of an N-formyl group enhances activity over the nonacylated tripeptides by some four orders of magnitude. The presence of a nonpolar residue in the C-terminal position is much more effective than a polar one. Hydrophobicity alone is not enough to account for the potency of f Met-Leu-Phe as its positional isomer, f Met-Phe-Leu, less effective by a factor of 10^3. It appears that an aromatic residue in the third position is of major significance since f Met-Met-Phe is almost as active as f Met-Leu-Phe. The very great specificity revealed in these studies, as well as the most potent activities of some of the synthetic attractants, strongly suggests that they act upon a stereospecific receptor at the cell surface.

THE ROLE OF PEPTIDASE IN LEUKOTAXIS

Using the peptide attractants, we studied their interaction with the cell. Previous work by Drs. Ward and Becker had implicated esterase activity in neutrophil

TABLE 1. *Chemotactic activity of synthetic peptides*

Peptide	ED_{50} + SE (M)
fMet-Leu-Phe	$7.0 \pm 1.7 \times 10^{-11}$
fMet-Leu-Glu	$1.3 \pm 0.38 \times 10^{-6}$
fMet-Leu-Arg	$3.6 \pm 1 \times 10^{-7}$
fMet-Leu-Leu	$4.8 \pm 1.3 \times 10^{-8}$
fMet-Phe-Leu	$5.4 \pm 1.9 \times 10^{-8}$
f-Met-Met-Phe	$2.1 \pm 0.49 \times 10^{-10}$
f-Leu-Trp-Met	$2.5 \pm 1.5 \times 10^{-8}$
Met-Leu-Phe	$6.7 \pm 1.9 \times 10^{-7}$
Met-Met-Phe	$9.0 \pm 3.9 \times 10^{-7}$

Cell migration was measured by a modified Boyden chamber technique. ED_{50} is that concentration of peptide giving 50% of the maximal activity obtained from dose-response curves. [Adapted from Showell et al. (12), with permission.]

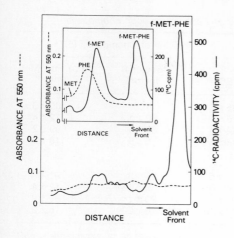

FIG. 2. Chromatographic analysis of products formed in the hydrolysis of ^{14}C-formyl-labeled fMet-Phe (1 mM) by neutrophils. Developed chromatograms were scanned for radioactivity (——), and, after reaction with ninhydrin, for absorbance at 550 nM (---). *Insert,* hydrolysis in *presence* of cells; *larger figure,* reaction in *absence* of cells. (From Aswanikumar et al., ref. 3.)

chemotaxis, since it was shown by them that both directed movement and hydrolytic activity were inhibited by low levels of organofluorophosphonates (13). Evidence was also presented for increased neutrophil esterase activity induced by chemoattractants (14). We therefore asked the qestion whether a chemotactic peptide was hydrolyzed by the cell. Incubation of ^{14}C-fMet-Phe (formyl-labeled) with neutrophils does indeed result in cleavage (3) with fMet and Phe as the principal products (Fig. 2). The cleavage is markedly reduced in cells treated with irreversible protease inhibitors, L-(1-tosylamido-2-phenyl) ethyl chloromethyl ketone (TPCK) and *N-α-p*-toysl-L-lysylchloromethyl ketone (TLCK), reagents that inhibit chymotrypsin and trypsin, respectively.

A correlation is seen between the potency of a chemoattractant and the rate at which it is cleaved (Fig. 3). For example, fMet-Phe, a good attractant, is hydrolyzed at a greater rate than fMet-His, a poor one. The correlation (correlation coefficient = 0.72) is apparently valid only for the formylated peptides, since the nonchemotactic, free peptides are all readily hydrolyzed.

Additional evidence for the role of peptide hydrolysis in chemotaxis is provided, since cell movement can be shown to be inhibited by the same reagents

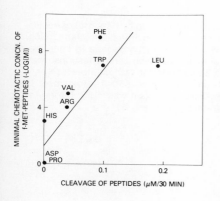

FIG. 3. Potencies of attractants and rates of their hydrolysis by neutrophils. Abbreviations refer to C-terminal residues of fMet dipeptides. Minimal chemotactic levels are those which produced a response greater than four times that of negative contol. (From Aswanikumar· et al., ref. 3.)

TABLE 2. *Effects of protease inhibitors and substrates upon chemotaxis*

		Inhibition of Chemotaxis (%) [a]		
Cell	Addition to cells	C5a [b]	Bacterial factor [c]	0.01 mM fMet-Phe [d]
Neutrophils	0.1 mM TPCK	95 ± 2	100	100 ± 3
	0.1 mM TLCK	75 ± 5	66 ± 1	12 ± 4
	0.1 mM BTEE	42 ± 5	60 ± 1	99 ± 2
	0.1 mM TAME	14 ± 6	0 ± 5	18 ± 2
Macrophages	0.1 mM TPCK	91 ± 5	65 ± 3	91 ± 3
	0.1 mM TLCK	4 ± 0	0 ± 14	12 ± 4
	0.1 mM BTEE	98 ± 1	90 ± 1	99 ± 2
	0.1 mM TAME	9 ± 10	0 ± 30	18 ± 2

[a] Results are the averages of triplicate samples. Activity in absence of attractants was 3 for neutrophils and 7 for macrophages as determined in Boyden assay.
[b] Positive control activity was 25 ± 4 for neutrophils, 87 ± 4 for macrophages.
[c] Positive control activity was 44 ± 11 for neutrophils, 52 ± 16 for macrophages.
[d] Positive control activity was 31 ± 5 for neutrophils, 85 ± 8 for macrophages. [Adapted from Aswanikumar et al. (3), with permission.]

that inhibit hydrolysis of the attractants. This is illustrated in Table 2, in which it can be seen that both TPCK and *N*-benzoyl-L-tyrosine ethyl ester (BTEE), the latter a substrate for chymotrypsin, inhibit chemotaxis by both neutrophils and macrophages to a synthetic peptide, fMet-Phe, and to two natural attractants, C5a and the bacterial factor. The reagents TLCK and *p*-tosyl-L-arginine methyl ester (TAME), the latter a substrate for trypsin, are much less effective. In related studies, we have found that phagocytes hydrolyze BTEE at greater rates than they do TAME. These results suggest that a peptidase with specificity for aromatic residues participates in chemotaxis, perhaps at the cell surface.

In the course of early studies on requirements for the position of methionine in chemotactic dipeptides, we found that the positional isomer of the attractant

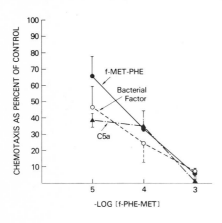

FIG. 4. The inhibition by fPhe-Met of neutrophil chemotaxis to three attractants: C5a, to which control response was 43 ± 11; bacterial factor, to which control response was 44 ± 2 and fMet-Phe (10 μM), to which control response was 55 ± 5. Response in *absence* of attractant was 4 ± 3. (From Aswanikumar et al., ref. 3.)

TABLE 3. *Typical attractants and inhibitors for leukotaxis* [a]

Attractants	ED_{50} (M)
fMet-Leu-Arg	4×10^{-7}
fMet-Leu-Phe	7×10^{-11}
fMet-Phe-TEMPA [b]	1×10^{-7}
fMet-Phe inulin	5×10^{-7}
fMet-Phe	4×10^{-7}

Inhibitor	Inhibition of chemotaxis to 0.01 mM fMet-Phe (%)
0.1 mM TPCK [c]	100
0.1 mM TLCK [c]	12
0.1 mM fPhe-Met	63

[a] Results were obtained principally with neutrophils; macrophages showed the same order of responsiveness.
[b] TEMPA refers to 1-oxyl-2,2,6,6-tetramethyl-4-aminopiperidine
[c] Corresponding substrates, BTEE and TAME, had similar effects to those of TPCK and TLCK, respectively.

fMet-Phe, namely fPhe-Met,[1] was an inhibitor of leukotaxis to the dipeptide as well as to C5a and the bacterial factor (Fig. 4). Both the attractant, its corresponding inhibitory positional isomer, and the two nonacylated dipeptides are all readily hydrolyzed by the cell, but the latter compounds do not affect cell migration. This suggests that the formylated peptides interact with a peptidase specific for the chemotactic process, while the nonacylated peptides are cleaved by unrelated enzymes.

At this point, it may be helpful to summarize the evidence in support of a specific chemotactic receptor at the cell surface of the leukocyte. In Table 3 are given representative data from the structure-activity relationships, discussed above, as well as information on other chemotactic compounds and on the nature of the putative peptidase that may play a role in directed cell movement. The markedly greater potency of hydrophobic compounds such as fMet-Leu-Phe over that of more polar attractants, the demonstration that the exceedingly hydrophobic spin-labeled fMet-Phe TEMPA [2] is chemotactic, and the fact that fMet-Phe linked to inulin, a compound not likely to be transported across the cell membrane, is an attractant—these all support the existence of a membrane-bound receptor on the cell. Also consistent with this is the specificity

---

[1] The properties previously reported for f-phe-met should be ascribed to carbobenzyloxy-phe-met, which is unequivocally an inhibitor of chemotaxis. This clarification has been inserted after it was determined that the supplier of some of our compounds had misinformed us about the identity of a compound. Evidence exists to suggest that f-phe-met on the other hand may be a weak attractant.

[2] TEMPA is 1-oxyl-2,2,6,6, tetramethyl-4-aminopiperidine, kindly provided by Drs. K. Fichter and R. Katz of the Mid-Atlantic Research Institute, Bethesda, Maryland. 20014.

for aromatic residues (part B of Table 3) of the hydrolytic enzyme which itself might be part of the receptor. Our suggestion, to be discussed more fully later, would be that such a receptor might consist of two sites: a binding site which, when occupied by a peptide ligand, initiates a signal to the cell's motility apparatus, and hydrolytic site which, as in the acetylcholine-cholinesterase system, cleaves the bound peptide and frees the receptor for successive cycles in responding to the gradient of attractant. If this model has validity, one might predict that enhanced binding of a labeled chemotactic peptide would be observed in cells treated with an irreversible peptidase inhibitor such as TPCK, compared to that in cells not subjected to this reagent.

DIRECT EVIDENCE FOR A SPECIFIC CHEMOTACTIC RECEPTOR ON THE NEUTROPHIL

Drs. Alan Day and R. Freer, with whom we have been collaborating, synthesized a new potent attractant, formylnorleucylleucylphenylalanine (fNLLP), which was labeled with tritium to a high specific activity (13 Ci/mM) in the *para* position of the *Phe* residue. The isosteric norleucine (Nle) was chosen to replace *Met* because the catalytic introduction of ^{3}H in the presence of that amino acid often results in poor yields and some desulfuration (A. Day et al., *unpublished data*). *Nle* can replace *Met* in initiating protein synthesis (5) and can also affect the synthesis of S-adenosylmethionine (6), suggesting that there is little discrimination between these two amino acids. Since this tripeptide was found to be highly active (10^{-10}M), we used it in studies to show specific binding with the aid of a rapid filtration technique (9). Dr. Candace Pert collaborated with us in these studies (3a). In Fig. 5, the kinetics of binding of fNLLP to rabbit neutrophils (PMNs) are given under a number of conditions, all performed at 0° in order to mininize transport and metabolism of the attractant (3). The

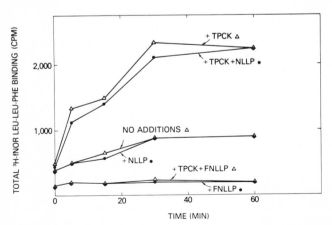

FIG. 5 Specific binding of [^{3}H] formylnorleucyleucylphenylalanine (fNLLP*) to rabbit neutrophils as a function of time at 0°. All samples contained the labeled attractant. Each point is the mean of triplicate samples with an SEM not greater than 10%. (From Aswanikumar et al., ref. 3a, with permission.)

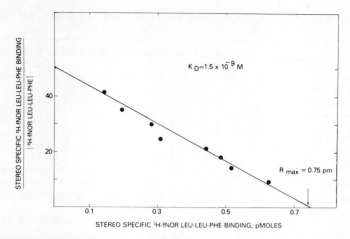

FIG. 6 Scatchard plot (bound/free vs. bound) of specific binding of fNLLP* to rabbit neutrophils at 0° as a function of concentration of labeled ligand (From Aswanikumar et al., ref. 3a, with permission.)

lowest curves show nonspecific, nonsaturable binding in the presence of at least 1,000-fold excess of unlabeled ligand. This binding is not altered with time, and when subtracted from total binding gives specific binding. The two pairs of upper curves indicate total binding of the undiluted ligand. It can be seen that the presence of TPCK (0.1 mM) even at 0° enhances binding (uppermost curves) by more than twofold, presumably by inhibiting peptidase activity. Binding is dependent upon time, reaching a maximum after 30 min. The presence of a 1,000-fold excess of Nle-Leu-Phe, the nonformylated peptide lacking chemotactic activity at the concentration used, did not alter the rate or extent of binding. This accords very well with the importance of an N-formyl group in conferring activity upon a peptide (10).

Scatchard analysis of specific binding (Fig. 6) indicated the presence of a binding site with an affinity of 1.5×10^{-9}M, a value close to that required to elicit a half-maximal chemotactic response: 7×10^{-10}M A. Day, et al., *unpublished data*). From these data, the number of receptors per cell has been estimated to be 10^5.

If a specific chemotactic receptor is being measured here, it should be possible to show a close correlation between the level of a given peptide necessary to displace 50% of specific binding and that required to elicit a half-maximal chemotactic response. Table 4 shows such a relationship. Two natural attractants, C5a and partially purified bacterial factor, were also tested for their abilities to displace labeled peptide, and it can be been (Table 5) that a chemotactically effective level of the bacterial factor did complete with the tritiated ligand while C5a did not, indicating different receptors for these two attractants. Also studied were the enantiomeric peptides f-L-Phe-L-Met, an inhibitor of chemotaxis (3), and f-D-Phe-D-Met (gift of Dr. E. D. Nicolaides, Park-Davis, Ann Arbor, Michigan), which was neither an attractant nor an inhibitor at the levels em-

TABLE 4. *Abilities of synthetic peptides to inhibit specific binding of [³H] F Nle-Leu-Phe to neutrophils in relation to their chemotactic potencies*

Peptide	Specific receptor ID_{50} (M)[a]	Chemotactic activity ED_{50} (M)[b]
fMet-Leu-Phe	3×10^{-10}	7×10^{-11}
fMet-Met-Met-Met	9×10^{-10}	3×10^{-10}
fNle-Leu-Phe	3×10^{-9}	7×10^{-10}
fMet-Leu	2×10^{-7}	4×10^{-7}
fMet-Leu-Arg	4×10^{-6}	3×10^{-7}
fMet-Leu-Glu	9×10^{-6}	2×10^{-6}
Nle-Leu-Phe	4×10^{-5}	1×10^{-6}
fMet-Pro	$> 1 \times 10^{-4}$	Nonattractant

[a] ID_{50} is the molar concentration required to displace 50% of specifically bound [³H] F Nle-Leu-Phe from cells at $0°$ C.

[b] Taken in part from Showell et al. (12), adapted from Aswanikumar et al. (3a) with permission.

TABLE 5. *Chemotactic activity and receptor binding inhibition of natural attractants and synthetic peptides*

Compound	Chemotactic activity[a]	Inhibition of	
		Chemotaxis (%)	Binding (%)
Bacterial factors	27	—	50
Bacterial factors treated with protease[b]	0	—	0
C5a	31	—	0
0.1mM F-L-Phe-L-Met[c]	0	63	50
0.1mM F-D-Phe-D-Met[c]	0	0	20

[a] Values for bacterial factor and C5a are close to those for maximal response.

[b] Bacterial factor was incubated with protease, heated to destroy enzymatic activity, and then tested. Factor itself is stable to heating.

[c] These compounds were tested against 0.01 mM fMet-Phe as attractant in the chemotactic assay. Adapted from Aswanikumar et al. (3), with permission.

ployed. The L isomer is more effective than the D compound in affecting binding. These results suggest that the receptor has stereospecificity. The receptor also appears to be specific to phagocytes, since neither erythrocytes, lymphocytes, platelets, nor rat brain cell membranes bound the ligand. It is also our contention that we are observing cell surface binding and not intracellular accumulation, since binding was not affected by ouabain added to whole cells, or by the homogenization of cells, or by freezing and thawing the cells.

A TWO-SITE MODEL FOR THE RECEPTOR

These results permit more detailed inferences on the nature of the receptor. Listed in Table 6 are properties of some compounds which affect the chemotactically responding PMN. fMet-Phe, a nonpolar compound, is more effective than

TABLE 6. *Properties of compounds affecting leukotaxis*

Compound	Chemotactic effect		Interaction with cell hydrolytic enzyme		Effects on binding
	Attractants	Inhibitor	Substrate	Inhibitor	
fMet-Phe	+	− [a]	+	−	Inhibits
fPhe-Met	−	+	+	−	Inhibits
BTEE	−	+	+	−	None
TPCK	−	+	−	+	Increases

[a] fMet-Phe competes with attractants when placed together with cell in Boyden chamber assay.

fMet-His, a fact suggesting that the attractant interacts at the cell membrane. This peptide is cleaved by the cell and inhibits specific binding by labeled attractant. fPhe-Met inhibits chemotaxis, is also hydrolyzed, and inhibits binding. BTEE on the other hand, while capable of inhibiting chemotaxis and being susceptible to hydrolysis, does not affect binding. This suggests that BTEE inhibits chemotaxis by competing with the attractant for the hydrolytic enzyme, while fPhe-Met may inhibit chemotaxis not only in this manner but also by forming an unproductive complex with the receptor—one incapable of generating a chemotactic signal. TPCK, the irreversible protease inactivator, inhibits both chemotaxis and hydrolysis, but enhances binding, suggesting that it protects the bound ligand from degradation. This reagent is more hydrophobic than TLCK, which has significantly less effect than TPCK upon the three parameters just cited.

It seems reasonable, therefore, to postulate that the chemotactic receptor on the neutrophil, which responds to the natural attractant from bacteria, has two functional sites at the cell surface: a binding site, at which the chemotactic signal is initiated, and an hydrolytic site, which, as indicated above, may allow the receptor to be freed of ligand in order to permit the cell to continue detection of the gradient.

OTHER CELL FUNCTIONS

As Dr. Becker and his colleagues have shown, there is an excellent correlation between peptide-induced lysosomal enzyme release and chemotaxis (14). Furthermore, the correlation between ID_{50}s and ED_{50}s for the enzymatic release is even closer than that between inhibition and chemotaxis, presumably because enzyme release may require occupancy of more receptors than would chemotaxis. In other studies to be reported by these investigators, fPhe-Met and TPCK, but not TLCK, are effective inhibitors of this cell function, providing additional support that similar receptors participate in both peptide-stimulated enzyme release and chemotaxis. Recently, Hook et al. (4) have demonstrated a good correlation between release of histamine from basophils and neutrophil chemotaxis by fMet peptides. This process is also inhibited, preferentially by TPCK and BTEE, compared to the effects of TLCK and TAME. Drs. M. Lett-Brown and E. Leonard, National Cancer Institute, NIH, have shown that basophils are also attracted by these peptides, and Drs. Goetzl and Becker have informed me *(personal communication)* that eosinophils respond to fMet peptides. While there are without a doubt important differences in the aforementioned cellular responses that may be mediated by receptors, it is worth noting that four major classes of phagocytes apparently are attracted to these small peptides. This gives credence to the suggestion that fMet peptides may indeed be closely related to natural attractants such as bacterial factors.

SUMMARY

Synthetic formylmethionyl peptides have been shown to attract phagocytes. These peptides may be related to bacterial products which are known to be potent chemotaxins. Hydrolysis of peptides may be an obligatory step in the induction of directed movement by cells, since the inhibition of peptide cleavage results in the inhibition of chemotaxis. A systematic study of the structure-chemotactic activity relations of synthetic peptides has led to the preparation of highly potent compounds (10^{-11}M), some of which have been used to demonstrate a specific chemotactic receptor on the neutrophil. The affinity of the binding site of this receptor has been determined to be 1.5 nanomoles per liter, and the number of sites per cell has been estimated to be 10^5.

REFERENCES

1. Adler, J. (1975): Bacterial chemoreception. In: *Functional Linkage in Biomolecular Systems,* edited by F. O. Schmitt, D. M. Schneider, and D. M. Crothers, pp. 279–290. Raven Press, New York.
2. Adler, J., Hazelbauer, G. L., and Dahl, M. M. (1973): Chemotaxis toward sugars in *Escherichia coli. J. Bacteriol.,* 115:824–827.
3. Aswanikumar, S., Schiffmann, E., Corcoran, B. A., and Wahl, S. M. (1976): Role of a peptidase in phagocyte chemotaxis. *Proc. Natl. Acad. Sci. U.S.A.,* 73:2439–2442.
3a. Aswanikumar, S., Corcoran, B. A., Schiffmann, E., Day, A. L., Freer, R. J., Showell, H. J., Becker, E. L., and Pert, C. B. (1977): Demonstration of a receptor on rabbit neutrophils for chemotactic peptides., *Biochem. Biophys. Res. Comm.,* 74:210–217.
4. Hook, W. A., Schiffmann, E., Aswanikumar, S., and Siraganian, R. P. (1976): Histamine release by chemotactic, formylmethionine containing peptides. *J. Immunol.,* 117:594–596.
5. Kerwar, S. S., and Weissbach, H. (1970): Studies in the ability of norleucine to replace methionine in the initiation of protein synthesis in *E. coli. Arch. Biochem. Biophys.,* 141:525–532.
6. Lombardini, J. B., Coulter, A. W., and Talalay, P. (1970): Analogues of methionine as substrates and inhibitors of the methionine adenosyltransferase reaction. *Mol. Pharmacol.,* 6:481–499.
7. Malchow, D., and Gerisch, G. (1974): Short-term binding and hydrolysis of cyclic 3: 5-adenosine monophosphate by aggregating dictyostelium cells. *Proc. Natl. Acad. Sci. U.S.A.,* 71:2423–2427.
8. Mesibov, R., and Adler, J. (1972): Chemotaxis toward amino acids in *Escherichia coli. J. Bacteriol.,* 112:315–326.
9. Pert, C. B., and Snyder, S. H. (1973): Opiate receptor: Demonstration in nervous tissue. *Science,* 179:1011–1014.
10. Schiffmann, E., Corcoran, B. A., and Wahl, S. M. (1975): *N*-formylmethionyl peptides as chemoattractants for leucocytes. *Proc. Natl. Acad. Sci. U.S.A.,* 72:1059–1062.
11. Schiffmann, E., Showell, H. J., Corcoran, B. A., Ward, P. A., Smith, E., and Becker, E. L.

(1975): The isolation and partial characterization of neutrophil chemotactic factors from *Escherichia coli. J. Immunol.,* 114:1831–1837.
12. Showell, H. J., Freer, R. J., Sigmond, S. H., Schiffman, E., Aswanikumar, S., Corcoran, B., and Becker, E. L. (1976): The structure-activity relations of synthetic peptides as chemotactic factors and inducers of lysosomal enzyme secretion for neutrophils. *J. Exp. Med.,* 143:1154–1169.
13. Ward, P. A., and Becker, E. L. (1967): Mechanisms of the inhibition of chemotaxis by phosphonate esters. *J. Exp. Med.,* 125:1001–1021.
14. Ward, P. A., and Becker, E. L. (1970): Biochemical demonstration of the activatable esterase of the rabbit neutrophil involved in the chemotactic response. *J. Immunol.,* 105:1057–1067.
15. Wilkinson, P. C. (1974): *Chemotaxis and Inflammation.* Churchill, Livingstone, Edinburgh and London, p. 54.

DISCUSSION

Dr. Ward: Do you have any evidence that in fact the hydrolase is an exoenzyme?

Dr. Schiffmann: No. We have attempted to get some information on this. About 50% of the hydrolytic activity remained with the cell pellet obtained from successive freezing and thawing of cells. We did not ascertain whether the granules were removed. We went a little further and put together some crude membrane preparations by differential centrifugation. Again, this was not too clean; however, the crude membrane fraction contained almost 50% of the hydrolytic activity. There does appear to be some bound hydrolytic activity.

Dr. Goetzl: My studies of the effects of the esterase inhibitors, TLCK and TPCK, on leukocyte random and chemotactic migration were published in *Immunology* in 1975. It is difficult to conclude that TLCK and TPCK are solely modulating the effects of the peptides, because the inhibitors themselves have potent effects on both the leukocyte chemotactic response to a variety of factors and their random migration. TLCK enhanced random migration and suppressed chemotaxis, with the latter effect predominating at the lower effective concentrations. TPCK suppressed both the chemotactic response and random migration. Thus, both inhibitors are clearly influencing a lot of esterase activities on the leukocyte surface. It currently is not possible to conclude that the effect of esterase inhibitors on the chemotactic response to the synthetic peptides is caused by a specific effect on esterases which selectively cleave the peptides.

Dr. Schiffmann: We have not demonstrated that conclusively. I agree.

Dr. Wilkinson: I am doubtful whether the effect of inhibitors of this type is really a result of their action in preventing hydrolysis of chemotactic factors by proteases. We have found that TPCK and TLCK inhibit leukocyte migration to lipid factors, which are not substrates for proteases, as well as to peptides, which may be. Also we found that we obtained the same amount of inhibition of locomotion even when the chemotactic factor was omitted completely.

Dr. Schiffmann: That is possible in a chemotactic assay, but when we did the binding assay, this was in the absence of any macromolecule.

With respect to the other comment, about TPCK affecting lipid chemotaxis,

I heartily agree with you. There may be some other events which involve some membrane rupture or perturbation, which involves proteases. I am very much impressed by the work on proteolytic control of cell regulation which has come out recently. There are a number of symposia on this topic. Not only chemotaxis, but mitogenic events, too, appear to be affected, especially in malignant cells. One can affect transformed cells by influencing proteolytic activities of the cells and restore them to normal. So it is likely that we are looking at a fairly complex phenomenon, which may involve proteolytic activity in membrane perturbation as well as removing the peptide. We conceive of chemoreception as a rough analogy to the acetylcholinecholinesterase system whereby the cells are restored to their responsive state by hydrolysis of the ligand after it has hit its target.

Dr. Wilkinson: That is the thing. Those proteases are acting in some kind of regulatory way, one of the problems being that they actually act to digest the chemotactic factor.

Dr. Schiffmann: The evidence we have presented is consistent, at least, with their acting in part, that way.

Dr. Becker: I would like to present some recent unpublished data obtained by Henry Showell, Richard Freer, and me. These data have bearing on the nature of the receptor for the synthetic oligopeptide chemotactic factors, and they deal with the requirement for a formyl group to acylate the amino-terminal residue of the peptide and the structural requirements with respect to the length of the alkyl chain of the amino-terminal amino acid.

What we have done is to look at the activity of a group of peptides with respect to movement, and lysozyme and betaglucuronidase release. Essentially they were in parallel, so I only refer to the stimulated movement. The unacylated Met-Leu-Phe gave us an ED_{50} for stimulated movement of 9×10^{-7} M instead of 7×10^{-11} M for the fMet-Leu-Phe, i.e., when the deacylated compound dropped, it dropped 10,000-fold in activity. Our initial hypothesis was that this drop was merely the uncovering of a positive charge on the Met-Leu-Phe; however, this is incorrect. Acetylation instead of formylation of the Met-Leu-Phe produced a compound with almost the same low activity as the Met-Leu-Phe. In other words, the substitution of a methyl for the hydrogen of the formyl group almost completely destroys the 10,000-fold enhancing activity of that group. Moreover, if one removes the amino group completely, as in the desamino Met-Leu-Phe, one again obtains a compound with the same low degree of activity as the Met-Leu-Phe.

In addition, one can show the same thing with fMet-Leu-Phe and related peptides, that there is also a 1,000- to 10,000-fold drop in activity on removing the formyl group, and substituting the hexanoic acid for the norleucine as the terminal residue (desamino-norleucine) does not restore activity. So that it is apparent from this and, as in our previous studies, there is a very great specificity of the structures required for activity. These results and other subsequent results mean, among other things, that although these peptides are obviously hydrophobic in nature, their activity does not depend specifically on their hydrophobicity, per se. In addition, this sort of exquisite specificity that one sees, one only sees really when a ligand reacts with a protein, whether that protein is an antibody or an enzyme, or that protein is the usual pharmacologist's receptor. On that basis, I would like to infer that, in fact, the oligopeptide receptor on the neutrophil is also a protein.

Dr. Lynn: Is it possible to have a biological molecule which does not have a receptor? I do not think it is possible to have a molecule that does something to a cell, that does not have a receptor.

Dr. Snyderman: I think that depends solely on affinity. It is well known that collagen agglutinates platelets. That does not mean that there is a collagen receptor on platelets. Such a phenomenon may occur on the basis of fairly low affinity interactions such as hydrophobic interactions; binding does not necessarily have to depend on high affinity receptor sites.

Dr. Wilkinson: I prefer to think that interactions of relatively low specificity do play an important part in the recognition of many chemotactic factors by cells. After all, there are many chemotactic factors, and I find it difficult to visualize stereospecific receptors for them all. I have recently been doing binding studies of alkali-denatured albumin to rabbit neutrophils and obtained linear Scatchard plots with association constants around 10^6 L/M, which is quite a bit lower than you get for fMet peptides. It depends a bit how you define a receptor and whether binding sites, which may be fairly catholic in their structural requirements, should be called receptors. Can a line meaningfully be drawn across the spectrum of affinities and structural specificities?

Dr. Becker: There are criteria for defining receptors, and these criteria in fact are being met by our structure activity studies on the one hand and by Dr. Snyderman's binding studies on the other.

Dr. Snyderman: I would like to go briefly over our evidence for a specific receptor site on the human polymorphonuclear leukocytes for the formulated peptide chemotactic factors. First, I would like to make an acknowledgement to Dr. Schiffmann for two things: (a) for one of the major contributions to the field of chemotaxis in the last 15 years in terms of providing highly defined chemotactic factors, and (b) for showing tremendous generosity with other investigators in sharing his peptides with us.

Williams, Pike, Lefkowitz, and I were interested in looking at binding sites on polymorphonuclear leukocytes of human beings, and we went after what we considered to be the best ligand that we were able to get; that is titrated fMet-Leu-Phe. The specific radioactivity of the material was 40 curies per millimole, so it was very highly labeled. Now to show that the chemotactic activity of the labeled material is the same as the cold material, we just looked at the dose effect of the chemotactic activity with the hot and with the cold material, and they are identical.

The binding of the tritiated fMet-Leu-Phe is saturable and that binding can be reversed by addition of large amounts of cold material. One definition of a specific binding site is that it is saturable. The kinetics of binding tends to be very rapid on and rapid off. The time for maximum is around 12 min. So it is very rapid on, and if a large amount of cold material is added, it is found to be very rapid off also. Again, the characteristics are similar to the insulin binding site and the beta-receptor. If one looks at the biological activity of the series of peptides as shown by Dr. Schiffmann and Becker, fMet-Leu-Phe is greater than f-trimet is greater than fMet-phe and fMet-leu. In our hands, fMet does not have chemotactic activity. So this is an order of potency series for chemotactic activity.

If one looks at the ability of the cold materials to block the binding of the hot material, one sees an identical order of potency. The cold fMet-Leu-Phe is the most effective in inhibiting binding of the hot material, and one sees an identical order of potency for the rest of the formylated peptides. If one does a correlation coefficient of EC-50 for inhibition of binding versus EC-50 chemotaxis dose, one sees a correlation of almost one; there is a correlation of about 0.998, again, indicating the specificity of the binding sites.

In our hands, C5a in a 10-fold greater amount than can produce the maximum chemotactic response had no effect on the binding of fMet-Leu-Phe. So our feeling is that in the human PMN there are specific binding sites for formylated peptide chemotactic factors. In addition, maximum chemotactic activity seems to occur when about 10% of the binding sites are occupied.

Dr. Gallin: Have you done the experiment in which you looked at the ability of the fMet peptides to block the C5a response?

Dr. Snyderman: We could get blocking of the C5a response with the fMet peptides, but I do not know if that agrees with anybody else's results. Dr. Ward, did you tell me once that you did not get blocking or were those experiments with the bacterial factors?

Dr. Ward: Blocking of binding?

Dr. Snyderman: No, of the chemotactic activity. Deactivation.

Dr. Ward: We had a very hard time showing deactivation with the low-molecular-weight peptides (bacterial factor and synthetic chemotactic peptides).

Dr. Snyderman: In the chemotaxis chamber, the fMet peptides inhibit the C5a response.

Dr. Van Epps: Dr. Snyderman and Dr. Schiffmann, do you have any evidence that all neutrophils will bind equally to this factor?

Dr. Schiffmann: We will be taking a look at that. We do not have any definite evidence on this point.

Dr. Van Epps: The reason I ask is because we have been doing some work with fluoresceinated casein and have been able to show that fluoresceinated casein binds to the polymorphonuclear leukocytes. Furthermore, only a certain percentage of cells bind casein, whereas other populations of cells do not bind casein.

Dr. Becker: From the Scatchard plot, there is not a large proportion of neutrophils that have a widely different dissociation constant. Otherwise, one would not get the linear plot. One can not rule out the possibility, however, that there might be a small proportion of cells with a small difference in the dissociation constant.

Dr. Van Epps: This still would not indicate whether there was a population of cells that failed to bind chemotactic factor.

Dr. Schiffmann: We have some very preliminary data that show if the incubation is done at 37°C instead of 0°, an increase in the number of receptors is obtained, but not an increase in the dissociation constant. This would suggest, as Dr. Becker said, a homogeneous population of cells that were binding.

Dr. Williams: Dr. Becker, are there a thousand different receptors for a thousand different chemotactic attractants? Or is there one receptor?

Dr. Becker: I think, from the work that has been presented so far, there is reasonable evidence that there is more than one receptor. So far, I do not think there are grounds for considering how many receptors there are.

Dr. Ward: Have any studies been done on binding of synthetic peptides to lymphocytes?

Dr. Snyderman: We have looked at mononuclear leukocytes from ficol-hypaque preparations and found roughly 30% of the binding compared to neutrophils on a per milligram protein basis. If we removed the adherent cells, binding fell down to levels below our ability to detect it. This may reflect the insensitivity of the system; however, it indicates that lymphocytes are not nearly as effective in binding as the PMNs and probably the monocytes.

Leukocyte Chemotaxis, edited by John I. Gallin
and Paul G. Quie. Raven Press, New York
© 1978.

Enzymes in Granulocyte Movement: Preliminary Evidence for the Involvement of Na$^+$, K$^+$ ATPase

Elmer L. Becker, Henry J. Showell, Paul H. Naccache, and Ramadan Sha'afi

Department of Pathology, University of Connecticut Health Center, Farmington, Connecticut 06032

The stimulation of neutrophil movement induced by chemotactic factors is a multistep, probably multisequential process involving a number of enzymatic reactions. The present evidence for the participation of any given enzyme is fragmentary and generally indirect. There is evidence for an activatable esterase (2) and an already activated esterase (4) and a protease(s) (1,7). I wish to present here the results of studies indicating the involvement of a Na$^+$, K$^+$-sensitive ATPase in neutrophil movement.

The concentration gradients of Na$^+$ and K$^+$ across mammalian cells are maintained by the so-called "Na$^+$, K$^+$ pump." The pump is driven by metabolic energy derived from the hydrolysis of ATP by an ouabain-inhibitable-membrane Na$^+$, K$^+$ ATPase. Recently, we have demonstrated the existence of ouabain-inhibitable, Na$^+$, K$^+$ ATPase activity in the membranes of rabbit peritoneal polymorphonuclear leukocytes (heterophil, neutrophils) (10). In what follows, I shall describe our recent evidence, as yet indirect, that the Na$^+$, K$^+$ pump is required to maintain optimal sensitivity for the movement of rabbit peritoneal neutrophils and that the pump is directly or indirectly activated by the chemotactic peptide, formylmethionylleucylphenylalanine, fMet-Leu-Phe. The conclusion is based on our published work on the requirement for extracellular K$^+$ and Na$^+$ for optimal effectiveness of factors chemotactic for neutrophils (11) and as yet, unpublished work on the effects of chemotactic factors on the transport properties of the neutrophil for Na$^+$ and K$^+$ (9). All the work to be described was performed on rabbit peritoneal polymorphonuclear leukocytes.

REQUIREMENT FOR EXTERNAL K$^+$ AND NA$^+$ IN NEUTROPHIL MOVEMENT

The stimulation of neutrophil movement was studied by means of a conventional Boyden chamber technique. The degree of stimulated movement when plotted against the logarithm of the concentration of chemotactic factor gives a sigmoid dose-response curve (11,12). K$^+$, in the external medium, shifts the curve to the left in a parallel manner relative to the curve obtained without

K^+. The concentration of K^+ required to give maximum enhancement of stimulated movement varies from 5 to 50 mM with different preparations of rabbit
peritoneal neutrophils. In 33 experiments performed in the presence of 5.5 mM
K^+, the activity of a butanol extract of *Escherichia coli* culture filtrates was
increased on the average 180% ± 2% (SE) compared to control cells stimulated
in the absence of K^+. In other words, K^+ essentially doubles the effectiveness
of the chemotactic factor. This same effect of K^+ was observed with all other
chemotactic factors tested, C5a, the pronase-sensitive, and the pronase-insensitive
fractions of a butanol extract of *E. coli* culture filtrates and the synthetic peptide,
formylmethionylleucylphenylalamine, fMet-Leu-Phe. K^+ also enhances the unstimulated random movement of neutrophils in the same concentration range.
This last observation suggests that the effect of external K^+ on the stimulation
by chemotactic factors is to facilitate the chemokinetic rather than the directed
or chemotactic response of the neutrophils; however, experiments directly testing
this point have not been carried out.

The hypothesis suggested to explain the enhancing effect of K^+ was that
external K^+ stimulates an increased influx of K^+ and possibly a coupled efflux
of Na^+ through the cell's Na^+, K^+ pump and that chemotactic factors enhance
the postulated K^+ influx. This hypothesis was mainly based upon the use of
the K-specific ionophore, valinomycin, and of ouabain (11).

Valinomycin specifically increases the permeability of the cell to K^+ by forming
a positively charged lipophilic complex with K^+. It induces in mitochondria
an intracellular influx of K^+ metabolically driven against the concentration gradient (8). In the presence of 5.5 mM K^+, valinomycin significantly and reproduci-
bly enhanced the responsiveness of the neutrophil to chemotactic factors by
43 ± 13% (9 experiments) but had no effect in the absence of K^+. This suggested
that an increase of K^+ transport might be responsible for the stimulatory effects
of extracellular K^+.

Ouabain completely abolishes the enhancing effect of K^+. In nine experiments
with 10^{-5} M ouabain and 5.5 mM K^+, the responsiveness of the peritoneal neutrophils to the butanol extract was 52 ± 2% (SE) of the activity found in the
absence of ouabain. This was the same as the 56 ± to 2% decrease in the response
to the chemotactic factor obtained when K^+ was deleted from medium. In
the absence of K^+, ouabain had no effect. The inhibitoiry activity of ouabain
was overcome by raising the K^+ concentration from 5.5 mM to 40 mM, suggesting
that the effect of ouabain was competitive.

Approximatley half the total influx of K^+ is inhibited by ouabain (5,6): the
portion inhibited being attributed to the action of the monovalent cation pump.
The fact that low concentrations (10^{-5} M to 5×10^{-6} M) of ouabain completely
abolish the enhancement of stimulated movement by K^+ suggests that this latter
effect, whatever its mechanism, depends upon the action of the monovalent
cation pump. This suggestion is supported by the apparent competitive nature
of the inhibition. In addition, the rank order of effectiveness of the different
monovalent cations $NH^+_4 = K^+ > Rb^+ > Cs^+ > Li^+ = Na^+$ does not differ essen-

tially from their rank order of effectiveness in activating the Na/K+ ATPase of nerve. Admittedly, the weight to be given the latter similarity is uncertain in view of the fact that these same cations affect a number of cellular and tissue processes and functions with roughly similar rank order (13).

Obviously, other explanations of the enhancing effects of K+ are possible. More direct evidence supporting the hypothesis has been obtained from measurements of the rates of influx and efflux of K+ in the presence and absence of chemotactic factor under varying circumstances.

EFFECT OF CHEMOTACTIC FACTORS ON THE TRANSPORT OF K+ AND NA+ BY THE NEUTROPHIL

The synthetic peptide, formylmethionylleucylphenylalanine was employed throughout (12).[1] This peptide is the most active that we have so far, its ED_{50} for chemotaxis, i.e., the concentration giving 50% of maximal movement is 7.0 ± 1.7 (SE) $\times 10^{-11}$ M (12); like other chemotactic agents, it can also induce random motility and lysosomal enzyme release and enhance phagocytosis by neutrophils (3,12). The radioactive tracers $^{42}K^+$ and $^{22}Na^+$ were used to study the fluxes of these ions. The fluxes were measured at 37°C using a fast reproducible technique involving the layering of a known volume of cell suspension over a layer of silicone oil in a microcentrifuge tube. The cells were separated from the suspending medium by centrifugation in an Eppendorf microcentrifuge that reaches 8,000 rpm in less than 10 sec. The radioactivity of the cell pellet or supernatant or both was measured. For influx studies, the cells were incubated in the presence of isotope and sampled at regular intervals. For efflux studies, the cells were preloaded with isotope and then incubated and sampled. Steady state, unidirectional fluxes were calculated using standard two-compartmental (extracellular and intracellular) analysis. The first-order rate constant, K, was determined using the equation

$$-\ln (1 - S/S_\infty) = Kt$$

where S and S_∞ refer to the radioactivity (counts per unit volume) in the cells at time t and at equilibrium, respectively. The cation fluxes were obtained by multiplying the rate constants by the intracellular concentrations per liter of cell of the respective cation.

The kinetics of steady state Na+ and K+ movements across rabbit polymorphonuclear leukocyte membranes were found to follow the two-compartment model. The movement of both ions is rapid, reaching virtual completion in less than 30 min. The value for the unidirectional steady state fluxes of K+ and Na+ is 7.4 mEq per liter cell min^{-1} and 3.0 mEq per liter cell min^{-1}, respectively. These values are about 50% higher than those reported by Cividalli and Nathan for human neutrophils (5). This probably reflects species differences.

Ouabain at 10^{-6} to 10^{-4} M was shown to inhibit the rate of influx of K+ and the efflux of Na+. The same concentrations of ouabain were without effect on the efflux of K^+ and the influx of Na^+. In addition, the rate of Na^+ efflux depended on the extracellular K^+ concentration, and removal of K^+ from the extracellular medium lowered the efflux of Na^+. Furthermore, the decrease in Na^+ efflux was about the same whether induced by ouabain or the removal of K^+. All these findings are what is expected if a Na^+, K^+ pump is operative in the rabbit neutrophil.

The effect of the chemotactic peptide fMet-Leu-Phe was next studied. The peptide causes a small but consistent increase in the influx of K^+ that at maximum is less than 20% of control. As shown in Fig. 1, the degree of increase depends on the concentration of fMet-Leu-Phe, and, furthermore, this concentration dependence, at least over the ascending limb of the curve, mirrors the concentration dependence of stimulated movement for the same peptide as determined previously (12). The increase in K^+ influx induced by fMet-Leu-Phe is ouabain-sensitive, 10^{-5} M ouabain completely abolishing it. There is no effect of fMet-Leu-Phe on the K^+ efflux.

The chemotactic factor induces a much larger concentration-dependent increase in the influx of Na^+. A slight enhancement of Na^+ influx is evident at 3×10^{-11} M, which increases slowly with concentration of peptide until 10^{-10} M, where it becomes linear with the concentration, reaching a value at 3×10^{-9} M fMet-Leu-Phe at least 4 times larger than that of the control. This influx is not affected by ouabain or removal of K^+. A much smaller dose-dependent efflux of Na^+ is also apparent over the same concentration range. In contradistinction to Na^+ influx, removing extracellular K^+ abolishes the enhancement of Na^+ efflux caused by 5×10^{-10} fMet-Leu-Phe. In five determinations in the

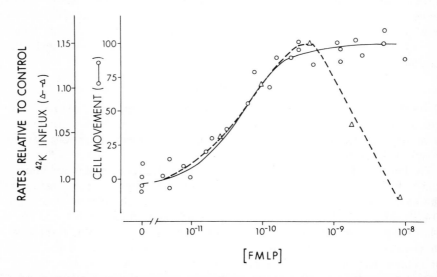

FIG. 1. The stimulation of neutrophil movement (O) and influx of K^+ (Δ) by varying concentrations of formylmethionylleucylphenylalanine (FMLP).

presence of 5.5 mM K$^+$, the ratio of ^{22}Na$^+$ efflux in the presence of peptide to that of the control was 1.25 ± 0.1 (SE); in the absence of K$^+$, the ratio was $1.05 + 0.1$.

In summary, the chemotactic peptide induces a small but consistent increase in K$^+$ influx and an equally small but consistent efflux of Na$^+$. Both of these fluxes are abolished by ouabain at the same concentrations. Moreover, the enhancement of the Na$^+$ efflux is critically dependent on the level of K$^+$ in the extracellular medium; in the absence of K$^+$ the increase of Na$^+$ efflux does not occur. These, as mentioned, are the characteristics of the Na$^+$, K$^+$ pump.

Although the evidence is indirect, and as yet we have not tested other chemotactic factors, nevertheless, it strongly supports the conclusion that interaction of chemotactic factors with the neutrophil membrane activates the Na$^+$, K$^+$ pump, i.e., the Na$^+$, K$^+$ ATPase of the neutrophil. Even if we accept this conclusion, we are still left with a number of questions. Among them are: Is the putative activation of the pump a direct or indirect action of chemotactic peptide? Is the activation of the pump directly or indirectly involved in the enhancement by K$^+$ of the effectiveness of the chemotactic factors, and, if so how?

There are at least two possibilities as to how the chemotactic peptide enhances the activity of the K$^+$, Na$^+$ pump. One mechanism would be a direct activation of the membrane K$^+$, Na$^+$ ATPase either through the peptide acting on the enzyme directly or, more likely, by perturbing the membrane and thus activating the enzyme. The other possibility is that the large increased influx of Na$^+$ into the cell consequent to the interaction of chemotactic factor and neutrophil raises the intracellular Na$^+$ concentration sufficiently to activate the Na$^+$, K$^+$ ATPase. Some plausibility is furnished this latter hypothesis by the finding that although the influx of Na$^+$ occurs extremely rapidly after the interaction of chemotactic factor with the cell, there is a lag of 5 to 7 min before the increase in K$^+$ influx begins; however, as yet, we have not been able to demonstrate an increase in the concentration of intracellular Na$^+$ following interaction of the neutrophil and chemotactic peptide. Measurement of the small amounts of intracellular Na$^+$ in the presence of large amounts of extracellular Na$^+$ presents certain difficulties, and these experiments are continuing.

We currently plan to attempt to differentiate between these hypotheses by testing whether the chemotactic factor can act on isolated membranes to activate their Na$^+$, K$^+$ ATPase. A positive result will strongly support the first hypothesis. Similarly, the finding that the chemotactic factor is unable to activate the Na$^+$, K$^+$ ATPase of the isolated membrane but that it does activate the same enzyme in intact cells will support the idea that chemotactic factors indirectly activate the Na$^+$, K$^+$ pump of the neutrophil.

The ability of K$^+$ to double the effectiveness of the chemotactic factor and of ouabain to abolish this leave little doubt that the action of Na$^+$, K$^+$ ATPase is required for optimal neutrophil responsiveness. Nevertheless, this still leaves the question whether the influx of K$^+$ and efflux of Na$^+$ induced by the chemotactic factor play any role in the stimulatory activity of the chemotactic peptides.

Here again, at least two possibilities present themselves. The first possibility is that the influx of K+ and efflux of Na+ stimulated by the chemotactic factor are merely signs that the Na+, K+ pump is acting to maintain the optimum Na+ and K+ gradients in the cell, but the enhanced fluxes are not per se involved in the stimulation of movement. The second hypothesis is that the K+ influx and coupled Na+ efflux play a direct role in the enhancement of the cell's responsiveness to chemotactic factor. In favor of the first hypothesis is that, as mentioned, K+ in the absence of chemotactic factor, increases the nonstimulated locomotion of the neutrophil. Moreover, the stimulated influx of K+ and efflux of Na+ are both quite small, especially relative to the Na+ influx. In favor of the second hypothesis is the exact correspondence between the ascending limb of concentration dependence of the stimulation of neutrophil movement by fMet-Leu-Phe and the ability of the same agent to induce K+ influx (Fig. 1). (Note, however, that inhibition of K+ influx apparently occurs at concentrations of chemotactic factor giving maximum movement.) In addition, valinomycin, in the presence of K+, and only in the presence of K+, increases the ability of chemotactic factors to stimulate movement. Obviously, further work is required to decide between these hypotheses.

SUMMARY

Extracellular K+ increases the random motility and the ability of all chemotactic factors tested to stimulate the locomotion of rabbit peritoneal neutrophils. The enhancement by K+ of the stimulatory activity of chemotactic factors is prevented by low concentrations of ouabain. This action of ouabain is reversed by increasing the concentration of K+. The K+-specific ionophore, valinomycin, enhances the activity of chemotactic factors in the presence of K+ but not in its absence; this suggested that K+ influx is stimulated by the chemotactic factor.

Na+ and K+ transmembrane fluxes of the neutrophil were measured in the absence and presence of the chemotactic peptide, formylmethionylleucylphenylalanine, fMet-Leu-Phe. Ouabain inhibited both K+ influx and Na+ efflux, the latter being also dependent on the presence of extracellular K+, indicating the presence of a Na+, K+ pump. In prior work, we have established the presence in the membranes of rabbit peritoneal neutrophils, the presence of a ouabain inhibitable, Na+, K+-sensitive ATPase, indicating that in the neutrophil, as in other cells, the Na+, K+ pump activity is caused by such an ATPase. fMet-Leu-Phe induced a large and rapid increase in the permeability of the neutrophil plasma membrane to Na+. Smaller and delayed enhancements of K+ influx and Na+ efflux were also noted. There was no effect of the peptide on K+ efflux. The enhanced K+ influx and Na+ efflux were prevented by ouabain, and omitting K+ from the medium prevented the enhanced Na+ efflux, indicating the peptide enhanced the Na+, K+ pump, i.e., the Na+, K+ ATPase. The possible ways this could be done, and the role of this enhancement in the stimulation of neutrophil movement were discussed.

ACKNOWLEDGMENT

The experimental work reported here was supported in part by NIH Research Grant A1 06948 to E. L. Becker.

REFERENCES

1. Aswanikumar, S., Schiffmann, E., Corcoran, B. A., and Wahl, S. M. (1976): Role of peptidase in phagocyte chemotaxis. *Proc. Natl. Acad. Sci. U.S.A.,* 73:2439–2442.
2. Becker, E. L. (1975): Enzyme activation and the mechanism of polymorphonuclear leukocyte chemotaxis. In: *The Phagocytic Cell in Host Resistance,* pp. 1–14. Raven Press, New York.
3. Becker, E. L. (1976): Some interrelations among chemotaxis, lysosomal enzyme secretion and phagocytosis by neutrophils. In: *Molecular and Biological Aspects of the Acute Allergic Reaction,* edited by S. G. O. Johansson, K. Strandberg, and B. Uvnäs, pp. 353–370. Plenum Pub. Corp., New York.
4. Becker, E. L., and Ward, P. A. (1967): Partial biochemical characterization of the activated esterase required in the complement dependent chemotaxis of rabbit polymorphonuclear leukocytes. *J. Exp. Med.,* 125:1021–1038.
5. Cividalli, G., and Nathan, D. G. (1974): Sodium and potassium concentration and transmembrane fluxes in leukocytes. *Blood,* 43:861–869.
6. Dunham, P. B., Goldstein, I. M., and Weissman, G. (1974): Potassium and amino acid transport in human leukocytes exposed to phagocytic stimuli. *J. Cell Biol.,* 63:215–226.
7. Goetzl, E. J. (1975): Modulation of human neutrophil polymorphonuclear leukocyte migration by human plasma alpha-globulin inhibitors and synthetic esterase inhibitors. *Immunology,* 29: 163–174.
8. Harold, F. M. (1972): Conservation and transformation of energy by bacterial membranes. *Bacteriol. Rev.,* 36:172–230.
9. Naccache, P. H., Showell, H. J., Becker, E. L., and Sha'afi, R. I. (1977): Sodium, Potassium and Calcium Transport Across Rabbit Polymorphonuclear Leukocyte Membranes: Effect of Chemotactic Factor. *J. Cell Biol.,* 73:428–444.
10. Sha'afi, R. I., Naccache, P., Raible, D., Krepcio, A., Showell, H., and Becker, E. L. (1976): Demonstration of (Na+ +K+) sensitive ATPase activity in rabbit polymorphonuclear leukocyte membranes. *Biochim. Biophys. Acta,* 448:638–641.
11. Showell, H. J., and Becker, E. L. (1975): The effects of external K+ and Na+ on the chemotaxis of rabbit peritoneal neutrophils. *J. Immunol.,* 116:99–105.
12. Showell, H. J., Freer, R. J., Zigmond, S. H., Schiffmann, E., Aswanikumar, S., Corcoran, B., and Becker, E. L. (1976): The structure-activity relations of synthetic peptides as chemotactic factors and inducers of lysosomal enzyme secretion for neutrophils. *J. Exp. Med.,* 143:1154–1169.
13. Skou, J. C. (1960): Further investigations of a Mg++ and Na+-linked activated transport of Na+ and K+ across the nerve membrane. *Biochim. Biophys. Acta,* 42:6–14.

DISCUSSION

Dr. Gallin: Dr. Becker, you showed us the data of the stimulated potassium influx by the fMet peptides. When one does unidirectional flux studies, as you have done, there is always the concern that a measured influx could be coupled with an efflux that might be occurring simultaneously. Have you done experiments looking at potassium efflux simultaneously with influx?

Dr. Becker: Yes. There is no effect of this chemotactic factor on potassium efflux that we could detect. This is not to say it does not occur, but it certainly is below our limits of detection.

Dr. Stossel: Isn't it necessary to be careful also about sodium-sodium exchange and potassium-potassium exchange? The only way to rule that out is to do measurement of total ion levels, is it not? In other words, isotopic movement measurements do not tell you about net flux.

Dr. Becker: I have deliberately not put the analysis in terms of how much of the Na^+ or K^+ fluxes are a result of the pump action; how much they are a result of facilitated diffusion; or how much they are a result of sodium-sodium interchange or potassium-potassium interchange. This is an analysis that is undoubtedly called for and which we are going to be doing, but we have not attempted it so far.

Dr. Wilkinson: I was just thinking about the analogies between neutrophil locomotion and smooth-muscle contraction, and one difference in the neutrophil is that there must be continued contractions and relaxations going on all the time to sustain locomotion. How is this affecting your measurements and your thinking about it?

Dr. Becker: I do not think this type of analysis, by itself, is going to give us the full answer, but, what it is going to do is put limits on the kinds of hypotheses that we will be able to make. Coupled with the sort of studies that Dr. Gallin is going to present, which I think complement ours very well, we will eventually be able to put this thing together. It is not going to give a full answer, but I think this approach will help answer the questions.

Dr. Leddy: Can you saturate the cell with chemotactic factor so that it is deactivated and unresponsive to the chemotactic agent, and then show that you cannot stimulate the ATPase? This would help determine if these events are necessarily related.

Dr. Becker: We intend to do this experiment to determine what deactivation is all about and why the cell no longer responds; for example, is deactivation a matter of a lack of ability to change ion permeability, i.e., an inability to reopen ion gates?

Dr. Leddy: In addition to showing that ouabain blocks the changes in sodium and potassium fluxes that are attributable to the ATPase in the membrane, have you shown that ouabain also inhibits the actual chemotactic response of the cells?

Dr. Becker: Yes. The stimulation by potassium of chemotactic effectiveness of the chemotactic factor was blocked by ouabain.

Dr. Leddy: But the basic response of the cells to chemotactic agent was not blocked?

Dr. Becker: Yes, in the absence of potassium we had no effect of ouabain.

Dr. Ward: Does this effect of chemotactic factors on the ion flux parallel the chemotactic activity of the peptide?

Dr. Becker: We do not know. We do not know whether other chemotactic factors do this. We are going to be surprised if we do find a difference, but obviously, these experiments have to be done.

Dr. Hill: What was the relationship again between calcium and sodium exchange?

Dr. Becker: It was pure postulate that with the increase in sodium influx, there is an exchange of Na^+ for calcium in the putative sequestered calcium compartment of the neutrophil, whatever that may be. The release of calcium with that exchange into the cytoplasm frees calcium to go into the exterior of the cell. In addition, there would be a prevention of Ca^{2+} efflux by the sodium-calcium exchange process. These are pure hypotheses, at present.

Dr. Snyderman: We have some experimental data on calcium movement. If the cells are equilibrated first with calcium so that there are the internal/external pools in equilibrium, and then chemotactic agents are added, there is a net calcium influx.

Dr. Becker: We have noted that too. But the change in steady state calcium stimulated by the chemotactic factor depends upon the level of external calcium. Addition of 5×10^{-10} molar, fMet peptide caused a very large increase in steady state level of calcium in the presence of 0.25 millimolar external calcium on the outside, suggesting that there was an increase in exchangeable calcium as Dr. Snyderman stated; however, we also did another experiment which was exactly the same, except with no added external calcium other than the calcium-45. The addition of chemotactic factor at the steady state resulted in transient actual displacement of calcium from the cell, a decrease in the steady state level. We think this calcium is coming from the membrane of the cell, although, again, we have no real evidence bearing on this, one way or the other.

But what these experiments are really saying is that the action of the chemotactic factors on calcium transport is quite complex, that an increase in the exchangeable calcium can be obtained and also a displacement of calcium from the cell.

Leukocyte Chemotaxis, edited by John I. Gallin
and Paul G. Quie. Raven Press, New York
© 1978.

Structural and Ionic Events During Leukocyte Chemotaxis

*John I. Gallin, **Elaine K. Gallin, *Harry L. Malech,
and †Eva B. Cramer

*Laboratory of Clinical Investigation, National Institute of Allergy and Infectious Diseases,
National Institutes of Health, Bethesda, Maryland 20014; **Division of Experimental
Hematology, Armed Forces Radiobiology Research Institute, Bethesda, Maryland 20014;
and †Department of Anatomy, Downstate Medical Center,
Brooklyn, New York 11203*

The mechanism by which leukocytes respond to chemotactic stimuli with directed locomotion (chemotaxis) has been an area of interest in our laboratory in recent years. In particular, our attention has focused on the ultrastructural and ionic events associated with cell orientation during chemotaxis. Ultrastructural analysis of neutrophils during conditions of directed migration has revealed a highly organized orientation of intracellular elements that is essential for maintaining direction during chemotaxis (33). In association with our evaluation of intracellular structure, certain surface events have also been studied during interaction of chemotactic factors with the cell. For example, it has been shown that the negative surface charge in human neutrophils was diminished after incubation with chemotactic factors (20). In this communication, surface charge changes caused by chemotactic factors are assessed at the ultrastructural level, using antimony deposition as an indicator of cation localization (46,47). Evidence will be presented that cations localize at the cytoplasmic side of the plasma membrane in advancing pseudopods during conditions of chemotaxis.

Studies of the electrophysiology of chemotactic factor interaction with leukocytes (15) have been helpful in understanding how the orientation process may be modulated by ionic events occurring during locomotion. Calcium and magnesium are both known to be required for directed migration (5,24). We previously demonstrated calcium release as a result of chemotactic factor interaction with leukocytes (24) and Boucek and Snyderman described a rapid calcium uptake when chemotactic factors interact with human neutrophils (8). Naccache et al. recently reported chemotactic factor-induced calcium exchange, and their data implicated a role for sodium and potassium during interaction of chemotactic factors with leukocytes (36). Observations using electrophysiological techniques combined with the ion flux data, and analysis of ultrastructural events occurring during leukocyte-directed migration, provide the basis for a hypothetical model of ionic control of cell orientation during chemotaxis.

NEUTROPHIL ORIENTATION DURING DIRECTED MIGRATION

During directed migration (chemotaxis), neutrophils assume an oriented morphology characterized by cell polarization with the nuclei toward the back of the cell and pseudopods toward the leading end (1,40–42). Based on data using the antitubulins, colchicine and vincristine, it has been postulated that microtubules are important for maintaining cell orientation (1,9,12,39). In support of this was the observation of Goldstein et al. that C5a induced microtubule assembly in cytochalasin B-treated neutrophils (27) and our observation that neutrophils migrating through micropore filters had increased polymerization of microtubules (24). It has been speculated that localized microtubule assembly in the leading end of the cell would stabilize the cell (24) and perhaps modulate sol-gel transformation, which has been postulated by others to be important in establishing the vector of locomotion (42). We have recently tested this hypothesis by ultrastructural analysis of neutrophils oriented on 0.45-μm micropore filters (33,34). During conditions of directed migration, neutrophil internal structures assumed a highly organized orientation. In the low-power electron micrograph shown in Fig. 1, the nuclei are toward the rear of the cell while the bulk of cytoplasm and granules are between the nuclei and advancing pseudopods. A high-power electron micrograph of a neutrophil oriented under conditions of directed migration is shown in Fig. 2. The centriole and its radial array of microtubules are located between the nucleus and advancing pseudopod. Bundles of a loose meshwork of microfilaments are found in the advancing pseudopod, with a thin veil of microfilaments on the sides and top of the cell.

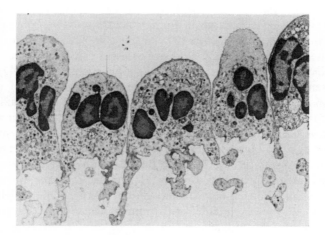

FIG. 1. Electron micrograph of human neutrophils at the surface of a 0.45-μm filter after 45 min incubation under conditions of chemotaxis with *Escherichia coli* endotoxin as the chemotactic stimulus. Cells were fixed in cold 2% glutaraldehyde, rinsed in sodium cacodylate buffer, pH 7.3, postfixed in Dalton's chrome osmium (1%), stained in 5.0% uranylacetate, dehydrated in graded series of alcohol, cleaned with propylene oxide, and imbedded in eponaraldite. ×3,000.

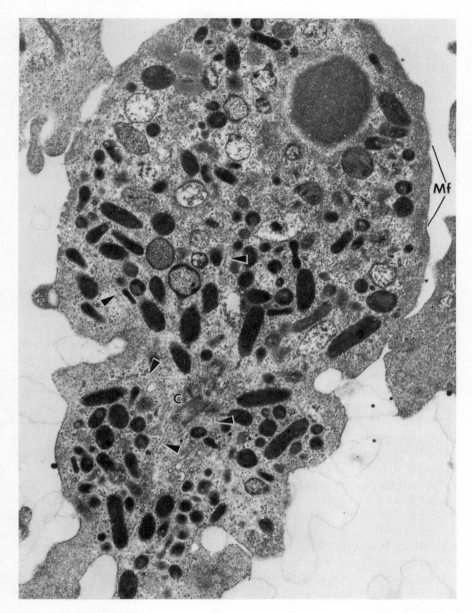

FIG. 2. Electron micrograph of a neutrophil oriented in a gradient of *Escherichia coli* endotoxin-activated serum with the source of 5% activated serum beneath a 0.45-μm pore filter. The nuclear lobes are toward the upper part of the cell, while the bulk of the granule containing cytoplasm lies beneath the nucleus. A thin layer of submembranous microfilaments (Mf) can be seen at the sides and top of the cell, while in the pseudopods, microfilaments aggregate in discrete areas (not clearly seen in this micrograph). The centriole is indicated by *C,* and radiating microtubules are indicated by *arrowheads*. Glutaraldehyde, osmium-pyroantimonate fixation. Uranyl acetate, lead citrate strain. ×15,000.

Dense bundles of microfilaments are noted at sites of attachment to the filter. Upon reversal of the gradient of chemotactic factor (placing chemotactic factor on top of the cell), a complicated but organized series of events ensues as the cell reorients (33). Initially, within 2 min, the centriole and associated array of microtubules migrate down toward, and often into, one of the pseudopods. The nucleus then migrates away from the new source of chemotactic factor, penetrating deep into one of the old pseudopods. A loose meshwork of microfilaments forms at the new leading end of the cell, and the centriole and its microtubule array reorient between the nucleus and the new leading end of the cell as the cell migrates toward the chemotactic factor. Orientation of internal structure during directed migration and reorientation of these structures in response to changes in location of chemoattractant, prior to changes in the direction of locomotion, suggested that the orientation process is critical for and not merely a consequence of directed migration (33).

Effect of Cytochalasin B and Colchicine on Neutrophil Orientation and Locomotion

To assess the role of microfilaments and microtubules in cell orientation, we studied the effects of cytochalasin B and cholchicine on these processes. Cytochalasin B at 3.0 μg/ml inhibits neutrophil migration (3,53). Addition of cytochalasin B (3.0 μg/ml) to oriented neutrophils caused pseudopod retraction but did not inhibit the ability of cells to orient their internal structure in a gradient of chemotactic factor or to reorient the internal structure by changing the location of the chemoattractant (33). Cytochalasin B, however, abolished microfilament bundles in advancing pseudopods and prevented migration of cells off the filter when the location of chemoattractant was reversed and placed above the cells. These experiments were compatible with the concept that the microfilament system is essential for locomotion but not orientation of internal structure or cell polarization.

Similar experiments were performed using cells incubated for 30 min in colchicine (33). As little as 10^{-8} to 10^{-7} M colchicine significantly affected neutrophil orientation. With 10^{-6} M colchicine, nuclei were randomly distributed within the cell, and there was no orientation of centrioles with respect to the nuclei. Pseudopod formation occurred with colchicine treatment but only if a filter matrix was provided for the pseudopod to adhere to. Direction-finding by pseudopods was impaired by colchicine. The inhibition of orientation was associated with inhibition of microtubule assembly. Functional studies of cells migrating under conditions of spontaneous random migration (in buffer), stimulated random migration (uniform concentration of chemoattractant), and directed migration (gradient of chemoattractant) demonstrated that colchicine (5 $\times$ 10^{-7} M) had no effect on spontaneous random migration, caused minimal inhibition of stimulated random migration, but markedly inhibited directed migration. As shown in Fig. 3, the effects of colchicine were detected over a wide

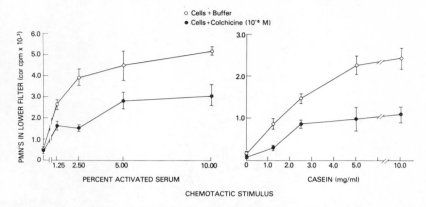

FIG. 3. Effect of colchicine on human neutrophil chemotaxis using the radioassay technique (19). Cells were incubated at 37°C in buffer or colchicine (10^{-6} M) for 30 min prior to being placed in chemotaxis chambers. The indicated concentrations of *Escherichia coli* endotoxin-activated serum *(left panel)* or sodium caseinate *(right panel)* were the chemoattractants. Mean ± SEM, four determinations.

concentration range of chemoattractants. Lumicolchicine (10^{-6} M) did not produce the colchicine effects. Based on these experiments, we concluded that the microtubule system is required for maintaining cell orientation and providing the vector of locomotion during chemotaxis, whereas the microfilament system provides the locomotory apparatus and contributes only indirectly, as a consequence of oriented assembly, to direction-finding (33).

Local Submembranous Cation Changes During Directed Migration

In order to delineate further the physiological events associated with chemotactic factor-induced decreases in surface charge (20), ultrastructural analyses of cation deposition in leukocytes prepared under conditions of directed and random migration were performed. The technique involves formation of electron-opaque precipitates of tissue cations with antimonate anions included in the osmium tetroxide fixation (31,46,47). For these experiments, human neutrophils were placed in chemotactic chambers under conditions of random or directed migration using *Escherichia coli* endotoxin-activated serum as the chemotactic stimulus (18) and employing 0.45 μM cellulose nitrate micropore filters (Millipore Corp., Bedford, Massachusetts 01730). After appropriate incubation, cells were fixed in osmium pyroantimonate and then analyzed by electron microscopy. As shown in Fig. 4A, cells prepared under conditions of random migration have antimony precipitates in the granules and in the heterochromatin of their nuclei, confirming a previous report (29). Little deposit was noted on the cytoplasmic membrane. Compared with randomly migrating neutrophils, cells oriented in a gradient of chemotactic factor (Fig 4B) had increased cytoplasmic pyroantimonate deposits. In addition, in the oriented cells, there was heavy deposition of antimonate

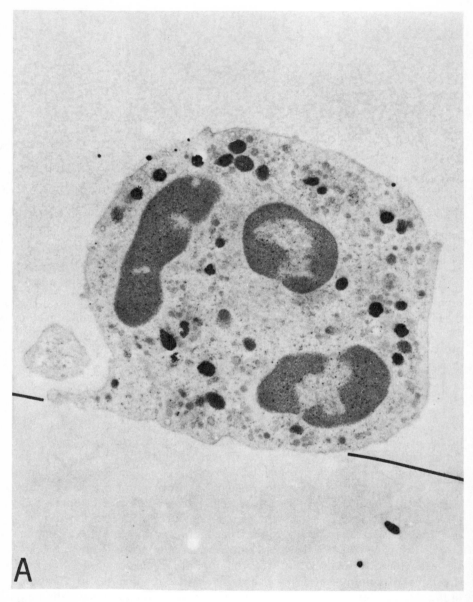

FIG. 4 A: A neutrophil under conditions of spontaneous migration on a 0.45-μm cellulose nitrate filter (Millipore) (*black line* is top of filter). Osmium-pyroantimonate fixation. Unstained. X10,000. Note deposits of pyroantimonate in some granules and in the nucleus. Virtually no deposit is seen associated with the plasma membrane. **B:** A neutrophil in fixed orientation on a 0.45-μm cellulose nitrate filter toward a gradient of chemoattractant (activated serum). Pyroantimonate fixation. Unstained. X8,500. *Inset:* unstained. X29,000. Note deposits of pyroan-

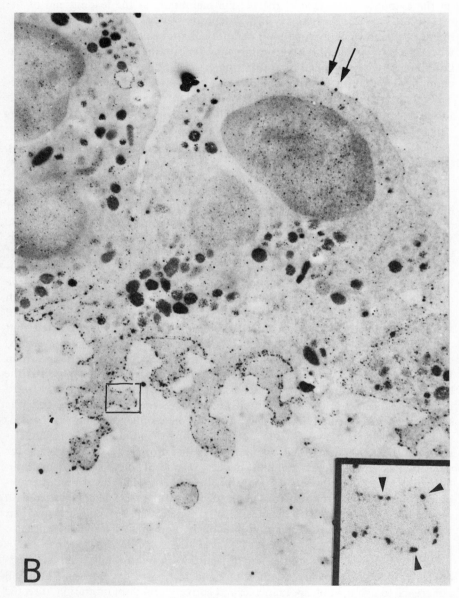

B

timonate in some granules, in the nucleus, and associated with the plasma membrane. The amount of deposit appears to be heavier on the leading end of the cell, in the region of the pseudopods. The *inset* is an enlargement of a portion of a pseudopod *(black rectangle)*. The bulk of the deposit in the pseudopods is inside the plasma membrane *(arrowheads)* in contrast to that seen at the rear of the cell where the deposit frequently lies outside the cell membrane *(arrows)*.

on the cytoplasmic surface of the plasma membrane at the leading end of the cell (inset, Fig 4B). Particularly heavy deposits were associated with the membrane of the advancing pseudopod. Additional studies are needed to determine whether these submembranous antimonate deposits in oriented cells represent unfolding of cationic membrane sites; increased binding of cations such as calcium, magnesium, or sodium; mobilization of positively charged membrane receptors to the leading end of the cell; or fusion of granule membranes with the cytoplasmic membrane during exocytosis.

Neutrophil Orientation in Patients with Defective Chemotaxis and Abnormal Microtubule Assembly

During our evaluation of patients with recurrent pyogenic infections, we have studied several groups of patients with abnormal chemotaxis as their major host defense abnormality (17,25). Clark and Kimball demonstrated that patients with the Chediak-Higashi syndrome (CHS) have defective neutrophil chemotaxis (10), and we have subsequently shown that these patients have a similar defect of mononuclear cells (22). Studies by Oliver have implicated abnormal microtubule assembly and cyclic nucleotide metabolism in the CHS (38). We have assessed orientation of neutrophils from a previously described patient with the CHS (50) under conditions of directed migration. In the middle panel of the low-magnification electron micrograph shown in Fig. 5, it is noted that neutrophils from this patient contain the large lysosomal granules *(arrowheads)* characteristic of this disease. As seen in Fig. 5 and quantitatively shown in Fig. 6, the nuclei in the CHS neutrophils did not orient normally toward the back of the cell. Although CHS nuclei orient away from midposition (0.5) toward the top of the cell (1.0), the position of the CHS nuclei within the cell was significantly less oriented than normal. In addition, compared to normal neutrophils, CHS cells had fewer pseudopods penetrating the filter (Fig. 5). In association with defective neutrophil orientation, the CHS nuclei had a tendency for decreased assembly of microtubules (mean $\pm$ SEM centriole associated microtubules of 6 ± 0.93 in CHS vs 10 ± 2 in normal, $p > 0.20$).[1] This decreased microtubule assembly in neutrophils from our patient with the CHS is compatible with reports by Oliver (38). The magnitude of the defect in our patient, however, was not as striking as that reported previously, and more data are required to establish significance.

We have also recently studied cell orientation in neutrophils from a 7-year-old girl (W.S.) with recurrent infections and leukocyte dysfunction (23). Cell adherence to nylon wool, spontaneous and activated random migration, directed migration, bactericidal activity for *Staphylococcus aureus,* and enzyme secretion

---

[1] Centriole-associated microtubules were the number of microtubules (structures with straight parallel sides, 250 Å apart, 100 nm long, and more electron-dense than the ground substance) counted in a 1 μm radius drawn around the centriole.

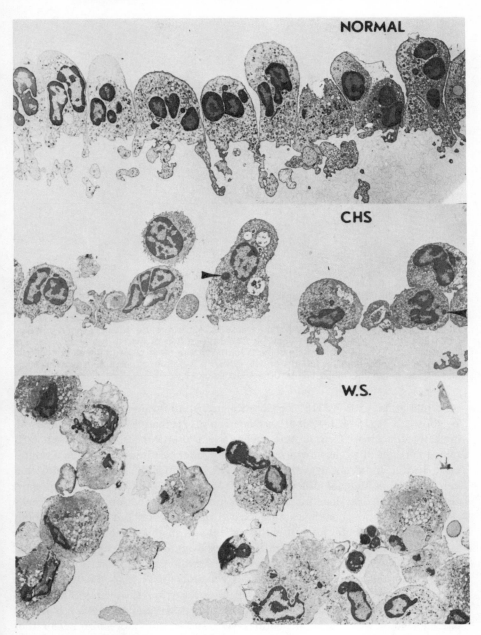

FIG. 5. Electron micrographs of neutrophils at the surface of 0.45-μm pore cellulose nitrate filters after 45 min incubation under conditions of directed migration (chemotaxis) with *Escherichia coli* endotoxin activated serum as the chemoattractant. Upper panel: neutrophils from a normal subject (X2,400); middle panel: from a patient with the Chediak-Higashi syndrome (X2,400); and lower panel: from a patient with recurrent infections (W.S.) (X2,400). Cells prepared as described in Fig. 1.

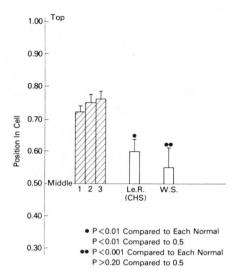

FIG. 6. Average position of the nucleus in the vertical axis of neutrophils with *Escherichia coli* endotoxin-activated serum as the chemoattractant. "1, 2, and 3" are normal subjects; a patient with the Chediak-Higashi syndrome (CHS) and another patient (W.S.) are indicated. Nucleus position was calculated with the formula B/B+T, where the distance from the portion of the neutrophil surface furthest from the filter surface (top of cell) to the nearest lobe of the nucleus is "T", and the distance from the lowest lobe of the nucleus to the part of pseudopods extending into the filter (bottom of cell) is "B." 0 is bottom of cell, 0.5 mid cell position, and 1.0 top of the cell. Mean ± SEM, 30 determinations.

on stimulation with A23187 or phorbol myristate acetate were all abnormal. As shown in Fig. 5 *(lower panel),* her neutrophils (Hypaque-Ficoll) were morphilogically abnormal. Cytoplasmic membrane protuberances, which often contained portions of nuclei *(arrow),* were seen. Under conditions of directed migration, the nuclei did not orient normally. The mean position of the nuclei within her neutrophils did not differ from midposition (0.5), and the large standard error of the nuclear location reflected a random distribution within the cells (Fig. 6). In addition, centrioles were located randomly without orientation about the nuclei. Of particular interest in this patient was an abnormality of microtubule assembly characterized by markedly increased numbers of centriole-associated microtubules under conditions of directed migration (10 ± 2 microtubules/centriole for normal vs 23 ± 1.5 microtubules/centriole for W. S., $p < 0.01$.[1] Because of recent associations between cyclic nucleotide levels and the degree of polymerization of microtubules (54), we also measured cAMP and cGMP levels in this patient's leukocytes. Cyclic nucleotides were studied in mononuclear cells rather than in neutrophils, since we have had difficulty measuring cyclic nucleotides

---

[1] Centriole-associated microtubules were the number of microtubules (structures with straight parallel sides, 250 Å apart, 100 nm long, and more electron-dense than the ground substance) counted in a 1 μm radius drawn around the centriole.

in neutrophils (43). In unstimulated cells, cGMP levels were markedly elevated (4.48 ± 0.6 $p$moles/10^7 cells from normals vs 16.15 ± 2.45 $p$moles/10^7 cells from W.S., $p < 0.001$). cAMP was normal.

Neutrophils from these two patients with abnormal chemotaxis, abnormal orientation, and abnormal microtubule assembly provide pathological models in support of the concept that normal microtubule function is critical for directed migration. More specifically, the data from these patients' cells suggest that proper polymerization and depolymerization of microtubules are critical for maintenance of directed migration. Whether the fundamental defect causing abnormal tubulin polymerization and cell orientation in neutrophils obtained from patients with the CHS and in W.S. is related to an abnormality of cyclic nucleotide metabolism, as the available data suggest, or another defect, perhaps involving abnormal membrane receptors, remains to be determined.

IONIC EVENTS DURING CHEMOTACTIC FACTOR INTERACTION WITH LEUKOCYTES

As part of our attempt to understand the physiological basis of leukocyte orientation in response to chemotactic factors, we have studied the role of divalent cations in the chemotactic response (24). Both calcium and magnesium are required for a normal chemotactic response (5,24). In addition, our studies of the uptake and release of ^{45}calcium demonstrated a C5a-induced calcium release (24). More recently, it was shown that chemotactic factors also induce a rapid calcium uptake (8). To evaluate ionic events occurring during chemotaxis in a more precise way, we have recently studied the electrophysiology of chemotactic factor-leukocyte interaction (15).

Cultivated human macrophages (3-week cultures of human peripheral blood mononuclear cells) are large enough (20 to 40 μm) to permit stable micropuncture studies. These cells remain differentiated, retain many of their *in vivo* characteristics under routine culture conditions, and have been used to study the role of the macrophage in immunological phenomema and other aspects of host defense (28,48). In response to *E. coli* endotoxin-activated serum, these cultivated macrophages migrated through 12-μm nucleopore polycarbonate filters, Neuro Probe, Bethesda, Maryland 20014, (2 ± 0.3 cells/hpf with buffer stimulus vs 25 ± 3 cells/hpf with activated sera stimulus, $p < 0.01$). In a uniform concentration of endotoxin-activated serum, random migration was stimulated (2 ± 0.3 cells/hpf for spontaneous random migration vs 13 ± 1 cells/hpf for stimulated random migration, $p < 0.01$).

Standard electrophysiological techniques were used to study the interaction of chemotactic factors with macrophages to determine if these agents triggered membrane potential changes (16). Initial studies were performed with *E. coli* endotoxin-activated human sera (18), since it had recently been shown that such sera cause membrane-ruffling and macrophage-spreading related to products of the complement- and the kinin-generating system (6). As shown in Fig.

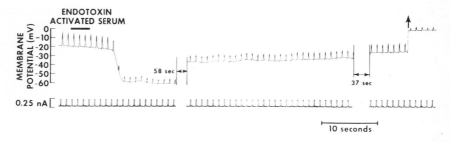

FIG. 7. Recording of membrane potential in a cultured human macrophage during addition of 5% endotoxin-activated serum to bath. The cell resting membrane potential = —24 mV. Small current pulses used to monitor membrane resistance are superimposed on the tracing. The vertical arrow (↑) indicates withdrawal of electrode from the cell.

7, addition of endotoxin-activated serum (final concentration of 5%) to a bath containing macrophages produced a large membrane hyperpolarization. This response was seen in 90% of cells studied. The hyperpolarization (—10 to —50 mV in amplitude) was associated with a decrease in membrane resistance as monitored by the decreased electrotonic potential produced by constant-current pulses. Nonactivated serum, or serum heated 30 min at 56°C prior to addition of endotoxin, produced small hyperpolarizations in only 40% of the cells. Moreover, endotoxin-activated human serum deficient in the third component of human complement, C3, did not cause potential changes unless the serum was first reconstituted with C3. These preliminary studies suggested that products of complement activation, perhaps C5a, initiated the membrane potential changes.

Additional studies were done with partially purified C5a (G-75 Sephadex), and the synthetic peptide chemotactic factor fmet-leu-phe (courtesy of Dr. Elliott Schiffmann). For each agent, a gradient of stimulus was applied by allowing the test stimulus to diffuse from a blunted microelectrode (10 to 20 μ tip diameter) placed adjacent to the cell with a micromanipulator. An electrical recording from a cell stimulated with C5a is shown in Fig. 8. Immediately following addition of C5a, there was a small brief depolarization followed by a more sustained hyperpolarization. Of cells stimulated with C5a, 80% responded

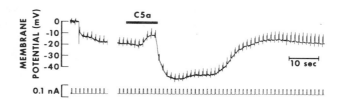

FIG. 8. Recording of membrane potential from a cultured human macrophage during exposure to C5a contained in a blunted microelectrode brought adjacent to the cell. Resting membrane potential = —20 mV.

with potential changes. In 49 responding cells, these changes were characterized by either a depolarization followed by a hyperpolarization (26%), a hyperpolarization alone (65%), or a depolarization without hyperpolarization (8%). The C5a-induced responses were not observed when C5a was pretreated with goat antisera to human C5, whereas antisera to C3 had no effect on the responses. Kallikrein and fmet-leu-phe, which have chemotactic activity for macrophages (21,45), produced similar potential changes.

The chemotactic factor-evoked potential changes were blocked by Mg^{++} (5 mM) − EGTA (10 mM), suggesting a role of calcium in the response. In one cell that responded to eight stimulations with C5a, the reversal potential[2] of the depolarizing and hyperpolarizing responses was determined to be O mV and −65 mV, respectively. A reversal potential of 0 for the depolarizing response is compatible with an increase in permeability to calcium or sodium, each of which have positive equilibrium potentials, as well as to potassium, which has a negative equilibrium potential. A reversal potential of −65 mV for the hyperpolarizing response could be accounted for by an increased permeability to potassium. In order to determine conclusively which ions are responsible for these potential changes, ion substitution experiments are planned. Based on these experiments, however, we concluded that the initial events resulting from macrophage interaction of chemotactic factors include a small transient depolarization, possibly related to an influx of calcium and perhaps sodium, followed by a much larger prolonged hyperpolarization related to potassium efflux (17). These initial membrane potential changes probably precede the calcium release we have observed previously (24).

In additional studies, changes in cell morphology were monitored while electrophysiological responses were recorded. Chemotactic factor-induced potential changes preceded pseudopod formation. Moreover, with constant stimulation by a gradient of C5a, only a single electrical event, characterized by a more prolonged hyperpolarization, accompanied pseudopod development. New potential changes were noted only if the blunted electrode containing the chemotactic factor was removed and then reintroduced, thus establishing a new gradient of chemotactic factor. Repeated stimulation of cells with a chemotactic factor resulted in desensitization of the response. Desensitization may be the electrical correlate of deactivation of chemotactic responsiveness of cells to chemotactic stimuli when they are pretreated with chemotactic factors (49).

Although the electrophysiological data are compatible with the concept that potential changes are related to pseudopod formation and locomotion, the potential changes may also be related to enzyme secretion stimulated by chemotactic factors when leukocytes are adherent to a substratum (4,45). In this regard, it is important to emphasize that the functions of locomotion and secretion may be integrally related to the amount of ionized calcium in the cell. We have

---

[2] The membrane potential at which the response disappears because no net current flows through the membrane.

recently provided evidence that the process of leukocyte enzyme secretion is related to termination of locomotion, and these two processes are dependently modulated by calcium but independently influenced by cyclic nucleotides (26). Additional studies are needed to understand how chemotactic factors interact with the cell membrane to initiate ion fluxes, activate enzymes (2), and initiate other intracellular processes involved in locomotion and enzyme secretion.

HYPOTHETICAL MODEL OF IONIC CONTROL OF LEUKOCYTE ORIENTATION DURING CHEMOTAXIS

We propose a model (Fig. 9) for the ionic control of neutrophil orientation during chemotaxis which is based on our data (15,16,24) as well as others (7,11,30,36,52). Chemotactic factor interaction with the leukocyte membrane results in an influx of calcium and possibly sodium ions, producing a membrane depolarization which may trigger the release of additional calcium from intracellular stores. An increase in ionized calcium may be important for microfilament function. Deposition of calcium (or sodium) on the cytoplasmic side of the plasma membrane could account for the local antimonate deposition (Fig. 3) and decreases in surface charge, we have observed (20). If occurring locally, these membrane changes may facilitate cell deformability (32) as well as adherence and particle ingestion (37).

Increased intracellular ionized calcium would increase the permeability of the cytoplasmic membrane to potassium, producing the observed membrane hyperpolarization in addition to possibly activating secretion. A potassium efflux coupled with an efflux of water would cause local cell contraction which may be involved in the orientation process. In support of this are reports that chemotactic factors induce contraction in cytochalasin B-treated rabbit neutrophils

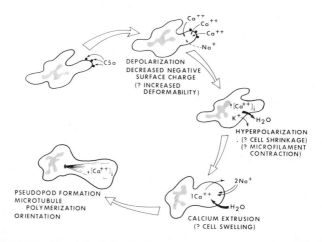

FIG. 9. Hypothetical model of ionic events occurring during neutrophil orientation in response to a gradient of chemotactic factor.

(30) and that A23187, which also causes a large membrane hyperpolarization in macrophages (15), causes potassium efflux and contraction of erythrocytes (13). As a consequence of the increase in intracellular calcium, cell recovery must involve the sequestration of calcium intracellularly and/or the extrusion of calcium from the cell. The increased antimonate deposition in the cytoplasmic ground substance noted in Fig. 4B in neutrophils exposed to a gradient of endotoxin-activated serum may represent intracellular calcium sequestration. Chemotactic factors also induce calcium release from both neutrophils (24) and mononuclear cells (26), which is sustained throughout 30 min. A sodium-calcium exchange, which has been demonstrated in a number of cells (7), may contribute to a decrease in intracellular ionized calcium. In this regard, it is of interest that Naccache et al. have reported increased sodium uptake by neutrophils incubated with chemotactic factors (36). An electroneutral exchange of sodium and calcium (2 Na^+ and 1 Ca^{++}) would result in water movement into the cell, although the resulting volume expansion would be small. Evidence exists for chemotactic factor-induced volume expansion in rabbit neutrophils (30). Decreases in intracellular calcium would provide an environment favorable to microtubule assembly (14,36,44,51). A sodium-potassium pump, such as described by Dr. Becker (Chap. 10) would contribute to recovery. If these events occurred at the leading end of the cell, orientation would then ensue.

SUMMARY

The mechanism of orientation of human leukocytes during directed locomotion or chemotaxis was studied. Ultrastructural analysis of leukocytes oriented on a 0.45-μm micropore filter during conditions of chemotaxis revealed highly organized orientation of the nucleus, centriole, and its radial array of microtubules and microfilaments. The centrioles and their radial array of microtubules orient between the nuclei and psuedopods, while microfilament assembly is localized to advancing psuedopods. The chemical probes cytochalasin B and colchicine, utilized to assess the importance of the microfilament and microtubule systems during locomotion and direction-finding, demonstrated that orientation and direction finding are stabilized by microtubule function. The microfilaments are essential for locomotion. In related studies designed to examine the role of cations in the orientation process, the pyroantimonate fixation technique provided evidence that submembranous cations localize at the leading edge of the cell during chemotaxis. Thus, neutrophil orientation during chemotaxis includes orientation of the nucleus, centriole, microtubules, microfilaments, and submembranous cations as well.

Clinically, neutrophils were studied from two patients with recurrent infections, abnormal chemotaxis, and defective cell orientation. Neutrophils from the first patient, with a Chediak-Higashi syndrome, had minimally decreased microtubule assembly. The second patient's neutrophils had markedly increased microtubule assembly and elevated cGMP. The leukocytes from both these patients provide pathological models in support of the concept that normal microtubule function is critical for directed migration. In addition, the morphological studies in these patients emphasize that in selected patients analysis of cell orientation and ultrastructure is necessary to define the basis of the chemotactic defect.

Ionic events occurring during leukcoyte activation by chemotactic factors were also investigated using electrophysiological methods to study the interaction of chemotactic factors with human macrophages. The results obtained revealed a rapid, brief depolarization, followed by a more prolonged hyperpolarization, in the majority of cells exposed to chemotactic factors. Chemotactic factor-induced membrane potential changes preceded pseudopod formation, during which time the transmembrane potential usually returned to prestimulation values. These studies, together with previous experiments using isotope tracers, provide the basis for a hypothetical model of ionic control of cell orientation during chemotaxis.

REFERENCES

1. Allison, A. C. (1974): Mechanism of movement and maintenance of polarity in leukocytes. In: *Chemotaxis: Its Biology and Biochemistry, Antibiotics and Chemotherapy,* Vol. 19, edited by E. Sorkin, pp. 191–217, S. Karger, Basel.
2. Becker, E. L. (1972): The relationship of the chemotactic behavior of the complement derived factors C3a, C5a, and C567, and a bacterial chemotactic factor to their ability to activate the proesterase 1 of rabbit polymorphonuclear leukocytes. *J. Exp. Med.,* 135:376–387.
3. Becker, E. L., Davis, A. T., Estensen, R. D., and Quie, D. G. (1972): Cytochalasin B: IV. Inhibition and stimulation of chemotaxis of rabbit and human polymorphonuclear leukocytes. *J. Immunol.,* 108:396–402.
4. Becker, E. L., Henson, P. M., Showell, H. J., and Hsu, L. S. (1974): The ability of chemotactic factors to induce lysosomal enzyme release: I. The characteristics of the release, the importance of surfaces and the relation of the enzyme release to chemotactic responsiveness. *J. Immunol.,* 112:2047–2054.
5. Becker, E. L., and Showell, H. J. (1972): The effect of Ca^{2+} and Mg^{2+} on the chemotactic responsiveness and spontaneous motility of rabbit polymorphonuclear leukocytes. *Z. Immunitaetsforsch.,* 143:466–476.
6. Bianco, C., Eden, A., and Cohn, Z. A. (1976): The induction of macrophage spreading: Role of coagulation factors and the complement system. *J. Exp. Med.,* 144:1531–1544.
7. Blaustein, M. (1974): The interrelationship between sodium and calcium fluxes across cell membrane. *Rev. Physiol. Biochem. Pharmacol.,* 70:34–82.
8. Boucek, M. M., and Snyderman, R. (1976): Calcium influx requirement for human neutrophil chemotaxis: Inhibition by lanthanum chloride. *Science,* 194:905–907.
9. Caner, J. E. Z. (1965): Colchicine inhibition of chemotaxis. *Arthritis Rheum.,* 8:757–764.
10. Clark, R. A., and Kimball, H. R. (1971): Defective granulocyte chemotaxis in the Chediak-Higashi syndrome. *J. Clin. Invest.,* 50:2645–2652.
11. Coza, E. P., Wright, T. E., and Becker, E. L. (1975): Lysosomal enzyme secretion and volume contraction induced in neutrophils by cytochalasin B, chemotactic factor and A23187. *Proc. Soc. Exp. Biol., Med.,* 149:476–479.
12. Edelson, P. J., and Fudenberg, H. F. (1973): Effect of vinblastine on the chemotactic responsiveness of normal human neutrophils. *Infect. Immun.,* 8:127–129.
13. Edmondson, E., and Li, Ting-Kai (1976): Effects of the ionophore A23187 on erythrocytes: Relationship of ATP, 2, 3 diphosphoglycerate to calcium binding capacity. *Biochem. Biophys. Acta,* 443:106–113.
14. Fuller, G. M., Ellison, J. J., McGill, M., Sordahl, L. A., and Brinkley, B. R. (1975): Studies on the inhibitory role of calcium in the regulation of microtubule assembly *in vitro* and *in*

vivo. In: *Microtubules and Microtubule Inhibitors,* edited by M. Borgers and M. De Brabander, pp. 379–392. North-Holland Publishing Co., Amsterdam.

15. Gallin, E. K., and Gallin, J. I. (1977): Interaction of chemotactic factors with human macrophages: Induction of transmembrane potential charges. *J. Cell Biol.,* 75 *(in press).*
16. Gallin, E. K., Wiederhold, M. L., Lipsky, P. E., and Rosenthal, A. S. (1975): Spontaneous and induced membrane hyperpolarizations in macrophages. *J. Cell Physiol.,* 86:653–661.
17. Gallin, J. I. (1975): Abnormal chemotaxis: Cellular and humoral components. In: *The Phagocytic Cell in Host Resistance,* edited by J. A. Bellanti and D. H. Dayton, pp. 227–248. Raven Press, New York.
18. Gallin, J. I., Clark, R. A., and Frank, M. M. (1975): Kinetic analysis of chemotactic factor generation in human serum via activation of the classical and alternate complement pathways. *Clin. Immunol. Immunopathol.,* 3:334–346.
19. Gallin, J. I., Clark, R. A., and Kimball, H. R. (1973): Granulocyte chemotaxis: An improved *in vitro* assay employing ^{51}Cr-labeled granulocytes. *J. Immunol.,* 110:233–240.
20. Gallin, J. I., Durocher, J. R., and Kaplan, A. P. (1975): Interaction of leukocyte chemotactic factors with the cell surface: I. Chemotactic factor-induced changes in human granulocyte surface charge. *J. Clin. Invest.,* 55:967–974.
21. Gallin, J. I., and Kaplan, A. P. (1974): Mononuclear cell chemotactic activity of kallikrein and plasminogen activator and its inhibition by C1 inhibitor and α2-macroglobulin. *J. Immunol.,* 1928–1934.
22. Gallin, J. I., Klimerman, J. A., Padgett, G. A., and Wolff, S. M. (1975): Defective mononuclear leukocyte chemotaxis in the Chediak-Higashi syndrome of humans, mink, and cattle. *Blood,* 45:863–870.
23. Gallin, J. I., Malech, H. L., Wright, D. G., Whisnant, J., and Kirkpatrick, C. H. (1977): Leukocyte dysfunction associated with increased microtubule assembly and elevated leukocyte cGMP. *Clin. Res.* 25:358A.
24. Gallin, J. I., and Rosenthal, A. S. (1974): The regulatory role of divalent cations in human granulocyte chemotaxis: Evidence for an association between calcium exchanges and microtubule assembly. *J. Cell Biol.,* 62:594–609.
25. Gallin, J. I., and Wolff, S. M. (1975): Leukocyte chemotaxis: Physiological considerations and abnormalities. *Clin. Haematol.,* 4:567–607.
26. Gallin, J. I., Sandler, J. A., Wright, D. G., and Manganiello, V. A. (1976): Calcium ionophore A23187 increases leukocyte Ca^{++} exchanges, inhibits chemotaxis, mobilizes neutrophil specific granules and increases cAMP. *Fed. Proc.,* 35:1580A.
27. Goldstein, I. M., Hoffstein, S., Gallin, J., and Weissmann, G. (1973): Mechanisms of lysosomal enzyme release from human leukocytes: Microtubule assembly and membrane fusion induced by a component of complement. *Proc. Natl. Acad. Sci. USA,* 70:2916–2920.
28. Gordon, S., and Cohn, Z. A. (1973): The macrophage. *Int. Rev. Cytol.,* 36:171–214.
29. Hardin, J. H., Spicer, S. S., and Greene, W. B. (1969): Ultrastructural localization of antimonate deposits in rabbit heterophil and human neutrophil leukocytes. *Lab. Invest.,* 21:214–224.
30. Hsu, L. S., and Becker, E. L. (1975): Volume changes induced in rabbit polymorphonuclear leukocytes by chemotactic factor and cytochalasin B. *Am. J. Pathol.,* 81:1–14.
31. Legato, M. J., and Langer, G. A. (1969): The subcellular localization of calcium ion in mammalian myocardium. *J. Cell Biol.,* 41:401.
32. Lichtman, M. A., and Weed, R. I. (1970): Electrophoretic mobility and *N*-acetyl neuraminic acid content of human normal and leukemic lymphocytes and granulocytes. *Blood,* 35:12–22.
33. Malech, H. L., and Gallin, J. I. (1977): Structural analysis of human neutrophil migration: centriole, microtubule, and microfilament orientation and function during chemotaxis. *J. Cell Biol.,* 75 *(in press).*
34. Malech, H. L., Root, R. K., and Gallin, J. I. (1976): Centriole, microtubule and microfilament orientation during human polymorphonuclear leukocyte chemotaxis. *Clin. Res.,* 24:314A. Abstract.
35. Mellon, M. G., and Rebhun, L. I. (1976): Sulfhydryls and the *in vitro* polymerization of tubulin. *J. Cell Biol.,* 70:226–238.
36. Nacchache, P., Freer, R. J., Showell, H. J., Becker, E. L., and Sha'afi, R. I. (1977): Transport of sodium, potassium, and calcium across rabbit polymorphonuclear leukocyte membranes: Effect of chemotactic factor. *J. Cell Biol.,* 73:428–444.
37. Nagura, H., Asai, J., Katsumata, Y., and Kojima, K. (1973): Role of electric surface charge of cell membrane in phagocytosis. *Acta Pathol. Jap.,* 23:279–290.

38. Oliver, J. M. (1976): Impaired microtubule assembly correctable by cyclic GMP and cholinergic agonists in the Chediak-Higashi syndrome. *Am. J. Pathol.,* 85:395–412.
39. Phelps, P. (1969): Polymorphonuclear leukocyte motility *in vitro:* IV. Colchicine inhibition of the formation of chemotactic activity after phagocytosis of urate crystals. *Arthritis Rheum.,* 13:1–9.
40. Ramsey, W. S. (1972): Analysis of individual leukocyte behavior during chemotaxis. *Exp. Cell Res.,* 70:120–139.
41. Ramsey, W. S. (1974): Leukocyte locomotion and chemotaxis. In: *Chemotaxis Its Biology and Biochemistry, Vol. 19, Antibiotics and Chemotherapy,* edited by E. Sorkin, pp. 179–180. S. Karger, Basel.
42. Ramsey, W. S. (1972): Locomotion of human polymorphonuclear leukocytes. *Exp. Cell Res.,* 72:489.
43. Sandler, J. A., Gallin, J. I., and Vaughan, M. (1975): Effects of serotonin, carbamylcholine and ascorbic acid on leukocyte cGMP and chemotaxis. *J. Cell Biol.,* 67:480–484.
44. Schliwa, M. (1976): The role of divalent cations in the regulation of microtubule assembly: *In vivo* studies on microtubules of the *Heliozoan axopodium* using the ionophore A23187. *J. Cell Biol.,* 70:527–540.
45. Showell, H. J., Freer, R. J., Zigmond, S. H., Schiffmann, S., Aswandumar, S., Corcoran, B., and Becker, E. L. (1976): The structure activity relations of synthetic peptides as chemotactic factors and inducers of lysosomal enzyme secretion for neutrophils. *J. Exp. Med.,* 143:1154–1169.
46. Simson, J. A. Z., and Spicer, E. S. (1975): Selective subcellular localization of cations with variants of the potassium (pyro) antimonate technique. *J. Histochem. Cytochem.,* 23:575–598.
47. Tomnick, H. (1962): Elektronenmikronzophische localization von Na^+ and Cl^- in Zellen und Gewebun. *Protoplasma,* 55:414–418.
48. Unanue, E. R. (1972): The regulatory role of macrophages in antigenic stimulation. *Adv. Immunol.,* 15:95–165.
49. Ward, P. A., and Becker, E. L. (1968): The deactivation of rabbit neutrophils by chemotactic factor and the nature of the activatable esterase. *J. Exp. Med.,* 127:693–709.
50. Weary, P. E., and Bender, A. S. (1967): Chediak-Higashi syndrome with severe cutaneous involvement. *Arch. Intern. Med.,* 119:381–386.
51. Weisenberg, R. C. (1972): Microtubule formation *in vitro* in solutions containing low calcium concentrations. *Science,* 177:1104–1105.
52. Wilkinson, P. C. (1975): Leukocyte locomotion and chemotaxis: The influence of divalent cations and cation ionophores. *Exp. Cell Res.,* 93:420–426.
53. Zigmond, S. H., and Hirsch, J. G. (1972): Cytochalasin B: Inhibiton of D-2-deoxyglycose transport into leukocytes and fibroblasts. *Science,* 177:1432–1434.
54. Zurier, R. B., Weissmann, G., Hoffstein, S., Kammerman, S., and Tai, H. H. (1974): Mechanisms of lysosomal enzyme release from human leukcoytes: II. Effects of cAMP and cGMP, autosomal antagonists, and agents which affect microtubule function. *J. Clin. Invest.,* 53:297–309.

DISCUSSION

Dr. Jensen: The sequence of events is reminiscent of smooth-muscle contractions caused by C5a in organ baths: There is a short lag period before the contraction, and a very definite tachyphylaxis afterward; then there is recovery after an hour or so. One question that comes to mind is can you overcome the nonresponsiveness (tachyphylaxis) to this high dosage of C5a?

Dr. Gallin: We have not done that specific experiment; however, in most cells, we have shown that the ability of one chemotactic factor to desensitize the electrical events cross-reacts with another chemotactic factor. For example, kallikrein, as well as the peptide fMet-Leu-Phe, which Elliott Schiffmann gave us, will each induce membrane potential changes and cross-desensitize each other.

Dr. Wilkinson: I very much like the ideas you put forth; however, I find it difficult to believe that the effect of colchicine is actually on the orientation of the cell. We see quite clearly orientation toward a gradient source in individual cells treated with colchicine, and we have seen the same thing in cells that are just sitting still and not translocating. To my mind, the effects of colchicine are on the arrangement of cytoplasmic structure and on the turning behavior of the cell, but not on its ability to polarize during movement.

Dr. Gallin: I don't think we really disagree. I am talking about the effect of colchicine on orientation of intracellular structure or cytoplasm. Our pictures show that colchicine clearly disorganizes intracellular orientation. Colchicine-treated cells lose some direction-finding or turning behavior as you have noted; however, some direction-finding persists presumably from oriented microfilament function.

Dr. Wilkinson: We have film of colchicine-treated cells, and there is a leading-edge on colchicine-treated cells. Even on cells showing abnormally wide angles of turn as they move toward Candida, the front can be distinguished from the back.

Dr. Gallin: If you looked at nuclear orientation, I am sure it would not be in its proper location. We believe that the microtubule system maintains proper cytoplasmic orientation and stability during locomotion.

Dr. Wilkinson: Yes. I am sure you are right, there.

Dr. Schiffmann: Would it make any sense to do water flux studies with deuterium oxide?

Dr. Gallin: Yes, we thought of doing that and we have also thought of using ^{14}C inulin and urea. We are going to perform these experiments.

Dr. Turner: Dr. Zigmond spoke of a leukocyte that polarized in an isotropic field of attractant. Does your model agree with this?

Dr. Gallin: What we propose is that the cells are polarized during random locomotion, whether it be spontaneous or stimulated. The difference between chemotaxis and random locomotion is the responsiveness of the population of cells or a given cell to its environmental stimulus. The orientation of a cell about its internal structure involves the same intracellular machinery for random or directed locomotion.

Dr. Wilkinson: Yes, that would be consistent with the persistent random-walk type of locomotion that our laboratory has shown.

Leukocyte Chemotaxis, edited by John I. Gallin and Paul G. Quie. Raven Press, New York © 1978.

The Mechanism of Leukocyte Locomotion

Thomas P. Stossel

Medical Oncology Unit, Massachusetts General Hospital, Boston, Massachusetts 02114; and Department of Medicine, Harvard Medical School, Boston, Massachusetts 02115

To explain leukocyte locomotion, the process must be broken down into its components. Venerable and repetitive descriptions of leukocyte locomotion over the years have led to a picture of these components (8,20,23,33,36). Even older and more abundant descriptions of the movement of cultivated mammalian cells and of the prototype wandering cells, the amoebas, are appropriate to add to this picture because of the similarities in the morphology of locomotion between most eukaryotic cells (1,5,27,32,38). The major features are:

(a) *Reversible adhesion.* The cells crawl; they do not swim. Therefore, adhesion to the substrate is essential for locomotion. This adhesion must be reversible, since excessive adhesion to the substrate, when focal, can alter the pattern of movement, and, when global, it can impede net movement.

(b) *Spreading.* Pseudopodia are the hallmarks of locomotion and include anterior blebbed and undulating tongues called *lamellipodia* and stubbier posterior pseudopodia called *uropods* or tails. The tails may or may not have arachnoid filopodia or retraction fibers associated with them. The features these diverse appendages have in common besides their picturesque names are:

(i) They are hyaline, i.e., organelle-excluding when seen in the phase contrast microscope.

(ii) They are evanescent.

(c) *Polarity.* Added to the asymmetry of pseudopod morphology during locomotion is the generally fusiform configuration of the cell body, parallel to the plane of movement.

(d) *Movement.* By direct observation alone, done usually from above but occasionally from the side, it is difficult to discern the wheels, treads, or paddles that yield movement. The amoebas classically studied, *Amoeba proteus* and *Chaos chaos,* feature rather sharp demarcations between hyaline ectoplasm and the endoplasm that streams anteriorly during locomotion. The streaming of endoplasm and the apparent gel-like consistency of ectoplasm in these creatures permit imaginative investigators to concoct mechanisms to explain cell translocation. On the other hand, another amoeba, *Hyalodiscus simplex,* although oriented as described above, reveals no streaming of endoplasm. Leukocytes locomote in a fashion between these extremes. They occasionally demonstrate endoplasmic flow from tail to cell anterior, especially where the tail has been stretched by what appears to be firm attachment to the substrate and either abruptly releases or is actually broken off. This pattern of locomotion is common in cultured fibroblasts, which seem to get more involved with the substrate than leukocytes; however, leukocytes can locomote with no apparent endoplasmic movement, save for a very characteristic scintillating vibration of cytoplasmic granules, which occurs just posterior to the lamellipod.

SPREADING AND ADHESION

Phenomena

Most cells cultivated *in vitro* on appropriate substrates stick and spread. Cells may stick to raw surfaces, e.g., glass, in salt solutions, but under the usual experimental conditions they adhere to and spread on surfaces that have first interacted with proteins, generally serum proteins. The physical forces that theoretically mediate adhesion have been much discussed over the years, but the chemistry and stereology that confer these forces to either cell or substrate remain elusive (16,26,27,56,60). At some level, adhesion involves the passive interaction of mutually active surfaces, but evidence points to adhesion and spreading as active events initiated by surface contact. Therefore, adhesion and spreading, like phagocytosis, are examples of cell surface-to-cytoplasm communication and activation. The receptors and signals for the activation are obscure, but the effector mechanism can be ascribed to the popular notion of activated "subplasmalemmal structural elements."

Figure 1 shows a coronal section of a human blood cell spread on glass in the presence of serum. The peripheral zone of organelle exclusion is largest at the leading edges of the presumptively spreading pseudopodia, as can be seen in numerous detailed renditions of the morphology of spread leukocytes and other cells seen with the electron microscope (12,13,25). The generic similarity

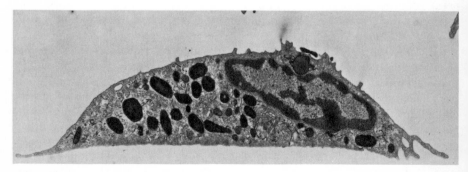

FIG. 1. Thin-section electron micrograph of a human eosinophil attached and spreading on a glass coverslip. Note the layer of organelle exclusion at the cell base and in the lateral pseudopodia. X13,000.

between the morphology of spreading and that of phagocytosis is that the area of organelle exclusion is also greatest in the tips of the advancing pseudopodia, which spread around a curved particle rather than on a flat surface. The comparison between spreading and phagocytosis is also not new (42).

The regions of organelle exclusion are composed of a rather nondescript amorphous matrix now well known to represent a randomly oriented collection of microfilaments. The microfilament lattice is a meshwork of actin filaments and associated contractile proteins. The evidence for this conclusion is compiled in innumerable current reviews of the burgeoning field of contractile proteins of nonmuscle cells (24,45,59). A "contractile" basis for leukocyte locomotion was first suggested by Lewis in 1939 (34). The report by Senda and co-workers concerning the isolation and definition of crude "contractile proteins" of horse leukocytes represented the first serious attempt to test this appealing idea in a meaningful way (47). Subsequent work by others on blood cells and other cell types permits construction of some working hypotheses to explain the mechanism of cell-spreading.

Contractile Protein Interactions in Blood Cells

The principal contractile protein of neutrophils and other blood cells studied in detail (which include human neutrophils, horse leukocytes, human chronic myelogenous leukemic granulocytes, and rabbit pulmonary macrophages; see Table 1) is actin (9,11,20,54). Actin extracted in cold buffers low in salt concentra-

TABLE 1. *Contractile proteins isolated from leukocytes*

Proteins	Properties	Cell types	Reference
Actomyosin	Enzymatic and rheologic properties suggestive of actomyosin complexes; filaments seen resembling muscle actin and myosin	Horse leukocytes	(47)
Myosin	Subunit composition and enzymatic activity resembling muscle myosin; formed bipolar filaments	Guinea pig neutrophils Horse leukocytes Rabbit lung macrophages Human leukemic granulocytes	(48) (54) (51) (11)
Actin	Subunit composition, myosin-activating, and assembly properties similar to muscle actin	Horse leukocytes Rabbit lung macrophages Human neutrophils Human leukemic granulocytes	(54) (30) (9) (11)
Cofactor	Required for activation of macrophage actomyosin Mg^{2+}-ATPase and contraction	Rabbit lung macrophages	(51) (52)
Actin-binding protein	Crosslinks actin filaments	Rabbit lung macrophages Human leukemic granulocytes	(30) (11)

tion from leukocytes may be largely depolymerized or monomeric G-actin (11,30); however, the actins, insofar as hitherto characterized, do not differ from skeletal muscle actin in any important structural or functional properties. Therefore, if actin monomer : filament interconversion occurs in these cells as a basis for gel-sol transformations, as has been speculated, it must be the consequence of factors other than the actin itself. Most evidence indicates that cytoplasmic actin would be polymerized (F-actin) in the presence of likely intracellular ions and metabolites.

Blood leukocytes and other nonmuscle cells have much higher ratios of actin to other contractile proteins, e.g., myosin, than the ratio in muscle. This fact plus the randomness of the actin filament arrangement in pseudopodia indicate that the performance of these proteins differs in that setting from their actions in muscle. One picture that has emerged is that a high-molecular-weight actin-binding protein (11,30,51,52) [and possibly other proteins or fragments of this protein (37)] reversibly stabilize actin filaments into a gel lattice. Reversible crosslinking of F-actin causes sol-gel transformations without any marked change in the polymerization state of the actin. Actin-binding protein has been localized by immunochemical techniques to the cell periphery of human neutrophils, inferentially suggesting an association with the plasma membrane (10). Phagocytosis alters the extractability of actin-binding protein from membranes of macrophages (52), a finding consistent with the idea that the prominence of hyalin in the pseudopodia is the result of increased gelation of actin by actin-binding protein "activated" somehow by phagocytosis. Gels composed of purified actin filaments plus actin-binding protein resemble the microfilament feltwork of phagocytizing (and spreading) leukocytes (11,30,51,52).

Myosin, the energy-transducing protein of skeletal muscle, is present and enzymatically and mechanically active in neutrophils and macrophages (11, 30,48,51,52,54), as well as in various other cells (24,45,59). Myosin molecules are distributed throughout the cytoplasm of leukocytes (22), but some recent evidence suggests that this protein may be concentrated near or on the plasma membrane (Jantzen, Hartwig, and Stossel, *unpublished data*). Purified myosin in the presence of $Mg^{++}ATP$ contracts gels of purified actin plus actin-binding protein. Such motile systems have been reconstituted from purified protein of granulocytes and macrophages (11,52).

The exact effect of actin gelation of movement is difficult to determine. On the one hand, cross-linkage of actin filaments could increase the efficiency of myosin contraction, a single actomyosin complex being able to move many actin filaments. This amplification idea is attractive, given the low myosin : actin ratios of nonmuscle cells. On the other hand, gelation might actually impede volume contraction of an actin meshwork by myosin if the gel were sufficiently rigid. Both increased and decreased movement of actin may obtain in different regions of the putative cortical gel. From the foregoing, it is apparent that the gel state of actin (and, indirectly, actin-binding protein) could control movement. Scholars of muscle, however, look for other factors that control the interaction between actin and myosin, in particular for factors that render calcium the ultimate regulator of this interaction. Thus far, no work has convincingly established that such calcium control of actin-myosin interaction obtains in leukocytes, fibroblasts, or amoebas (24). Hence the effect of calcium on locomotion or whether calcium moves in or out of the cell in response to chemotactic factors cannot be interpreted. Protein cofactors and phosphorylation reactions appear to be relevant for the activity of nonmuscle actomyosins (3,44,52), but this knowledge is not yet readily translatable into an explanation for the activation of contraction in living cells.

In any case, the sketchy information available can be synthesized to claim that cell surface contact somehow activates actin-binding protein and myosin located on the cytoplasmic face of the plasmalemma. The activation causes these proteins to engage, gel, and contract subplasmalemmal actin filaments. The tension on the gel, parallel to and now attached via myosin, actin-binding protein and possibly other proteins to the plasmalemma, causes the membrane to (a) pucker and (b) establish additional contact points with the substrate.[1] The membrane, now firmly adherent to the substrate, is moved centrifugally by the action of the contractile protein gel.[2]

Contractile Protein Translocation in Cell Spreading

If one accepts that surface contact activates the contractile proteins by a mysterious process and that actin-binding protein and/or myosin are the primary targets of this activation, it is still necessary to explain how this activation propagates itself sequentially with spreading. Two alternatives seem most likely (Fig. 2). The activating proteins could be randomly and continuously distributed in fixed positions around the membrane. In response to contact, they would become turned on and subsequently be switched off by metabolic or other means. The signal to turn "on" would be strongest at the advancing pseudopod tips, and the "off" setting most pronounced in the middle of the attached surface where cytoplasmic granule secretion could occur. The second alternative is that the activator proteins are mobile and themselves move into the pseudopod tips in response to the activating signals. Wherever actin-binding protein and myosin are most concentrated along the membrane would be the region of most intense gelation and contraction. Recent experiments designed to decide the question resulted in favor of the second mechanism. Macrophages spread on nylon wool

---

[1] It may be that filopodia first must engage the substrate (4,25). These excrescences might provide the source of force vectors that actually bring more membrane in contact with the substrate rather than simply puckering the cells at that site.

[2] From morphology alone, one could argue that the spreading pseudopod is not "contraction" at all but rather "relaxation," that cytoplasm in the periphery is less gel than sol, and that the cell spreads like a broken egg in a pan under the influence of gravity. As described below, there is evidence that pseudopodia are more "gel" than "sol." Furthermore, flat pseudopodia form when cells contact surface *above* them, i.e., against the force of gravity.

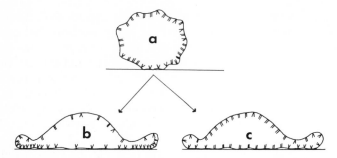

FIG. 2. Alternative mechanisms to explain prominence of filaments in advancing pseudopodia of spreading cells. **(a)** Cell initiating contact with substrate. Contractile activation proteins, e.g., myosin, in resting (‖) or activated (v) state randomly distributed about membrane. With spreading, these proteins could **(b)** become activated and move into pseudopodia, or **(c)** remain fixed but become activated and remain activated only in advancing pseudopodia tips, becoming inactivated elsewhere.

fibers and when removed by shear, yield peripheral pseudopodia in the form of filament-filled plasmalemma-bounded sacs, or "podosomes" (19) and residual cell bodies. Extracts of the cell bodies have markedly reduced concentration of actin-binding protein and myosin, whereas these proteins are enriched in podosomes, indicating translocation (Table 2). Only a small quantity of actin flows from the cell body to the pseudopodia as determined by this approach (31). This result is not surprising, because actin is so richly concentrated in motile cells. For example, one can estimate that if all the actin of one pulmonary macrophage were polymerized into a single filament, that filament would be 60 mm long! Hence it is more reasonable to control the state of actin (gel vs viscous liquid) than to move it. The concept of contractile protein translocation is essential to the theory of locomotion to be introduced later in this chapter.

Impaired Spreading

If contractile proteins are relevant for spreading, inhibition of the functions of contractile proteins should deter spreading. Two examples corroborate this prediction.

1. *Neutrophil actin dysfunction.* Pseudopod spreading was abortive in the neutrophils of a human infant, and the extent of polymerization of the actin of these neutrophils was about 15% of that of normal neutrophil actin (24). Recent experiments show that the extent of actin polymerization in extracts of the neutrophils of this patient's parents is about 40 to 60% of normal, suggesting that the underlying defect is genetic and transmitted as an autosomal recessive trait. Furthermore, the impaired polymerization cannot be ascribed to the presence of an inhibitor or to excessive proteolysis. The findings do not prove that actin polymerization must occur during spreading, but they do show that its failure impedes spreading.

TABLE 2. Effect of macrophage spreading on the distribution and functions of contractile protein

	Distribution					
	Actin-binding protein[c]		Myosin		Actin	
	Cell body extract[d]	Podosomes[e]	Cell body extract	Podosomes	Cell body extract	Podosomes
Control[a]	117 ± 20	6 ± 1	332 ± 39	19 ± 3	3,820 ± 97	117 ± 10
Spread[b]	39 ± 4	33 ± 3	118 ± 20	113 ± 13	3,080 ± 136	600 ± 53

	Function			
	Gelation and aggregation of sucrose extracts			
	Visual	Protein sedimented[f] (%)	Viscosity (dL/G)	Protein sedimented[g] (%)
Control[a]	4+gel	17.2 ± 0.2	1.0 ± 0.2	30.0 ± 0.2
Spread[b]	± gel	7.5 ± 2.0	0.6 ± 0.3	25.7 ± 3.3

[a]Rabbit pulmonary macrophages incubated in suspension for 5 min at 37°C.
[b]Macrophages incubated for 5 min at 37°C with nylon wool fibers.
[c]Total amount of indicated protein in each fraction in μg. The values are derived from total protein (Folin) determinations and quantitative densitometry of sodium anazotene (Coomassie Blue®) stained polyacrylamide gels after electrophoresis of fractions in sodium dodecyl sulfate. All values are means ±SD ≥3 experiments.
[d]Particle-free sucrose extract of cells.
[e]Hyaline blebs removed from all cells by mechanical agitation (used to shear spread cells from Nylon wool).
[f]Percent of total protein sedimented at $10^4 \times$ g, 10 min after warming macrophage extracts. A fibrous gel that forms in the warmed extract is sedimentable at low speed (29).
[g]Percent of total protein sedimented at $10^5 \times$ g, 60 min after warming cell extracts indicates the assembly (polymerization) of actin (29).

2. *Cytochalasin B.* This drug was long thought to inhibit cell motility by impairing microfilament function, but interpretation of its effects was complicated by (a) an action on membrane transport at concentrations lower than those affecting motility (62), (b) a variable influence of the drug on motility, i.e., it inhibited some movements but not others (61), and (c) the effects of cytochalasin B on purified contractile protein functions at concentrations that inhibited motility were unimpressive (49). Recently, some of these inconsistencies have been reconciled by the discovery that low concentrations of cytochalasin B dissolve gels of actin plus actin-binding protein (29) and crude cytoplasmic actin gels (58). These concentrations do not depolymerize actin filaments or interfere with actin-myosin interaction. These findings can explain why (a) cytochalasin B inhibits many cell movements including phagocytosis, spreading, and locomotion; (b) why microfilaments and some movements persist in cytochalasin B-treated cells; and (c) why morphologists inferred that cytochalasin B promoted changes interpreted as "hypercontraction" and filament aggregation in regions of drug-treated cells (40). Release of actin lattice rigidity permits exuberant focal aggregation by activated and unimpaired myosin. The motile functions altered by cytochalasin B, which include spreading, can be inferred to depend on actin gelation.

CELL ORIENTATION

Phenomena

As discussed above, spreading is not uniform during locomotion, which implies that the signals activating the actin-binding protein and/or myosin act asymmetrically. An important point is that polarization of individual cells occurs whether or not the investigator exogenously imposes a chemotactic factor. This fact suggests that either the activation system always has a fluctuating noise level of varying intensity around the cell or that activating factors always assault the cell surface from without. These factors could be medium molecules focally concentrated by convection or they could be substances released from other cells.

If binding of a chemotactic factor to surface receptors is the first step in activation of directed locomotion and the chemotactic factor is subsequently hydrolyzed (6), two possibilities follow, to permit the interaction to repeat itself with new molecules in the chemotactic gradient. The receptor could remain stationary while the chemotactic factor is hydrolyzed on the spot (see Chap. 9). Alternatively, the receptor-ligand complex could be internalized and subsequently replaced. Evidence to follow favors the second choice.

The similarity between the morphology of the "capped" lymphocyte and any locomoting cell is striking (33). It is agreed that the "uropod" of the capped lymphocyte represents the site of congregation of external surface molecules swept to that location during capping (21,35,55). There is some confusion as to the relationship between capping and locomotion,[3] but it is fair to say that while all capped cells need not locomote, cells probably must "cap" in order to locomote. Some work concerning neutrophil "capping" has shown that under appropriate conditions lectins of fluorescein bound to the cell surface collects in the cell's tail to be subsequently shed or endocytosed (43,46). It is logical to extend the effect of cap inducers to include chemotactic factors, which may also be perturbing surface receptor molecules. The precise correlation between chemoattractiveness and hydrolysis rates of different chemotactic factors is consistent with this idea (6). Capping, endocytosis, and hydrolysis of chemotactic factors provide a means for disposing of the cell's "memory" when a new gradient is encountered. Shedding of the capped factors accomplishes the same purpose.

Mechanism

What is the relationship between the "flow" of external molecules and the asymmetry of spreading? One simple explanation is that contractile proteins directly move the external molecules.[4] The external molecules are swept through the membrane posteriorly with clumps of gelled actin motored by myosin and the external ligands indirectly connected to the motor by membrane-spanning proteins. The colocalization of microfilaments with external surface molecules at capping sites is consistent with (but does not prove) this idea (Fig. 3). The collection of these contractile proteins at the tail promotes vigorous contraction, hence the narrowing of the tail. The direction of a surface gel movement is dictated by the site of initial membrane activation, possibly the major site of assault by a chemotactic factor. The gel material originates in and breaks off from the anterior lamellipod. Repletion of anterior actin gel could occur by one of the following: (a) *de novo* synthesis of contractile proteins; (b) recycling of the proteins, possibly by endoplasmic flow; or (c) both mechanisms. A choice among these alternatives cannot presently be made.

The density and continuity of actin gel in the periphery of the cell body is presumed to be less than in the pseudopodia, but nevertheless it is finite, so that some tension is developed. This tension plus uropod contraction is further

---

[3] This confusion arises from the rather diverse agents employed to induce or promote capping, some of which may affect locomotion by mechanisms unrelated to orientation and from the obscurity previously surrounding the molecular sites of action of cytochalasin B. Cytochalasin B always inhibits locomotion but does not always inhibit capping (55). As related above, not all contractile events related to cell movement need be impaired by this drug.

[4] Explanations for this movement based on "lipid flow" (14) and "protein flow" (28) suffer from failing to provide a biologically plausible motive force for the "flow." There seems to be agreement that metabolic energy is required for capping (57). Although not conclusive by any means, this fact favors a "contractile" (in the sense of myosin-transduced) rather than, say, a differential solubility mechanism (28). On the other hand, some of the movement of membrane molecules, e.g., "patching" may be independent of metabolic energy, and influenced principally by structural restraints or lack thereof in the membrane (21,35,55).

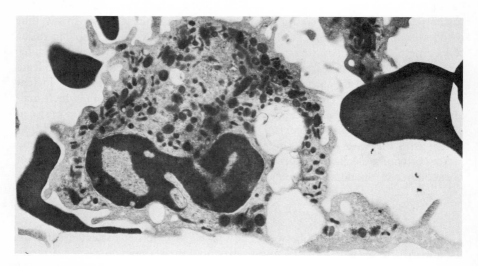

FIG. 3. Thin-section electron micrograph of a human neutrophil migrating on glass toward zymosan (on the right). Note the organelle excluding anterior lamellipod and cell base, and contiguity of granules with membrane folds in the anterior cell body. X13,000.

presumed to create the fusiform configuration of the cell body and maintain posterior → anterior endoplasmic flow that lines up other structural elements such as microtubules and intermediate filaments in the axis of locomotion.[5]

Membrane Turnover in Polarity Maintenance

If translocation and endocytosis of surface receptors were required for locomotion, the cell would rapidly deplete itself of receptors. The idea of membrane turnover has been frequently considered in theories of amoeboid (32) and fibroblast (2) movement, but has received little attention in the field of blood cell locomotion. The reason may be the common knowledge that neutrophils are "end" cells, and the evidence that inhibitors of RNA or protein synthesis do not impair phagocytosis (17). However, Carruthers reported in 1966 that high concentrations of puromycin and actinomycin D inhibited chemotaxis of neutrophils (15). Table 3 shows that cycloheximide inhibits chemotaxis [and the confirmation that the drug inhibits protein synthesis by leukocytes (41)]. Exogenous protein, either albumin or serum, has long been known to activate locomotion (see Chap. 1). Table 3 also shows that dialyzed serum promotes the incorporation

---

[5] Microtubules: hollow 125-nm fibers made up of the protein tubulin and associated proteins. Intermediate filaments: 100-nm wavy filaments of unknown composition in leukocytes, most prominent in the perinuclear region. The theory being propounded contradicts earlier ones, which suggested that the arrangement of these structures might be the cause rather than the result of cell orientation.

TABLE 3. *Effect of cycloheximide and serum protein on locomotion, phagocytosis, adherence, and ³H-leucine incorporation by human neutrophils*

	Locomotion	Adherence (mg protein)	Phagocytosis (μg/oil ingested/ 10^7 cells/min)	³H-Leucine incorporation (cpm/10^6 cells[e])
Control	9 ± 1^a	0.5 ± 0.1^c	85 ± 4^d	$2,218 \pm 206$
—serum	5 ± 1^a	0.4 ± 0.1	90 ± 3	990 ± 156
Control	15 ± 7^b	1.5 ± 0.8	90 ± 3	—
Cyclohex- imide (2 μg/ml)	2 ± 2^b	1.8 ± 0.4	96 ± 2	448 ± 56

[a]Distance (μ) of cell farthest after 45 min into 25-μ micropore filter of 3-μ pore size (63) in Krebs-Ringer phosphate medium with or without 10% human serum. All values are means ±SD.

[b]Cells hpf traversing 25-μ micropore filter of 3-μ pore size toward zymosan-activated human serum for 45 min.

[c]Cell protein adherent to glass coverslips after 45 min of incubating followed by rinsing with Krebs-Ringer phosphate medium.

[d]Initial rate of ingestion assayed for 5 min (18). Cells were preincubated with serum or cycloheximide for 45 min.

[e]Trichloroacetic acid-precipitable radioactivity of cells settled onto 0.45-μ size millipore filters and incubated with 8.3×10^4 cpm of ³H-leucine.

of ³H-leucine into protein by blood leukocytes. The addition of cycloheximide or the depletion of exogenous albumin or serum does not constitute nonspecific cytotoxic insults because neither of these maneuvers inhibits the initial rate of phagocytosis, another energy-dependent contractile protein-driven event. Cycloheximide does not impair leukocyte adhesion to a substrate (Table 3) nor its assumption of an oriented configuration. These findings can be interpreted to indicate that protein synthesis is essential for leukocyte locomotion, which differs from the requirements concerning phagocytosis. This divergence is not surprising, since the cell has enough membrane to sustain an initial burst of phagocytosis but then ceases to ingest, presumably because of membrane depletion (39,53). Extending this interpretation, the protein synthesis represents the rebuilding of membrane capped, shed, and interiorized during locomotion (Fig. 4).

The recognition of membrane turnover in neutrophil chemotaxis potentially brings to order the observation that chemotactic factors promote lysosomal enzyme release (7). Although this release could simply be a sloppy concomitant of endocytosis at the uropod ["regurgitation during the feeding" (64)], the fact that violent granule movement [resembling the movements associated with degranulation during phagocytosis (31)] occurs at the anterior of the cell body suggests that lysosomal fusion could be a vehicle for inspection of new membrane plus receptors.

A cycle of endocytosis and secretion, dependent upon constituents provided by serum or albumin, is reminiscent of the mechanism of membrane turnover emerging from studies of cultivated mouse macrophages (50). The integration of macromolecule synthesis and secretion into the mechanism of leukocyte loco-

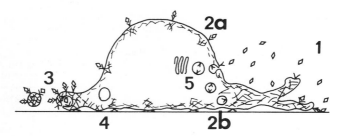

FIG. 4. Hypothetical mechanism of leukocyte locomotion. **1.** Chemotactic factors (◊) engage membrane receptors, activating contractile proteins (criss-crossed lines). Factors plus substrate maintain flat configuration of lamellipod. **2a.** Factors plus receptors on the free cell edge are moved to the tail with bits of contractile gel. **2b.** Substrate attachment sites are also moved tailward yielding movement of cell. **3.** Convergence of activated receptors at the tail promotes blebbing and endocytosis. **4.** Interiorized receptors plus factors are hydrolyzed. This hydrolysis activates synthesis of new receptors **5.**

motion obviously widens the scope for interpreting the action of diverse pharmocological agents which influence locomotion, particularly drugs affecting microtubules. Equally obvious is the demand to identify the molecules involved in the turnover process.

MOVEMENT

I have hitherto proffered explanations for movement of cytoplasm and movement of surface receptors, but have provided no explanation for movement of the cell. So much theory has gone into the explanations thus far that the synthesis of these hypotheses, required for an exegesis of locomotion, however vague, piles speculation upon speculation.

The posterior sweep of surface molecules will include molecules adherent to the substrate as well as those which have bound chemotactic factors (Fig. 4). In other words, the cell tries to "cap" the substrate. These substrate adherent molecules, linked to the contractile meshwork, will act like tank treads to propel the cell forward. For such propulsion to occur: (a) the adherent ligands must slither through the lipid bilayer of the membrane, and (b) counter torque must be provided to some other aspect of the cell. This torque could arise if units of moving contractile proteins at the base of the cell are attached to other proteins in the gel lattice which in turn are fixed, immobile, to membrane at the sides of the cell. Intermediate filaments and microtubules could be part of the stabilizing complex. The reversal of adhesion is accomplished in this scheme simply by having the cell ingest or bleb off the adhesive sites at the tail. The association between intensive endocytosis and blebbing is interesting, both possibly reflecting destabilization of membrane. This destabilization is the result of extensive actin gel contraction which frees patches of membrane from association with the cytoskeleton. It is inferred that this destabilized membrane then vesiculates, either outward (bleb) or inward (pinosome).

CONCLUSION

Whether any of the above "explanations" for the components of locomotion and for locomotion per se turns out to be correct remains to be seen. In any case, there are interesting biochemical and physiological data bearing on these points, sometimes more, sometimes less. A systematic dissection of what clinical states and drugs do to each of these components in addition to cataloging what these do to the overall rate of locomotion, and the systematic isolation and characterization of molecules involved in locomotion, will hasten the resolution of the mechanisms of leukocyte movement.

ACKNOWLEDGMENTS

Supported by a Grant HL 19429 from the U.S. Public Health Service and a grant from the Edwin S. Webster Foundation.

REFERENCES

1. Abercrombie, M., Heaysman, J. E. M., and Pegrum, S. M. (1970): The locomotion of fibroblasts in culture: II. "Ruffling." *Exp. Cell Res.,* 60:437–444.
2. Abercrombie, M., Heaysman, J. E. M., and Pegrum, S. M. (1970): The locomotion of fibroblasts in culture: III. Movements of particles on the dorsal surface of the leading lamella. *Exp. Cell Res.,* 62:389–398.
3. Adelstein, R. S., and Conti, M. A. (1975): Phosphorylation of platelet myosin increases actin-activated myosin ATPase activity. *Nature,* 256:597–598.
4. Albrecht-Bühler, G., and Lancaster, R. M. (1976): A quantitative description of the extension and retraction of surface protrusions in spreading 3T3 mouse fibroblasts. *J. Cell Biol.,* 71:370–382.
5. Allen, R. D., and Kamiya, N. (eds.), (1964): *Primitive Motile Systems in Cell Biology.* Academic Press, New York.
6. Aswanikumar, S., Schiffmann, E., Corcoran, B. A., and Wahl, S. M. (1976): Role of a peptidase in phagocyte chemotaxis. *Proc. Natl. Acad. Sci. U.S.A.,* 73:2439–2442.
7. Becker, E. L., Showell, M. J. (1974): The ability of chemotactic factors to induce lysosomal enzyme release: II. The mechanism of release. *J. Immunol.,* 112:2055–2062.
8. Bessis, M. (1973): *Living Blood Cells and Their Ultrastructure.* Transl. R. I. Weed. Springer Verlag, Berlin, Heidelberg, New York.
9. Boxer, L. A., Hedley-Whyte, E. T., Stossel, T. P. (1974): Neutrophil actin dysfunction and abnormal neutrophil behavior. *N. Engl. J. Med.* 291:1093–1099.
10. Boxer, L. A., Richardson, S., and Floyd, A. (1976): Identification of actin-binding protein in membrane of polymorphonuclear leukocytes. *Nature,* 263:259–261.
11. Boxer, L. A., and Stossel, T. P. (1976): Interactions of actin, myosin and an actin-binding protein of chronic myelogenous leukemia leukocytes. *J. Clin. Invest.,* 57:964–976.
12. Bragina, E. E., Vasilev, J. M., and Gelfand, I. M. (1976): Formation of bundles of microfilaments during spreading of fibroblasts on the substrate. *Exp. Cell Res.,* 97:241–248.
13. Breton-Gorius, J. (1968): Étude des leucocytes étalés par coupes sériées parallèles et perpendiculaires au plan d'étalement. *J. Microsc. (Oxf.),* 7:95–106.
14. Bretscher, M. S. (1976): Directed lipid flow in cell membranes. *Nature,* 260:21–22.
15. Carruthers, B. M. (1967): Leukocyte motility: II. Effect of absence of glucose in medium; effect of presence of deoxyglucose, dinitrophenol, puromycin, actinomycin D, and trypsin on the response to chemotactic substance; effect of segregation of cells from chemotactic substance. *Can. J. Physiol. Pharmacol.,* 45:269–280.
16. Chambers, R., and Fell, H. B. (1932): Microoperations on cells in tissue cultures. *Proc. R. Soc. Lond. [Biol.],* 149:380–402.

17. Cline, M. J. (1966): Phagocytosis and synthesis of ribonucleic acid in human granulocytes. *Nature,* 212:1431–1433.
18. Cox, J. M., and Stossel, T. P. (1976): Measurement of phagocytosis by macrophages. In: *In Vitro Methods in Cell-Mediated and Tumor Immunity,* edited by B. R. Bloom and J. R. David, pp. 363–368. Academic Press, New York.
19. Davies, W. A., and Stossel, T. P. (1977): Peripheral hyaline blebs ("Podosomes") of macrophages. *J. Cell Biol. (in press).*
20. DeBruyn, P. P. H. (1946): The amoeboid movement of the mammalian leukocyte in tissue culture. *Anat. Rec.,* 95:177–191.
21. Edidin, M., and Weiss, A. (1972): Antigen cap formation in cultured fibroblasts: A reflection of membrane fluidity and of cell motility. *Proc. Natl. Acad. Sci. U.S.A.* (1972): 69:2456–2459.
22. Fujiwara, K., and Pollard, T. D., (1976): Fluorescent antibody localization of myosin in the cytoplasm, cleavage furrow, and mitotic spindle of human cells. *J. Cell Biol.,* 71:848–875.
23. Fukushima, K., Senda, N., Ishigami, S., Murakami, Y., and Nishian, K. (1954): Dynamic pattern in the movement of leukocyte: II. The behavior of neutrophils immediately after commencement and removal of stimulation. *Med. J. Osaka Univ.,* 5:47–56.
24. Goldman, R., Pollard, T., and Rosenbaum, J. (eds.), (1976): *Cell Motility,* Cold Spring Harbor Conferences on Cell Proliferation, Vol. 3. Cold Spring Harbor, New York.
25. Grinnel, F., Tobleman, M. Q., and Hackenbrock, C. R. (1976): Initial attachment of baby hamster kidney cells to an epoxy substratum: Ultrastructural analysis. *J. Cell Biol.,* 70:707–713.
26. Harris, A. (1973): Location of cellular adhesions to solid substrata. *Dev. Biol.,* 35:97–114.
27. Harris, A. K. (1973): Cell surface movements related to cell locomotion. In: *Locomotion of Tissue Cells,* pp. 3–20. Ciba Foundation Symposium 14 (New Series). Elsevier, North Holland.
28. Harris, A. K. (1976): Recycling of dissolved plasma membrane components as an explanation of the capping phenomenon. *Nature,* 263:783–786.
29. Hartwig, J. H., and Stossel, T. P. (1976): Interactions of actin, myosin and an actin-binding protein of rabbit pulmonary macrophages: III. Effects of cytochalasin B. *J. Cell Biol.,* 71:295–303.
30. Hartwig, J. H., and Stossel, T. P. (1975): Isolation and properties of actin, myosin and a new actin-binding protein in rabbit alveolar macrophages. *J. Biol. Chem.,* 250:5699–5705.
31. Hartwig, J. H., Davies, W. A., and Stossel, T. P. (1977): Evidence for contractile protein translocation in macrophage spreading, phagocytosis, and phagolysosome formation. *J. Cell Biol. (in press).*
32. Kominick, H., Stockem, W., and Wohlfarth-Bottermann, K. E. (1973): Cell motility: Mechanisms in protoplasmic streaming and ameboid movement. *Int. Rev. Cytol.,,* 34:169–249.
33. Lewis, W. H. (1934): On the locomotion of the polymorphonuclear neutrophils of the rat in autoplasma cultures. *Bull. Johns. Hopkins Hosp.,* 55:273–279.
34. Lewis, W. H. (1939): The role of a superficial plasmagel layer in changes of form, locomotion and division of cells in tissue cultures. *Z. Exp. Zellforsch.,* 23:1–7.
35. Loor, F., Forni, L., and Pernis, B. (1972): The dynamics of the lymphocyte membrane: Factors affecting the distribution and turnover of surface immunoglobulin. *Eur. J. Immunol.,* 2:203–206.
36. McCutcheon, M. (1946): Chemotaxis in leukocytes. *Physiol. Rev.,* 26:319–336.
37. Maruta, H., and Korn, E. (1977): Purification from *Acanthamoeba castellanii* of proteins that induce gelation and syneresis of F-actin. *J. Biol. Chem.,* 252:399–402.
38. Mast, S. O. (1926): Structure, movement, locomotion and stimulation in amoeba. *J. Morphol.,* 41:347–425.
39. Michell, R. H., Pancake, S. J., Noseworthy, J., and Karnovsky, M. L. (1969): Measurement of rates of phagocytosis: The use of cellular monolayers. *J. Cell Biol.,* 40:216–224.
40. Miranda, A. F., Godman, G. C., and Tannenbaum, S. W. (1974): Action of cytochalasin D on cells of established lines: II. Cortex and microfilaments. *J. Cell Biol.,* 62:406–423.
41. Neth, R., and Winkler, K. (1972): Proteinsynthese in menschlichen leukocyten: II. Wirkung einiger antibiotica auf die proteinsyntheseleistung von zellsuspensionen und auf die peptidyl-transferase-aktivität in zellfreien systemen. *Klin. Woschenschr.* 50:523–524.
42. North, R. J. (1970): Endocytosis. *Semin. Hematol.* 7:161–171.
43. Oliver, J. M. (1976): Impaired microtubule function correctable by cyclic GMP and cholinergic agonists in the Chediak-Higashi syndrome. *Am. J. Pathol.* 85:395–418.
44. Pollard, T. D., and Korn, E. D. (1973): *Acanthomoeba* myosin: II. Interaction with actin and a new cofactor protein required for actin activation of Mg^{2+}-adenosine triphosphatase activity. *J. Biol. Chem.,* 248:4691–4697.

45. Pollard, T. D., and Weihing, R. R. (1974): Actin and myosin and cell movement. *CRC Crit. Rev. Biochem.*, 2:1–65.
46. Ryan, G. B., Borysenko, J. Z., and Karnovsky, M. J. (1974): Factors affecting the redistribution of surface-bound concanavalin A on human polymorphonuclear leukocytes. *J. Cell Biol.*, 62:351–365.
47. Senda, N., Shibata, N., Tatsumi, N., Kondo, K., Hamada, K. (1969): A contractile protein from leucocytes: Its extraction and some of its properties. *Biochim. Biophys. Acta*, 181:191–200.
48. Shibata, N., Tatsumi, N., Tanaka, K., Okamura, Y., and Senda, N. (1975): Leucocyte myosin and its location in the cell. *Biochim. Biophys. Acta*, 400:222–243.
49. Spudich, J. A., Lin, S. (1972): Cytochalasin B, its interaction with actin and actomyosin from muscle. *Proc. Natl. Acad. Sci. U.S.A.*, 69:442–446.
50. Steinman, R. M., Brodie, S. E., Cohn, Z. A. (1976): Membrane flow during pinocytosis: A stereologic analysis. *J. Cell Biol.*, 68:665–687.
51. Stossel, T. P., and Hartwig, J. H. Interactions between actin, myosin and a new actin-binding protein of rabbit alveolar macrophages: Macrophage myosin Mg^{++}-adenosine triphosphatase requires a cofactor for activation by actin. (1975): *J. Biol. Chem.*, 250:5706–5712.
52. Stossel, T. P., and Hartwig, J. H. (1976): Interactions of actin, myosin and a new actin-binding protein of rabbit pulmonary macrophages: II. Role in cytoplasmic movement and phagocytosis. *J. Cell Biol.*, 68:602–619.
53. Stossel, T. P., Mason, R. J., Hartwig, J. H., and Vaughan, M. (1972): Quantitative studies of phagocytosis by polymorphonuclear leukocytes: Use of emulsions to measure the initial rate of phagocytosis. *J. Clin. Invest.*, 51:615–624.
54. Stossel, T. P., and Pollard, T. D. (1973): Myosin in polymorphonuclear leukocytes. *J. Biol. Chem.*, 248:8288–8294.
55. Taylor, R. B., Duffus, P. H., Raff, M. C., and De Petris, S. (1971): Redistribution and pinocytosis of lymphocyte surface immunoglobulin molecules induced by antiimmunoglobulin antibody. *Nature* [New Biol.], 233:225–227.
56. Terry, A. H., and Culp, L. A. (1974): Substrate-attached glycoproteins from normal and virus-transformed cells. *Biochemistry*, 13:414–425.
57. Unanue, E. R., Ault, K. A., and Karnovsky, M. J. (1974): Ligand-induced movement of lymphocyte surface macromolecules: IV. Stimulation of cell motility by anti-Ig and lack of relationship to capping. *J. Exp. Med.*, 139:295–312.
58. Weihing, R. R. (1976): Cytochalasin B inhibits actin-related gelation of HeLa cell extracts. *J. Cell Biol.*, 71:303–307.
59. Weihing, R. R. (1976): Occurrence of microfilaments in non-muscle cells and tissues. *Biological Handbooks. Cell Biology*, Vol. 1, edited by P. L. Altman and D. D. Katz, pp. 341–356. FASEB Publications, Bethesda, Md.
60. Weiss, L. (1971): Biophysical aspects of initial cell interaction with solid surfaces. *Fed. Proc.*, 30:1649–1657.
61. Wessels, N. K., Spooner, B. S., Ash, J. F., Bradley, M. O., Ludeña, M. A., Taylor, E. L., Wrenn, J. T., and Yamada, K. M. (1971): Microfilaments in cellular and developmental processes. *Science*, 171:135–143.
62. Zigmond, S., and Hirsch, J. G. (1972): Cytochalasin B: Inhibition of D-2-deoxyglucose transport into leukocytes and fibroblasts. *Science*, 176:1432–1434.
63. Zigmond, S. H., and Hirsch, J. G. (1973): Leukocyte locomotion and chemotaxis: New methods for evaluation and demonstration of a cell-derived chemotactic factor. *J. Exp. Med.*, 137:387–410.
64. Zurier, R. B., Weissmann, G., Hoffstein, S., Kammerman, S., and Tai H. H. (1974): Mechanisms of lysosomal enzyme release from human leukocytes: II. Effects of cAMP and cGMP, autonomic agonists, and agents which affect microtubule function. *J. Clin. Invest.*, 53:297–309.

DISCUSSION

Dr. Jensen: Dr. Keller in Bern, Switzerland, showed that isolated pseudopods not only do what you show, but also respond to chemotactic stimuli. They must have the whole complement of receptors.

Dr. Stossel: Yes, they are interesting. I would like to see how far they really move and to know more details about their composition.

Dr. Becker: What is the relationship between the concentration of cyclohexi-mide that is required for depression of protein synthesis and locomotion?

Dr. Stossel: The relationship is directly proportional. This was also found with puromycin, shown previously to inhibit chemotaxis by Ward (*Biochem. Pharmacol. Suppl.,* 99:105, 1968).

Dr. Zigmond: These are very nice observations, but I wonder how you know that there is an increase in myosin and in actin-binding protein in the pseudopods.

Dr. Stossel: The amounts are not expressed as percent of total cellular protein. They are expressed as concentration of actin-binding protein relative to actin. There is loss of those particular proteins from the cell body to the podosome.

Dr. Gallin: Are you saying that your system explains the directional component of locomotion, without environmental influence? How do you explain the effects of colchicine on locomotion?

Dr. Stossel: I think the cells are always oriented. There may be intrinsic noise in the system that causes that. There may be potassium flux, or chronic calcium flux, or whatever, and you impose some kind of order on it when you add chemotactic factors. I do not believe that microtubules hold the cell oriented and that when colchicine is added the cell does not orient anymore. All that is certain about colchicine is that it disrupts microtubules.

Dr. Gallin: Where are the granules located in the cells during locomotion?

Dr. Stossel: As you watch the cell crawling around, the characteristic thing that you see is tails, head, and a little scintillating movement of granules right behind the lamellipod. I think that is because the gel is being pulled in both directions at that point. There is endoplasmic streaming movement sometimes, but often, very little. The only internal movement that you see routinely is a scintillating movement of the granules. And it is just like the movement when the cell degranulates during phagocytosis.

Dr. Gallin: Do you think microtubules have something to do with orientation?

Dr. Stossel: Certainly, it might help the granules get organized. I am just saying this, however; I do not really know.

Dr. Schiffmann: Dr. Stossel, I like your idea about capping and endocytosis and replacement of receptors with respect to what may be necessary for locomotion. How long do you incubate your cells during this micropore assay? The reason I am asking is because we found that cycloheximide most of the time stimulates chemotaxis at 10^{-4} M, a concentration at which there is not going to be much protein synthesis. It either stimulates or does not inhibit locomotion. Our observations are upon cells which have moved all the way through a filter after a 2-hr incubation.

It is conceivable that if your studies had been done any longer you might have started to get some degenerative effects.

Dr. Stossel: These cells were in the incubator 45 min. It is not just a nonspecific toxic effect. We looked at phagocytosis after a comparable interval, but we did not find any inhibition. It does not seem to affect orientation. So I would postulate it is effecting translational locomotion.

Dr. Schiffmann: We were using cycloheximide also, for another reason. We were attempting to study some of the subsequent events to chemoreception as well as the involvement of protein synthesis in interaction between cell and attractant. In the latter case, there appears to be more. To emphasize, we have not found an inhibition of chemotaxis.

Dr. Stossel: And you have looked at protein synthesis concomitantly?

Dr. Schiffmann: Incorporation of leucine was reduced, but it does not appear to damage the cell. We did not really do an exhausting examination of cell viability. But the cells look very nice, and they do travel.

Dr. Stossel: Protein synthesis may not be the best way to look at membrane turnover, which is the way we are trying to get it. I like the theory better than the experiments. Also, there may be differences in susceptibility to inhibitors of protein synthesis between cells, e.g., exudate vs blood, etc.

Dr. Wilkinson: About the localization of fluorescence on cell membranes, we have some data on fluorescein-labeled chemotactic factors (mostly with FITC-alkali-denatured serum albumin at a fluorscein-to-protein ratio of about 1.5 : 1 and using membrane fluorescence on moving cells). When the cells are moving around, the fluorescence is essentially uniform and not localized. Where the cell is rounded, it appears bright; where the cell is spread, it appears dull, simply because you are looking through different thicknesses. Later, at one to two hr, the fluorescence becomes localized as a bright spot, usually at the tail. Such cells no longer show translocations; they are usually well stuck down by that fluorescent tail, although they may break away leaving fluorescent material behind on the slide. An hour or two later, the whole population of cells has endocytosed the fluorescent protein, which now appears in intracellular vacuoles. In summary, capping and endocytosis of the chemotactic factor have taken place, but they have occurred *after* the chemotactic events and do not seem to be playing a direct role in locomotion.

Dr. Stossel: Of course, the endocytosis does not start movement again.

Dr. Wilkinson: No, that population is just rounded up. I have never seen them moving. All seem to be rounded. I do not know if they are saturated or deactivated or anything, but they are rounded up, and they are not responding any more.

Dr. Ward: Can your model be applied completely to the neutrophil, because, it is said by some that in neutrophils there is little or no measurable pinocytic activity.

Dr. Stossel: Others say that neutrophils do engage in pinocytosis (8). This cycle is being proffered simply to explain how you would account for loss of membrane and still sustain locomotion over a period of time.

Dr. Ward: The question is, do you necessarily have to internalize just to get the cell to respond (as in enzyme release)? That is really what it comes down to.

Dr. Stossel: There are no data.

Dr. Quie: Dr. Wilkinson's figures seem to be consistent with Dr. Stossel's impression that there is a kind of a movement backward of cytosol as cells locomote toward an object. The cell is crawling along in response to chemotactic factors, and as the cell moves forward, it looks as though cytoplasm is flowing toward the back.

Dr. Stossel: Dr. Quie, you would also have to get your contractile proteins up front again, too, and that could be synthesis or that could be an endoplasmic flow kind of thing; I do not know.

Dr. Snyderman: Cycloheximide at 10 μg per ml did not inhibit the human monocytes' chemotactic response. These may be much less of a challenge with the polycarbonate filter than with the nitrocellulose filter. I wonder if you have ever looked at what inhibitors of protein synthesis do to locomotion in the visual assay.

Dr. Stossel: We looked at adhesion just by letting the cells stick in monolayers, coverslips; and they seemed, if anything, to stick better in the presence of cycloheximide.

Dr. Snyderman: When you look at mononuclear cells crawling along the glass, you are essentially looking at a two-dimensional model, i.e., walking on a flat surface. In a three-dimensional environment, as exists in the body, are any differences expected?

Dr. Stossel: No; in fact, a study was done by Bard and Hay (*J. Cell Biol.,* 67:400–418, 1975) with fibroblasts, in collagen meshworks and looking at orientation, etc., and the morphology was the same as with cultivated cells on flat surfaces. It is clear that the basic pattern of locomotion for all cells is very similar.

Leukocyte Chemotaxis, edited by John I. Gallin and Paul G. Quie. Raven Press, New York © 1978.

Regulation of the Polymorphonuclear Leukocyte Chemotactic Response by Immunological Reactions

Edward J. Goetzl

Departments of Medicine, Harvard Medical School, Boston; and the Robert Breck Brigham Hospital, Boston, Massachusetts 02120

Polymorphonuclear (PMN) leukocytes of the eosinophil and neutrophil series are characteristic constituents of the tissue responses evoked by immediate and subacute immunological reactions. The eosinophil predominates in both the early and late cellular infiltrates of immediate-type hypersensitivity reactions (9,21), while neutrophils are more frequently associated with the subacute reactions initiated by non-IgE immune complexes (7,48). The *in vitro* demonstration of specific stimulatory or inhibitory leukotactic activities for a variety of factors derived from either mast cells or immune complexes and their effector pathways has provided the basis for further detailed analyses of mechanisms underlying preferential tissue accumulation of eosinophils or neutrophils. While high-molecular-weight neutrophil chemotactic factors (NCF) are released by IgE-dependent activation of mast cells and mast cell-rich tissues (1), the predominant eosinophil chemotactic activity of anaphylactic fluids favors eosinophils and is attributable to both the low-molecular-weight eosinophil chemotactic factor of anaphylaxis (ECF-A) and histamine (5,18). A distinct mast cell-derived peptide chemotactic factor having a molecular weight of 2,000 to 3,000 is also more active for eosinophils than neutrophils, although it is not as selective as ECF-A (1,15).

Humoral chemotactic stimuli generated by subacute immunological reactions include fragments of the third and fifth components of complement with C5a being the latter fragment (32), as well as the trimolecular complex $C\overline{567}$ (30), and the C3 convertase of the alternative pathway, $C\overline{3B}$, which expresses a leukotactic activity that is dependent on the integrity of the convertase active site (39). The complement component fragments are equally chemotactic for neutrophils and eosinophils, while $C\overline{567}$ and $C\overline{3B}$ are more active for neutrophils than eosinophils (18,30,39). Activation of Hageman factor on immunologically altered basement membranes and other surfaces, a reaction markedly facilitated by small quantities of kallikrein (35), generates kallikrein from prekallikrein resulting in the appearance of leukotactic activity that favors neutrophils over eosinophils (25,26).

Several leukocyte-directed activities have been discovered which may relate to both immediate and subacute hypersensitivity reactions, but the molecular bases of these activities have not yet been precisely defined. A potent lipid chemotactic activity which attracts eosinophils and neutrophils is generated by antigen challenge of rat peritoneal cavities previously prepared with IgGa-rich hyperimmune antiserum and by reversed challenge of human lung tissue fragments with anti-IgE (45). A possibly related lipid chemotactic activity, elaborated by antigen challenge of perfused lungs from sensitized guinea pigs, has been tentatively identified as thromboxane B_2 (20). Polymeric IgA alone, and possibly in immune complexes, is intrinsically inhibitory for PMN leukocyte chemotaxis, an activity not found with monomeric IgA, but its specificity within the PMN leukocyte series remains to be defined (46). Elevated serum levels of IgE in some patients may be associated with frequent bacterial infections and with a profound *in vitro* chemotactic hyporesponsiveness of neutrophil PMN leukocytes (24). It has not been determined whether IgE at high concentrations or present in immune complexes, or an inhibitory mediator generated in a chronically heightened state of immediate hypersensitivity accounts for the defect in neutrophil chemotactic function.

Although occasional delayed hypersensitivity reactions manifest an infiltrate containing eosinophils or neutrophils, the more characteristic cellular population is devoid of PMN leukocytes. Immunological stimulation of lymphocytes leads to the appearance of discrete chemotactic activities for neutrophils as well as monocytes (51), and it releases factors which become chemotactic for eosinophils after the addition of homologous immune complexes (41). Potent inhibitors of PMN leukocyte chemotaxis are also elaborated concomitantly which block PMN leukocyte influx into sites of delayed hypersensitivity reactions in response to the chemotactic factors. The leukocyte inhibitory factor (LIF), a protein having a molecular weight of 65,000 to 70,000 which is released by concanavalin. A treatment of lymphocytes and antigen challenge of sensitized lymphocytes, selectively inhibits PMN leukocyte migration (36,37). LIF alone or in combination with other inhibitors may be responsible for preventing a PMN leukocyte chemotactic response to lymphocyte-derived stimuli. The preferential accumulation of eosinophils in immediate hypersensitivity reactions and of neutrophils in subacute immunological reactions, and the absence of PMN leukocytes from most delayed hypersensitivity reactions, represent the net balance of activities of multiple stimuli and inhibitors in each instance, rather than the predominant action of a single mediator of leukocyte mobility.

IMMEDIATE HYPERSENSITIVITY

Primary Mediators

ECF-A, a primary mediator of immediate-type hypersensitivity reactions, is present preformed in mast cell granules and is released rapidly along with histamine by IgE-dependent activation of mast cells and mast cell-rich tissues (27,

29,52,53). The preferential eosinophil chemotactic activity of ECF-A in diffusates from immunologically challenged fragments of guinea pig or human lung tissue was initially attributed to a peptide having a molecular weight of 300 to 1,000 (18,27,29). Extraction of fragments of human lung tissue, under conditions minimizing endogenous proteolytic activity, and filtration of the supernatant on Sephadex G-25, revealed considerable heterogeneity in the size of the preformed eosinophil chemotactic factors (1,14,15). The material resembling ECF-A in size and preferential eosinophil chemotactic activity was selected for further purification by sequential chromatography on Dowex-1, Sephadex G-10, and paper, which resolved two distinct factors of amino acid sequences Ala-Gly-Ser-Glu and Val-Gly-Ser-Glu (14). The activity released by IgE-mediated stimulation of human lung tissue was resolved into two comparable peaks which co-chromatographed with the acidic hydrophobic tetrapeptides in the lung extracts during parallel isolation procedures. Purified natural and synthetic tetrapeptides exhibited comparable maximum eosinophil chemotactic activity at concentrations of 3×10^{-8} M to 10^{-6} M *in vitro*, and accounted for 30 to 40% of the activity obtainable at optimal doses of the initial Sephadex G-25 low-molecular-weight peak from anaphylactic diffusates (11). The synthetic tetrapeptides attracted eosinophils into marmoset and human skin in *in vivo* studies, with peak activity at levels of 10^{-3} M to 10^{-4} M (42).

ECF-A tetrapeptides can effectively modulate eosinophil chemotaxis *in vitro* by way of deactivation (49,50), a process rapidly leading to complete chemotactic unresponsiveness of eosinophils preincubated in the absence of a gradient with synthetic tetrapeptides at concentrations as low as 1/1000 the optimal chemotactic level (14,54). The secondary specificity of ECF-A tetrapeptides for human neutrophils, which is maximally expressed at peptide concentrations of 3- to 10-fold the optimal level for eosinophil chemotaxis, is also manifested by their rapid chemotactic deactivation of neutrophils (Fig. 1). Pretreatment of neutrophils with 10^{-8} M Val-Gly-Ser-Glu for 2 min, followed by a thorough washing of the cells, resulted in complete unresponsiveness to a subsequent challenge with the homologous stimulus. The same deactivating exposure had only a marginal effect on their response to purified plasma kallikrein, complete inhibition of which required either more prolonged treatment or an increase in the level of Val-Gly-Ser-Glu to 10^{-6} M. Stimulus-dependent deactivation was also observed after preincubation of neutrophils for 8 min with 10^{-10} M Val-Gly-Ser-Glu (Fig. 1). As the substituent NH_2-terminal tripeptides Val/Ala-Gly-Ser and the common COOH-terminal tripeptide Gly-Ser-Glu exhibited only marginal *in vitro* chemotatic activity for eosinophils, their ability to regulate eosinophil responses to the parent tetrapeptide was studied in detail (16). Such functional data indicated that the NH_2-terminal residue interacts reversibly with a hydrophobic domain on the eosinophil, while the COOH-terminal residue perturbs a polar domain on the cell to activate, or deactivate, directed migration (16). The relative chemotactic inactivity of the NH_2-terminal and COOH-terminal substituent tripeptides for neutrophils indicates that both end-groups of

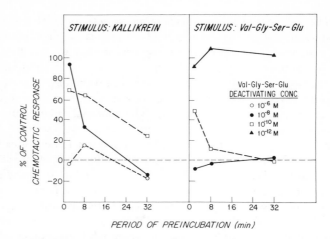

FIG. 1. Chemotactic deactivation of neutrophil PMN leukocytes by Val-Gly-Ser-Glu. Neutrophils purified on Ficoll-Hypaque cushions were pretreated at 37°C, washed twice, and resuspended in Hanks' solution, 0.4 g/100 ml ovalbumin prior to assessment of residual responsiveness to 3×10^{-6} M Val-Gly-Ser-Glu or purified kallikrein (25,26). Background migration of control leukocytes was 6.2 leukocytes/high-power field (hpf), and their chemotactic response to Val-Gly-Ser-Glu was 14.7; and to kallikrein it was 26.8 net leukocytes/hpf.

the tetrapeptides are also critical for directed stimulation of neutrophils, and it suggests the presence of a neutrophil-tetrapeptide receptor analogous to that of the eosinophil.

Histamine, a primary mediator of immediate-type hypersensitivity reactions by virtue of its ability to contract smooth muscle and alter microvascular permeability, has potent *in vitro* effects on eosinophil migration. At concentrations ranging from 3×10^{-7} M to 1.25×10^{-6} M in the stimulus compartment, histamine exerted a chemotactic influence that was preferential for eosinophils as compared to neutrophils (5). Although the eosinophil chemotactic activity of histamine was abrogated by the elimination of a concentration gradient, the presence of 10^{-5} M histamine on both sides of the micropore filter enhanced the random migration of a fraction of the target pool of eosinophils (5). Further, an optimal chemotactic concentration of histamine appeared less able than the tetrapeptides of ECF-A to stimulate a true wave of eosinophil movement into cellulose acetate micropore filters (15). Finally, the introduction of histamine into the eosinophil compartment modulated their random and directed migration in a dose-dependent fashion (6,15).

The addition of histamine to the responding cells, at concentrations below the peak chemotactic range, enhanced both eosinophil random migration and responsiveness to other chemotactic stimuli, while histamine at levels above the chemotactic range inhibited random and chemotactic migration (15). The low-dose enhancing effects were blocked by H_1-type receptor antagonists, while the high-dose inhibitory effects were prevented by H_2-type receptor antagonists

(6). Since the dose-response curve of histamine modulation of leukocyte migration is likely to include additive as well as competitive regions of H_1- and H_2-dependent effects, and as pharmacological inhibitors rarely exert selective antagonism in the absence of some agonist function, studies were performed with analogs of histamine which exhibit predominantly H_1- or H_2-receptor activity (3). Neutrophils were selected for initial studies as neither histamine nor its analogs possessed substantial chemotactic activity for this type of PMN

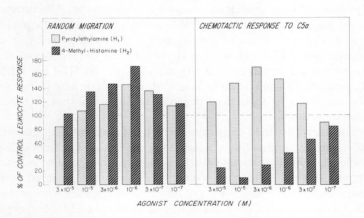

FIG. 2. Effect of histamine analogs on human neutrophil PMN leukocyte migration. Analogs at varying concentrations were added to the cell compartment to assess their effect on both random migration, which had a control level (100%) of 18.2 leukocytes/hpf (left-hand frame), and the chemotactic response to C5a (13,18), which had a control level (100%) of 24.6 net leukocytes/hpf (right-hand frame).

leukocyte. The addition to neutrophils of pyridylethylamine, which preferentially stimulates H_1 receptors, or 4-methyl-histamine, which stimulates H_2 receptors with comparable specificity, enhanced their random migration in micropore filters (Fig. 2). Peak enhancement reached 50 to 100% of unstimulated random migration with either histamine analog at concentrations of 3×10^{-7} M to 10^{-5} M. Similar treatment of neutrophils profoundly altered their chemotactic response to C5a (Fig. 2). Suppression of chemotaxis by the H_2-predominant agonist was dose-related and reached 50% inhibition at a level of approximately 10^{-6} M. The H_1-specific agonist enhanced the neutrophil chemotactic response to C5a by 50 to 100%, with a peak effect at a concentration of approximately 10^{-6} M to 10^{-5} M. Thus, both H_1- and H_2-directed histamine agonists enhanced random migration, but stimulation of H_1 and H_2 receptors achieved opposite effects on directed migration, as the former facilitated and the latter inhibited chemotaxis. These results suggest that histamine induction of eosinophil chemotaxis, which is not blocked by H_1 or H_2 antagonists alone (5,6), may result from a concomitant stimulation of both types of histamine receptors.

Secondary Mediators

The perturbation of cell surfaces induced by primary mediators of immediate hypersensitivity leads to the elaboration of secondary products including prostaglandins and the more labile endoperoxides and thromboxanes (20,34). Although the prostaglandins lack substantial intrinsic chemotactic activity, they can modulate the response of PMN leukocytes by a cell-directed action. The addition of $PGF_{2\alpha}$ at concentrations of 10^{-8} M to 10^{-7} M to human neutrophil suspensions markedly enhanced their chemotactic response, while comparable concentrations of PGE_1 were inhibitory (8,23). As PMN leukocytes engaged in phagocytosis generate and release a variety of prostaglandins (22), a continuing modulation of chemotaxis by the prostaglandins may derive from the leukocytes that have accumulated and are activated at a site of inflammation. The net influence of leukocyte-generated prostaglandins could be stimulatory or inhibitory, depending on the nature of the synthetic and degradative pathways that predominate in the cellular infiltrate.

Nonprostanoate fatty acid derivatives, which are elaborated as secondary mediators of immediate immunological reactions, may exhibit chemotactic activity for PMN leukocytes or modulate their chemotactic response to other stimuli. Both antigen challenge of rat peritoneal cavities passively prepared with IgGa-rich antisera and anti-IgE stimulation of human lung fragments led to the release of lipid factors chemotactic for neutrophil and eosinophil PMN leukocytes (45). The lipid chemotactic activity released from the rat peritoneal cavity was separated from less hydrophobic material by adsorption to Amberlite-XAD and subsequent elution in 80% ethanol, and was then further purified on a silicic acid column sequentially developed with hexane, methylene chloride, acetone, *n*-propanol, and ethanol:concentrated ammonium hydroxide:water (6:3:1, v/v) (45). The bulk of the chemotactic activity was recovered in the acetone fraction, and was thus completely resolved both from the slow-reacting substance of anaphylaxis (SRS-A) and a lipid platelet activating factor (PAF), which appeared in the last pool, and from a neutral lipid in the hexane fraction, which enhanced PMN leukocyte random migration irrespective of a gradient in its concentration (45).

The rat lipid factor(s) in the acetone fraction has chromatographic characteristics on thin-layer plates comparable to 12-L-hydroxy-5,8,10,14-eicosatetraenoic acid, designated HETE, which is strikingly chemotactic for human PMN leukocytes of the neutrophil and eosinophil series (19,43,44). HETE is generated from arachidonic acid by the action of a platelet-derived lipoxygenase that is not blocked by cyclo-oxygenase inhibitors such as indomethacin (33). HETE is selectively chemotactic *in vitro* for human PMN leukocytes, as compared to human mononuclear leukocytes, with a preference for eosinophils (19). As for nonlipid chemotactic principles, preincubation of PMN leukocytes with HETE at peak chemotactic concentrations reduced their random and chemotactic migration (Fig. 3) and concomitantly stimulated the activity of their hexose mono-

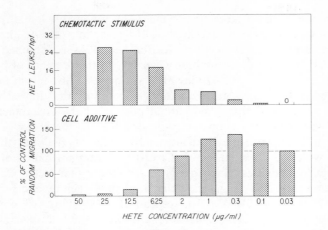

FIG. 3. Influence of HETE on human neutrophil PMN leukocyte migration. Highly purified HETE (19) was employed in the stimulus compartment or added to the cell compartment at varying concentrations. Background migration in the former protocol (top frame) was 4.9 leukocytes/hpf and control random migration (100%) in the latter protocol (bottom frame) was 16.2 leukocytes/hpf.

phosphate shunt (13,19). Exposure of PMN leukocytes to minimally chemotactic levels of HETE enhanced random migration (Fig. 3), an effect rarely observed with nonlipid leukotactic factors. HETE and possibly other structurally related lipids released by immediate and subacute hypersensitivity reactions may not only augment random migration, but also enhance the chemotactic responses of eosinophil and neutrophil PMN leukocytes to other stimuli.

Subacute Immunological Reactions: Activation of Complement Pathways

Activation of the classical or alternative complement sequences generates fragments of C3 and C5 which are chemotactic for PMN as well as mononuclear leukocytes (18,32,40,47). The chemotactically active fragments derived from C3 and C5 by *in vitro* tryptic cleavage exhibit considerable structural and functional heterogeneity, and the relationship of such products to the anaphylatoxins, C3a and C5a, elaborated by the complement cascade, has not been well established. Highly purified and synthetic C5a is chemotactic for PMN leukocytes, while C3a lacks *in vitro* leukotactic activity (32). Tryptic cleavage of purified C5 yielded polydisperse fragments chemotactic for PMN leukocytes which ranged in molecular weight from approximately 5,000 to 12,000 (38). The smaller fragments were also chemotactic for tumor cells, and further digestion of the larger products with aminopeptidases enhanced their tumor cell chemotactic activity while concomitantly reducing their effect on PMN leukocytes (38). The leukotactic activity of fragments of C3 and C5 is rapidly eliminated upon enzymatic digestion. The α-globulin chemotactic factor inactivator, CFI, degrades both C5a and the chemotactic principles of C3 by an aminopeptidaselike action

(2). Inactivation of the leukotactic fragments by the anaphylatoxin inactivator proceeds by way of its carboxypeptidase B-like action (4). As the ability of $\overline{C567}$ to prepare bystander erythrocytes for hemolysis is inhibited by serum factors, which exhibit greater inhibitory capacity in the presence of polycations, the chemotactic activity of $\overline{C567}$ may also be suppressed by serum factors (31).

Initial studies of the leukotactic factors generated by the alternative complement pathway revealed that a substantial portion of the chemotactic activity was labile, with a marked temperature-dependence for the decay process (39). Interaction of the chemotactically inactive purified factors B and $\overline{D}$ (the activated form of D) with cobra venom factor (CoVF) led to the formation of hemolytic and chemotactic activities which persisted far longer than when C3b was employed in place of CoVF, suggesting that the labile chemotactic principle was the C3 convertase $CoVF\overline{B}$ or $\overline{C3B}$, respectively (39). This was confirmed by the dose-response and kinetic correlations of the hemolytic and chemotactic activities generated in varying mixtures of CoVF, B and $\overline{D}$ as well as the absence of both activities from control mixtures reacted in the absence of Mg^{++}. The magnitude and duration of the chemotactic and deactivating activities of $\overline{C3B}$ may be potentiated by the presence of either activated properdin or C3 nephritic factor; these stabilize $\overline{C3B}$ hemolytic capacity by retarding the intrinsic decay of the convertase and preventing both displacement of B by β_{1H} and inactivation of C3b by C3bINA (10).

Delayed Hypersensitivity Reactions: Generation of Factors Inhibitory to PMN Leukocyte Migration

A variety of factors elaborated by immunologically stimulated lymphocytes are either directly chemotactic for PMN leukocytes or acquire activity after incubation with immune complexes. Gel filtration of supernatants derived by antigen challenge of sensitized lymphocytes has resolved two leukotactic factors, one preferentially chemotactic for monocytes and the other predominantly chemotactic for PMN leukocytes (51). Preferential eosinophil chemotactic activity has been recognized in supernatants from cultured lymph node cells of patients with Hodgkin's disease; this activity comprised four peaks of molecular weight ranging from approximately 500 to greater than 20,000 by gel filtration (28). Specific antigen stimulation *in vitro* of lymphocytes from guinea pigs with delayed hypersensitivity generated a precursor macromolecule that developed preferential chemotactic activity for eosinophils when mixed with homologous immune complexes (41).

As the predominant effect of supernatants from stimulated lymphocytes is inhibition of leukocyte migration, efforts have focused on nonchemotactic principles capable of suppressing PMN leukocyte migration. Leukocyte inhibitory factor, LIF, is a protein of molecular weight, approximately 68,000 which is elaborated along with other lymphokines following concanavallin A treatment of lymphocytes or antigen challenge of sensitized lymphocytes (36,37). LIF

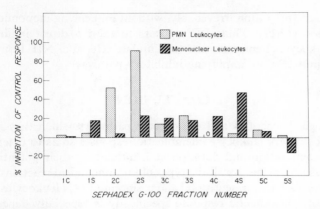

FIG. 4. LIF inhibition of human leukocyte chemotaxis. PMN and mononuclear leukocytes, separated by centrifugation of mixed leukocytes on Ficoll-Hypaque cushions, were preincubated for 5 min at 25°C with portions of LIF fractions prior to their loading into cell compartments. Background migration in leukocytes/hpf was 5.7 for PMN leukocytes and 4.3 for monocytes. The chemotactic response of PMN leukocytes to kallikrein was 19.3 net leukocytes/hpf and of monocytes to C5a was 16.2 net leukocytes/hpf. Sephadex G-100 fractions 1 to 5 of the control series (C) and of the concanavalin A-stimulated series (S) were pooled according to markers of known molecular weight with fraction 2 encompassing the peak of human serum albumin and fraction 4 the peak of chymotrypsinogen. (Modified from R. E. Rocklin and E. J. Goetzl, *manuscript in preparation.*)

lacks chemotactic activity and selectively inhibits the migration of PMN leukocytes from glass capillary tubes, without influencing migration of monocytes or guinea pig peritoneal macrophages (36). In addition to its size and functional capability, LIF also differs from MIF with respect to the susceptibility of its activity to diisopropyl fluorophosphate (36,37). Preincubation of human neutrophils with Sephadex G-100 fractions of human lymphocyte supernatants containing LIF, as assessed by their capacity to inhibit PMN leukocyte migration in the capillary tube assay, resulted in suppression of their chemotactic response in micropore filter chambers (Fig. 4). At the dilution assayed for inhibition of chemotaxis, none of the LIF-rich fractions exhibited chemotactic activity. Although spontaneous inhibitory activity which co-chromatographed with LIF and the serum albumin marker was present in fraction 2C from untreated control lymphocytes, the corresponding activity in fraction 2S from lymphocytes stimulated with concanavalin A was substantially greater and resulted in over 90% suppression of neutrophil chemotaxis to C5a (Fig. 4). The inhibition of monocyte chemotaxis to C5a produced by fraction 4S from stimulated lymphocytes is of appropriate size to represent macrophage migration inhibitory factor (MIF). Incubation of human PMN leukocytes, but not mononuclear leukocytes, with the LIF-rich fractions from Sephadex G-100 gave rise to a second inhibitor of PMN leukocyte chemotaxis of a molecular weight of 4,000 to 5,000. The low-molecular-weight inhibitor resembled the neutrophil-immobilizing factor (NIF) with respect to both its size and ability to suppress PMN leukocyte random and chemotactic migration irreversibly, without influencing mononuclear leukocyte migration (12,17). Thus, LIF appears to exert a direct inhibitory effect on PMN leukocyte chemotaxis and to stimulate release of NIF from the target leukocytes, initiating an amplifying inhibitory pathway.

CONCLUSION

Immunological reactions and the effector pathways which they initiate can modulate local PMN leukocyte chemotactic responses so as to determine their magnitude, composition and duration and, ultimately, their potential for host defense or tissue damage. As all the types of immunological reactions can generate factors chemotactic for neutrophil and eosinophil PMN leukocytes, the ability to regulate the chemotactic response specifically is especially dependent on a variety of nonchemotactic principles which selectively modify the responsiveness of the available pool of PMN leukocytes (Fig. 5). With the exception of NCF, the major chemotactic stimuli released by mast cells during immediate hypersensitivity reactions are preferentially chemotactic for eosinophils, including the primary mediators ECF-A and histamine, as well as some secondary lipid products similar to HETE. The predominant actions of histamine represent cell-directed modulation of chemotactic responses with inhibition by way of prototype H_2 receptors and enhancement through interaction with H_1 receptors (Fig. 2). Marginally chemotactic levels of HETE may enhance leukocyte migration in the absence of a concentration gradient (Fig. 3), while the nonchemotactic prostanoate derivatives $PGF_{2\alpha}$ and PGE_1, enhance and inhibit PMN leukocyte migration, respectively.

The complement-derived stimuli generated by subacute immunological pathways exhibit a chemotactic preference for neutrophils which extends to their chemotactic deactivating activity. The major controls of the principles from these pathways are not solely leukocyte-directed, but center on the mechanisms of inhibition or inactivation of the stimuli. C5a and the fragments of C3 are degraded by the anaphylatoxin inactivator and CFI, while other serum inhibitors suppress the activity of the trimolecular complex $C\overline{567}$. The chemotactic activity of the alternative pathway convertase, $C\overline{3B}$, is labile and may depend for its effectiveness on stabilizing factors such as $\overline{P}$ or C3NeF, which also retard the actions of the control proteins C3bINA and β_{1H}. Although stimulated lymphocytes elaborate several factors chemotactic for PMN leukocytes, the overwhelming inhibitory activity generated concomitantly may explain the usual absence of PMN leukocytes from delayed hypersensitivity reactions (Fig. 5). LIF, purified by gel filtration from supernatants of activated lymphocytes, selectively inhibits PMN leukocyte chemotaxis (Fig. 4) and secondarily leads to the generation of NIF from the PMN leukocytes. LIF thus both directly inhibits and recruits an inhibitor from the target cells to amplify its suppressive effect on PMN leukocyte migration. Modulation of PMN leukotaxis, therefore, varies with the type of immunological reaction: stimulus specificity and cell-directed controls

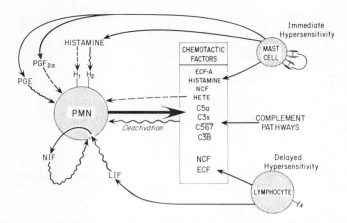

FIG. 5. Modulation of PMN leukocyte chemotactic response by immunological factors. → = generation or release; ➜ = chemotactic response; ----➤ = enhancement; ∿∿➤ = inhibition; x, on lymphocyte receptor = antigen or concanavalin A; C3x = chemotactic fragment of C3.

predominant in immediate hypersensitivity, stimulus specificity, and subsequent stimulus inactivation are critical to the complement pathways, and cell-directed inhibitors of chemotaxis are the major controls in delayed hypersensitivity (Fig. 5). Further purification of mediators of immunological reactions and the development of more sophisticated *in vitro* models of leukocyte migration will permit a better understanding and possibly allow for specific manipulation of immunological modulation of PMN leukocyte responses.

ACKNOWLEDGMENTS

Dr. Goetzl is an Investigator and Director of the Laboratories for the Study of Immunological Diseases, Howard Hughes Medical Institute.

This research was supported in part by NIH grant HL-19777.

The author is very grateful for the expert secretarial assistance of Ms. Catherine Owens and the skilled laboratory work of Ms. Catherine Camp.

REFERENCES

1. Austen, K. F., Wasserman, S. I., and Goetzl, E. J. (1976): Mast cell-derived mediators: Structural and functional diversity and regulation of expression. In: *Molecular and Biological Aspects of the Acute Allergic Reaction,* edited by S. G. O. Johansson, K. Strandberg, and B. Uvnäs, pp. 293–320. Plenum, New York.
2. Berenberg, J. A., and Ward, P. A. (1973): Chemotactic factor inactivator in normal human serum. *J. Clin. Invest.,* 52:1200–1206.
3. Black, J. W., Duncan, W. A. M., Durant, C. J., Cannellin, C. R., and Parson, E. M. (1972): Definition and antagonism of histamine H_2-receptors. *Nature,* 236:385–390.
4. Bokisch, V. A., and Müller-Eberhard, H. J. (1970): Anaphylatoxin inactivator of human plasma: Its isolation and characterization as a carboxypeptidase. *J. Clin. Invest.,* 49:2427–2436.

5. Clark, R. A., Gallin, J. I., and Kaplan, A. P. (1975): The selective eosinophil chemotactic activity of histamine. *J. Exp. Med.,* 142:1462–1476.

6. Clark, R. A., Sandler, J. A., Gallin, J. I., and Kaplan, A. P. (1977): Histamine modulation of eosinophil migration. *J. Immunol.,* 118:137–146.

7. DeShazo, C. V., McGrade, M. T., Henson, P. M., and Cochrane, C. G. (1972): The effect of complement depletion on neutrophil migration in acute immunologic arthritis. *J. Immunol.,* 108:1414–1419.

8. Diaz-Perez, J. L., Goldyne, M. E., and Winkelmann, R. K. (1976): Prostaglandin and chemotaxis: Enhancement of polymorphonuclear leukocyte chemotaxis by prostaglandin $F_{2\alpha}$. *J. Invest. Dermatol.,* 66:149–152.

9. Dolovich, J., Hargreave, F. E., Chalmers, R., Shier, K. J., Gauldie, J., and Bienenstock, J. (1972): Late cutaneous allergic responses in isolated IgE-dependent reactions. *J. Allergy Clin. Immunol.,* 49:43–53.

10. Fearon, D. T., Daha, M. R., Weiler, J. M., and Austen, K. F. (1976): The natural modulation of the amplification phase of complement activation. *Transplant. Rev.,* 32:12–15.

11. Goetzl, E. J. (1976): Modulation of human eosinophil polymorphonuclear leukocyte migration and function. *Am. J. Pathol.,* 85:419–436.

12. Goetzl, E. J., and Austen, K. F. (1972): A neutrophil immobilizing factor derived from human leukocytes: I. Generation and partial characterization. *J. Exp. Med.,*136:1564–1580.

13. Goetzl, E. J., and Austen, K. F. (1974): Stimulation of human neutrophil leukocyte aerobic glucose metabolism by purified chemotactic factors. *J. Clin. Invest.,* 53:591–599.

14. Goetzl, E. J., and Austen, K. F. (1975): Purification and synthesis of eosinophilotactic tetrapeptides of human lung tissue: Identification as eosinophil chemotactic factor of anaphylaxis. *Proc. Natl. Acad. Sci. USA,* 72:4123–4127.

15. Goetzl, E. J., and Austen, K. F. (1976): Specificity and modulation of the eosinophil polymorphonuclear leukocyte response to the eosinophil chemotactic factor of anaphylaxis (ECF-A). In: *Molecular and Biological Aspects of the Acute Allergic Reaction,* edited by S. G. O. Johansson, K. Strandberg, and B. Uvnäs, pp. 417–435. Plenum, New York.

16. Goetzl, E. J., and Austen, K. F. (1976): Structural determinants of the eosinophil chemotactic activity of the acidic tetrapeptides of eosinophil chemotactic factor of anaphylaxis. *J. Exp. Med.,* 144:1424–1437.

17. Goetzl, E. J., Gigli, I., Wasserman, S. I., and Austen, K. F. (1973): A neutrophil immobilizing factor derived from human leukocytes: II. Specificity of action of polymorphonuclear leukocyte mobility. *J. Immunol.,* 111:938–945.

18. Goetzl, E. J., Wasserman, S. I., and Austen, K. F. (1974): Modulation of the eosinophil chemotactic response in immediate hypersensitivity. In: *Progress in Immunology II, Vol. 4,* edited by L. Brent and J. Holborow, pp. 41–50. North-Holland Publ. Co., Amsterdam.

19. Goetzl, E. J., Woods, J. M., and Gorman, R. R. (1977): Stimulation of human eosinophil and neutrophil polymorphonuclear leukocyte chemotaxis and random migration by 12-L-hydroxy-5,8,10,14-eicosatetraenoic acid. *J. Clin. Invest.,* 59:179–183.

20. Hamberg, M., Svensson, J., Hedqvist, P., Strandberg, K., and Samuelsson, B. (1976): Involvement of endoperoxides and thromboxanes in anaphylactic reactions. In: *Advances in Prostaglandin and Thromboxane Research,* edited by B. Samuelsson and R. Paoletti, pp. 495–501. Raven Press, New York.

21. Hargreave, F. E., and Pepys, J. (1973): Allergic respiratory reactions in bird fanciers provoked by allergen inhalation provocation test: Relation to clinical features and allergic mechanism. *J. Allergy Clin. Immunol.,* 50:157–173.

22. Higgs, G. A., McCall, E., and Youlten, L. J. F. (1975): A chemotactic role for prostaglandins released from polymorphonuclear leukocytes during phagocytosis. *Br. J. Pharmacol.,* 53:539–546.

23. Hill, H. R., Estensen, R. D., Quie, P. G., Hogan, N. A., and Goldberg, N. D. (1975): Modulation of human neutrophil chemotactic responses by cyclic 3',5'-guanosine monophosphate and cyclic 3',5'-adenosine monophosphate. *Metabolism,* 24:447–456.

24. Hill, H. R., and Quie, P. G. (1974): Raised serum IgE levels and defective neutrophil chemotaxis in three children with eczema and recurrent bacterial infections. *Lancet,* 1:183–187.

25. Kaplan, A. P., and Austen, K. F. (1970): A pre-albumin activator of prekallikrein. *J. Immunol.,* 105:802–808.

26. Kaplan, A. P., Kay, A. B., and Austen, K. F. (1972): A prealbumin activator of prekallikrein:

III. Appearance of chemotactic activity for human neutrophils by the conversion of human prekallikrein to kallikrein. *J. Exp. Med.,* 135:81–97.

27. Kay, A. B., and Austen, K. F. (1971): The IgE-mediated release of an eosinophil leukocyte chemotactic factor from human lung. *J. Immunol.,* 107:899–902.

28. Kay, A. B., McVie, J. G., Stuart, A. E., Krajewski, A., and Turnbull, L. W. (1975): Eosinophil chemotaxis of supernatants from cultured Hodgkin's lymph node cells. *J. Clin. Pathol.,* 28:502–505.

29. Kay, A. B., Stechschulte, D. J., and Austen, K. F. (1971): An eosinophil leukocyte chemotactic factor of anaphylaxis. *J. Exp. Med.,* 133:602–619.

30. Lachmann, P. J., Kay, A. B., and Thompson, R. A. (1970): The chemotactic activity for neutrophil and eosinophil leukocytes of the trimolecular complex of the fifth, sixth, and seventh components of human complement (C$\overline{567}$) prepared in free solution by the "reactive lysis" procedure. *Immunology,* 19:895–899.

31. Lint, T. F., Behrends, C. L., Baker, P. J., and Gewurz, H. (1976): Activation of the complement attack mechanism in the fluid phase and its control by C$\overline{567}$-INH: Lysis of normal erythrocytes initiated by zymosan, endotoxin and immune complexes. *J. Immunol.,* 117:1440–1446.

32. Müller-Eberhard, H. J. (1976): The anaphylatoxins: Formation, structure, function and control. In: *Molecular and Biological Aspects of the Acute Allergic Reaction,* edited by S. G. O. Johansson, K. Strandberg, and B. Uvnäs, pp. 339–352. Plenum, New York.

33. Nugteren, H. (1975): Arachidonic lipoxygenase in blood platelets. *Biochem. Biophys. Acta,* 380:299–307.

34. Piper, P. J., and Vane, J. R. (1971): The release of prostaglandins from lung and other tissues. *Ann. N.Y. Acad. Sci.,* 180:363–385.

35. Revak, S. D., and Cochrane, C. G. (1976): The relationship of structure and function in human Hageman factor: The association of enzymatic and binding activities with separate regions of the molecule. *J. Clin. Invest.,* 57:852–860.

36. Rocklin, R. E. (1974): Products of activated lymphocytes: Leukocyte inhibitory factor (LIF) distinct from migration inhibitory factor (MIF). *J. Immunol.,* 112:1461–1466.

37. Rocklin, R. E. (1975): Partial characterization of leukocyte inhibitory factor by concanavalin A-stimulated human lymphocytes (LIF con A). *J. Immunol.,* 114:1161–1165.

38. Romualdex, A. G., Jr., Ward, P. A., and Torikata, T. (1976): Relationship between the C5 peptides chemotactic for leukocytes and tumor cells. *J. Immunol.,* 117:1762–1766.

39. Ruddy, S., Austen, K. F., and Goetzl, E. J. (1975): Chemotactic activity derived from interaction of factors $\overline{D}$ and B of the properdin pathway with cobra venom factor of C3b. *J. Clin. Invest.,* 55:587–592.

40. Snyderman, R., Shin, H. S., and Hausman, M. H. (1971): A chemotactic factor for mononuclear leukocytes. *Proc. Soc. Exp. Biol. Med.,* 138:387–390.

41. Torisu, M., Yoshida, T., Ward, P. A., and Cohen, S. (1973): Lymphocyte derived eosinophil chemotactic factors: II. Studies on the mechanism of activation of the precursor substance by immune complexes. *J. Immunol.,* 111:1450–1458.

42. Turnbull, L. W., Evans, D. P., and Kay, A. B. (1977): Human eosinophils, acidic tetrapeptides (ECF-A) and histamine: Interactions *in vitro* and *in vivo. Immunology,* 32:57–62.

43. Turner, S. R., Campbell, J. A., and Lynn, W. S. (1975): Polymorphonuclear leukocyte chemotaxis toward oxidized lipid components of cell membranes *J. Exp. Med.,* 141:1437–1441.

44. Turner, S. R., Tainer, J. A., and Lynn, W. S. (1975): Biogenesis of chemotactic molecules by the arachidonate lipoxygenase system of platelets. *Nature,* 257:680–681.

45. Valone, F. H., Leid, R. W. Jr., and Goetzl, E. J. (1977): Immunologic release of lipid factors chemotactic for human eosinophil and neutrophil polymorphonuclear leukocytes. *Fed. Proc.,* 36:1328A.

46. Van Epps, D. E., and Williams, R. C., Jr., (1976): Suppression of leukocyte chemotaxis by human IgA myeloma components. *J. Exp. Med.,* 144:1227–1242.

47. Ward, P. A. (1967): A plasmin-split fragment of C3 as a new chemotactic factor. *J. Exp. Med.,* 126:189–206.

48. Ward, P. A. (1971): Complement-derived leukotactic factors in pathological fluids. *J. Exp. Med.,* 134(Suppl.): 109S–113S.

49. Ward, P. A., and Becker, E. L. (1968): The deactivation of rabbit neutrophils by chemotactic factor and the nature of the activatable esterase. *J. Exp. Med.,* 127:693–709.

50. Ward, P. A., and Becker, E. L. (1970): Biochemical demonstration of the activatable esterase of the rabbit neutrophil involved in the chemotactic response. *J. Immunol.,* 105:1057–1067.

51. Ward, P. A., Remold, H. G., and David, J. R. (1969): Leukocyte chemotactic factors produced by sensitized lymphocytes. *Science,* 163:1079–1083.
52. Wasserman, S. I., Goetzl, E. J., and Austen, K. F. (1974): Preformed eosinophil chemotactic factor of anaphylaxis (ECF-A). *J. Immunol.,* 112:351–358.
53. Wasserman, S. I., Goetzl, E. J., Kaliner, M. A., and Austen, K. F. (1974): Modulation of the immunologic release of the eosinophil chemotactic factor of anaphylaxis from human lung. *Immunology,* 26:677–684.
54. Wasserman, S. I., Whitmer, D., Goetzl, E. J., and Austen, K. F. (1975): Chemotactic deactivation of human eosinophils by the eosinophil chemotactic factor of anaphylaxis. *Proc. Soc. Exp. Biol. Med.,* 148:301–306.

DISCUSSION

Dr. Lynn: Dr. Goetzl, were you able to isolate an enzyme from the mast cell for producing HETE, and also did you find HETE in your experimental peritoneal exudates?

Dr. Goetzl: The material, which has been highly purified, was derived from the peritoneal cavity of the rat, which is rich in mast cells but certainly has other cell types. This lipid chemotactic material has been generated both by IgG and IgE mechanisms and, in both cases, HETE was present but did not account for the bulk of the chemotactic activity. No experiments have been carried out with isolated mast cells.

Dr. Becker: You presented evidence that HETE was chemokinetic. What evidence do you have that it is chemotactic?

Dr. Goetzl: The chemotactic analysis has been carried out in several ways. If HETE is put on the cell side or both sides of the micropore filter, at the peak chemotactic concentrations, stimulation of leukocyte migration is eliminated. Thus, in the concentration range from approximately 3 to 25 μg/ml, the HETE effect depends on a concentration gradient. Enumeration of the cells stimulated by HETE at various levels within filters revealed that a characteristic wave of migration was achieved within the filters. HETE has other effects on PMN leukocytes which are independent of a concentration gradient, including enhancement of hexose monophosphate activity, chemotactic deactivation, and enhancement of random migration at concentrations below the chemotactic peak. It is the last effect that makes HETE a unique chemotactic stimulus.

Dr. Wilkinson: We have done quite a number of checkerboard analyses with lipids. They are rather difficult, because the lipids do not form very good gradients. I think this is because of their poor solubility. There is certainly a chemotactic effect with such checkerboard studies but in the case of individual lipids, there is considerable variation. So possibly a bit more care is necessary here than when working with soluble peptides.

Dr. Goetzl: Which lipids were you using?

Dr. Wilkinson: Fatty acids such as linoleic acid and also bacterially derived lipids which were not characterized. What effect do your peptides have on the binding of other peptides? Have you looked at them? Are the binding sites the same or different?

Dr. Goetzl: We have just recently synthesized a material that is sufficiently radioactive to use in examining the binding of the tetrapeptides, but we have no data to report at this time.

Dr. Zigmond: I am interested in your deactivation. You showed that 10^{-8}M tetrapeptide could deactivate. I do not understand that. How can you possibly get a chemotactic effect when a 10-fold lower concentration is causing 30% deactivation?

Dr. Goetzl: First, the earliest points of a deactivation protocol obviously include time for processing and washing the treated leukocytes prior to assessing chemotactic responses, while a standard chemotactic experiment involves instantaneous exposure of target cells to the stimulus. Thus, deactivation of leukocyte suspensions is a time-dependent process which currently cannot be examined at zero time.

Second, any deactivation in a chemotactic chamber during a chemotactic experiment would be occurring in a concentration gradient of the stimulus. It is, however, still possible that blocking deactivation in a chamber may enhance chemotactic activity. In a series of analogs of ECF-A tetrapeptides, some are less capable of deactivating and may have either decreased or increased chemotactic activity compared to the natural peptides. Chemotaxis and deactivation do not have totally overlapping characteristics and requirements.

Dr. Miller: Dr. Goetzl: what is your concept of preferential chemotaxis? Is that selectivity or is that sensitivity?

Dr. Goetzl: It can exhibit both features. In my studies, I adjust the concentration of various factors in a matrix type of experiment, so that a concentration of each factor can be selected which attracts a comparable number of one type of leukocytes, for example, neutrophils. I then look at the effect of these same concentrations on other cell types. This functional approach can be employed for chemotaxis or deactivation even if the absolute concentrations of the frequently unpurified factors are not known.

Dr. Gallin: Several investigators have had difficulty demonstrating activity of commercially produced tetrapeptides of ECF-A. Would you comment briefly on (a) the stability of these peptides and (b) problems of contamination by tripeptides of the tetrapeptides during synthesis?

Dr. Goetzl: Several commercial preparations have been examined by thin-layer and high-pressure liquid chromatography which revealed multiple peaks of small quantities of contaminating peptides. As you have demonstrated in your experiments with the material I sent you, a 10% contamination with substituent tripeptide will substantially reduce the moderate activity of the tetrapeptide. Our preparations are purified through two or three columns; this has been critical to eliminate any contaminants.

There is particular difficulty in coupling the NH_2-terminal valine, and the use of radioactive valine has revealed five or six radioactive spots on thin-layer chromatography of unpurified material from most solid-phase synthetic preparations.

Dr. Snyderman: You use the term *moderate activity.* I was just wondering what you mean by that. It looked from your dose-response curve that you were having activity at 10^{-8} M, which is really not very modest. In terms of the total number of cells that could respond to the tetrapeptides, as compared to the C5a, are you suggesting that there is a different maximum number of cells that could respond?

Dr. Goetzl: The ECF-A tetrapeptides are indeed quite potent, although not as potent as the fMet peptides; however, the peak leukocyte responses are lower than for C5a or HETE. Further, if we obtain eosinophils from different patients and examine the dose-response for the tetrapeptides and other factors, the optimal concentration and the response at that peak concentration vary from patient to patient more with the tetrapeptides than with other stimuli.

Dr. Miller: In other words, you cannot get a maximum response in any dose with this material?

Dr. Goetzl: That is right, not compared to other peptides and other chemotactic factors.

Dr. Schiffmann: Have you examined what the cell does to the tetrapeptide? Is it hydrolyzed?

Dr. Goetzl: Extracts of either eosinophils or neutrophils can rapidly cleave both tetrapeptides to either of their substituent tripeptides. I think the peptides are rapidly cleaved *in vivo* whether or not this is a membrane-associated phenomenon as you have suggested for your peptides.

Dr. Lynn: Is the serine in the tetrapeptide required for activity as you indicated?

Dr. Goetzl: If we substitute alanine for serine or make a similar substitution, it reduces the chemotactic activity by about 30% and increases by about 10-fold the dose for a maximum effect. While free alanine and valine were only marginally active in blocking either the deactivating or chemotactic activity of the tetrapeptides, their amides as well as leucine amide acted like Val-Gly-Ser, but required 10-fold higher concentrations. Thus, both substitutions and the greater activity of the NH_2- terminal tripeptides compared to smaller peptides or free amides of NH_2- terminal amino acids have convinced us that serine has a role in the overall activity of the tetrapeptides.

Dr. Turner: Have you looked at the tetrapeptide amides?

Dr. Goetzl: No.

Dr. Williams: You originally got this material from lung extracts. Eosinophils go to the lungs, but they also go to the skin. Have you looked at extracts of skin involved with dermatitis and so forth to see if you could get similar peptides?

Dr. Goetzl: These are mast cell-related peptides, and we have found comparable peptides in two other mast-cell-rich sources, including small bowel and skin biopsy specimens from patients. The other point we have made is that ECF-A accounts for less than half the activity in the initial supernatant, so that other peptides and functionally related active principles are left to be delineated in mast cells and basophils. Quantitatively, the two peptides I discussed are probably the predominant peptides, but there are others present at much lower concentrations which are far more active.

Dr. Williams: If you make stereo models, 3-D models, of your peptides, and look at them, is there anything similar? It is conceivable that if they were all really similar, there would be only one site.

Dr. Schiffmann: This could be determined by the competitive binding studies with a radio-labeled ligand.

Dr. Goetzl: While the binding studies will be useful, it is clear that the different laboratories are already postulating more than one site of interaction of chemotactic peptides with the cells, so that such data may not be definitive.

Dr. Leddy: Did you say that the arachidonic-acid-derived HETE was liberated following antigen challenge of reasonably pure preparations of mast cells?

Dr. Goetzl: It was obtained as a minor component in the rat peritoneal cavity by either an IgG or an IgE reaction, and I am postulating that the mast cells are a possible source.

Dr. Stossel: I wonder if the reason that the monocytes do not respond to HETE is because they make their own. Monocytes are more unsaturated and have more arachidonic acid than polys (*J. Clin. Invest.,* 54:638,1974).

Dr. Goetzl: The critical determinant is, as Drs. Lynn and Turner have discussed in their publications, the distribution of lipoxygenase. They would feel, if I may say this, that the platelet is the only human cell that definitely produces the 12-hydroxy product.

Dr. Lynn: Alveolar macrophages certainly produce no HETE.

Dr. Turner: We found that alveolar macrophages respond to a crude HETE preparation using the polycarbonate filter assay.

Dr. Goetzl: You have not found HETE being synthesized by any cell other than the platelet, aside from the photo-oxidation procedures?

Dr. Turner: We have not, but Hamberg (*Biochem. Biophys. Acta,* 431:651, 1976) has published that lung, spleen, kidney, and whole blood produce HETE when they are incubated at 37°C.

Dr. Goetzl: Could they be sure that those whole-tissue preparations were platelet-depleted?

Dr. Turner: They tested the blood as a control for platelets but it turned out that the lung and spleen produced more HETE than whole blood or kidney. Further more, lipoxygenase inhibitors blocked production of HETE from all four tissues.

Leukocyte Chemotaxis, edited by John I. Gallin and Paul G. Quie. Raven Press, New York © 1978.

Cyclic Nucleotides as Modulators of Leukocyte Chemotaxis

Harry R. Hill

Division of Clinical Immunology, Department of Pediatrics, and the Department of Pathology, University of Utah, Salt Lake City, Utah 84132

A large volume of material continues to accumulate suggesting that in a number of tissues cyclic 3′, 5′ adenosine monophosphate (cAMP) and cyclic 3′, 5′ guanosine monophosphate (cGMP) exert opposing regulatory influences (16,17,18). Such diverse processes as cardiac and smooth-muscle contraction, platelet aggregation, bacterial metabolism, and cell proliferation have been shown to be influenced by these agents (16,17). Bourne and co-workers (5) and Parker and associates (39) have reviewed the effects of cAMP on the immune response. Allergic mediator and lysosomal enzyme release, T-cell mediated cytotoxicity, antibody production, lymphocyte blastogenesis, and initial antigen lymphocyte interaction have been found to be impaired by cAMP and agents causing cellular accumulation of this compound. More recently, additional work has indicated that cGMP has an enhancing effect on many of these same cellular processes (16,17,18). The concept of regulation through opposing actions of the two cyclic nucleotides has been termed the *Yin-Yang Hypothesis of Biological Control* by Goldberg and associates (18). The purpose of this chapter is to review the effects of cAMP and cGMP on leukocyte motility and to discuss the role of cyclic nucleotides in the actions of chemoattractants and chemotactic modulators. Finally, I will speculate on the clinical significance of altered cyclic nucleotide metabolism in patients with severe or recurrent infections.

EFFECTS OF CYCLIC NUCLEOTIDES ON LEUKOCYTE CHEMOTAXIS

Rivkin and Becker (40) reported in 1972 that cAMP, histamine, epinephrine, isoproterenol, and prostaglandin E exert an inhibitory effect on rabbit polymorphonuclear leukocyte (PMN) chemotaxis and random migration. Subsequently, in that same year, Tse and co-workers (47) found that caffeine and cAMP also inhibited human PMN-directed and random motility. I first became interested in the effects of cyclic nucleotides on leukocyte locomotion later in 1972, while working in the laboratory of Dr. Paul Quie at the University of Minnesota. At that time, Dr. Richard Estensen of the Department of Pathology and Dr. Nelson Goldberg of the Department of Pharmacology were investigating the effects of a compound, phorbol myristate acetate (PMA), in a number of cell

TABLE 1. *Effect of phorbol myristate acetate (PMA) on human PMN chemotactic responses to the* E. coli *bacterial factor (BF)*

Agent[a]	Chemotactic index	BF alone (%)
Medium 199	12	22
1.0 ng PMA	28	52
10 ng PMA	30	56
BF	54	100
BF + 1 ng PMA	380	704
BF + 10 ng PMA	388	719

[a] Agents added to attractant side of Boyden chamber. (From *Nature,* 245:458, 1973.)

systems. This agent, the active principle of croton oil, is a co-carcinogen which acts to promote the development of tumors in animals treated with a carcinogenic agent such as benzpyrene. After attempting unsuccessfully for some time to detect an effect of the drug on PMN phagocytosis and intracellular killing, I suggested that we put the drug into the modified Boyden chamber chemotaxis assay (24), on which I had been working. The effects (Table 1) were dramatic (11). The agent possessed some inherent chemotactic activity when added to the attractant side of the chemotactic chamber. This activity amounted to approximately one-half the chemotactic activity of a standard 5% solution of *Escherichia coli* bacterial culture filtrate (BF) described by Ward et al. (48). Addition of 1 to 10 ng of the PMA to the attractant side of the chamber, along with 5% BF, resulted in a profound enhancement of the chemotactic response (up to 700%). We next performed experiments in which the leukocytes were preincubated in 0.01 to 1.0 ng of PMA for 10 min, washed gently, and then assayed for chemotactic responsiveness to the BF. Again, a marked enhancement (up to 460%) of the chemotactic response was observed (Table 2). Since PMA had been reported to increase cellular cGMP levels in other tissues, we went on to explore the possibility that the chemotactic enhancement resulted from an effect on the cellular level of this cyclic nucleotide. In these studies, involving both preincubation experiments (11) and experiments in which the test agent

TABLE 2. *Effect of leukocyte preincubation with PMA on chemotactic responses to the bacterial factor*

Preincubation solution[a]	Chemotactic index	Chemotactic activity BF control (%)
Medium alone	31	100
0.01 ng PMA	63	203
0.1 ng PMA	286	923
1.0 ng PMA	300	967

[a] Leukocytes incubated with agent for 10 min, washed once, and tested for chemotactic activity. (From *Nature,* 245:458, 1973.)

TABLE 3. *Effect of cGMP on human PMN chemotactic responses to bacterial factor*[a]

cGMP (M)	Control chemotaxis (%)
10^{-5}	130 ± 29
10^{-6}	214 ± 26
10^{-7}	223 ± 12
10^{-8}	263 ± 56
10^{-9}	223 ± 15
10^{-10}	97 ± 10

[a]Agents added to upper or cell side of Boyden chamber during 3-hr assay. (From *Metabolism,* 24:447, 1975.)

was added directly to the cell side of the chemotactic chamber during the assay (22), cyclic GMP and agents reported to cause its accumulation in other tissues were found to enhance the chemotactic response. These included such diverse agents as phenylephrine, prostaglandin $F_{2\alpha}$, imidizole and, as mentioned, cGMP itself. Interestingly, it was observed that an intermediate or low concentration of these agents often had a more pronounced effect than a higher level of the compound. This was especially true with cGMP itself, the effect of which was most pronounced at concentrations of 10^{-6} to 10^{-9} M (Table 3). Higher levels resulted in either no enhancement of the chemotactic response or much less. Prostaglandin $F_{2\alpha}$ actually had a biphasic dose-response effect on PMN chemotaxis. At a 10^{-6} M concentration, the chemotactic response to 5% BF was inhibited by 50%. A marked enhancement of up to 200% occurred, however, when the cells were exposed to $PGF_{2\alpha}$ in concentrations of 10^{-7} and 10^{-8} M. The exact reason for this effect is unknown. It may be that higher concentrations of $PGF_{2\alpha}$ elevate cAMP in addition to cGMP. As will be shown later with isoproterenol, we believe that the effects of an increase in cAMP are dominant over the effects of a simultaneous increase in cGMP. If so, this fact could help in explaining the biphasic response to $PGF_{2\alpha}$.

Additional studies by other investigators have tended to confirm our findings that agents which increase cellular cGMP have a stimulatory effect on cell movement. Goetzl and co-workers (15) have reported that ascorbic acid enhances chemotaxis and random migration of PMNs, eosinophils, and monocytes. In addition, ascorbate was found to stimulate hexose monophosphate shunt activity. (We have found that cGMP and phorbol myristate acetate, but not acetylcholine, significantly enhance ^{14}C-1 glucose oxidation to $^{14}CO_2$ in phagocytizing PMNs (Table 4). In addition, a correlation often exists between hexose monophosphate shunt activity, as measured by reduction of nitroblue tetrazolium, and chemotactic responsiveness (23). It appears that both functions are stimulated or enhanced by similar conditions but that neither function is dependent upon the other. This is best illustrated by the fact that patients with chronic granulomatous disease have normal to increased chemotactic activity in the absence of a function-

TABLE 4. *Effect of acetylcholine (A_c), phorbol myristate acetate (PMA), and cGMP on $^{14}CO_2$ generation from ^{14}C-1 glucose by PMNs phagocytizing latex particles*

Agent tested	Concentration	Generation of $^{14}CO_2$ control (%)[a]
Ac	10^{-5} M	110
	10^{-4} M	97
	10^{-3} M	105
PMA	1 ng/ml	108
	10 ng/ml	100
	100 ng/ml	262
cGMP	10^{-8} M	107
	10^{-7} M	123
	10^{-6} M	152

[a]Control was PMNs and latex particles alone.

ing hexose monophosphate shunt. Recently, Sandler and co-workers (42) have shown that ascorbate increases cGMP levels in monocytes and enhances chemotaxis of both PMNs and mononuclear cells. (These authors were unable to demonstrate a change in PMN cGMP levels in response to ascorbate, carbamylcholine, or serotonin). Schreiner and Unanue (45) have found that the cholinergic agents acetylcholine and carbamylcholine, as well as cGMP, markedly enhance motility of T and B lymphocytes.

Further studies by our group (22) on the effects of cAMP and its agonists on chemotactic function tended to confirm the results already reported by Rivkin and Becker (40) and Tse and co-workers (47). We found that epinephrine, isoproterenol, prostaglandin E_1, histamine, and cholera toxin had a depressive effect on PMN chemotaxis. (In contrast to Rivkin et al. (41), we also found that norepinephrine inhibited chemotaxis. Rivkin et al. reported that norepinephrine increased PMN cAMP but did not alter chemotactic function.) Studies employing specific receptor blocking agents including the beta adrenergic blocker propranolol, the alpha blockers phenoxybenzamine and phentolamine, and the H_2 histamine receptor blocking agents burimamide and metramide suggested that a number of receptors for these individual mediators were present on PMNs (23,40,41). In each instance, exogenous cyclic nucleotide continued to exert an effect on leukocyte function in the presence of the above-named blocking agents. This suggests that the cyclic nucleotides act at a step beyond that involving hormone-receptor interaction.

EFFECT OF CYCLIC NUCLEOTIDES ON RANDOM MOTILITY

We were unable to demonstrate an effect of cAMP or cGMP on human PMN random motility but this may well have been because of the methodology employed. Initially, we used a modification of the migration inhibition factor assay to determine random motility (35). Leukocytes were placed in glass capillary tubes, centrifuged, and the tube cut at the cell-fluid interface. The capillary tubes were then placed in Sykes-Moore tissue culture chambers and the agent to be tested was added in medium 199. The leukocytes were allowed to migrate for 4 hours, and the area of migration of the leading edge of granulocytes was then determined. No effects on random migration, as measured by this technique, were observed for cGMP, cAMP, or their agonists. Limited experiments measuring random motility in the Boyden chamber in the absence of a chemotactic gradient also failed to show an effect of added cyclic nucleotides (22). Sandler and co-workers (42) were also unable to demonstrate an effect of serotonin, an agent which increases cGMP, on leukocyte random migration. In contrast, Rivkin and co-workers (41) have reported that theophylline, PGE_1, epinephrine, isoproterenol, and cholera toxin inhibit, while Goetzl et al. (15) have shown that ascorbic acid increases random PMN locomotion. The former authors utilized a Boyden chamber technique to measure random motility that takes into account the number of cells that move away from the starting layer rather than the number that pass completely through the filter. It is likely that this technique is more sensitive in detecting changes in random motility than the one we used.

ASSOCIATION OF CYCLIC NUCLEOTIDE CHANGES WITH ALTERATION OF LEUKOCYTE CHEMOTACTIC FUNCTION

While it has been assumed that cyclic nucleotides are important in the action of the chemotactic modulators mentioned above, few direct measurements of the levels of cAMP and especially cGMP have been made in leukocytes in response to these agents. The results that have been obtained are often confusing and somewhat contradictory. Rivkin and co-workers (41) found that prostaglandin E_1 and A_1 but not $F_{2\alpha}$ increased PMN cAMP levels and inhibited chemotaxis. A quantitative relationship between prostaglandin stimulation of cAMP and inhibition of chemotaxis could not be found, however. In a similar manner, epinephrine and isoproterenol increased cellular cAMP and inhibited chemotaxis, but the relationship was not quantitative. Norepinephrine, in contrast, increased PMN cAMP but did not inhibit cell motility. Sandler and co-workers (42) found that ascorbic acid and serotonin enhanced monocyte chemotactic responses and increased cGMP levels but, as in Rivkin's studies, the relationship was often not quantitative. Moreover, they could not demonstrate an effect of these agents on PMN cGMP levels in concentrations which enhanced chemotaxis of these cells. The confusing results obtained thus far may well be caused by the complexity and sensitivity of the assays presently being utilized to measure cAMP and especially cGMP. Recently, Dr. Gary Hatch, working in my laboratory, has developed a useful modification (19) of the procedure for assaying cAMP and cGMP in leukocytes, which we hope will help to shed further light on this difficult problem. Standard procedures for preparing samples for radioimmunoassay of cyclic nucleotides require the use of denaturants such as trichloroacetic or perchloric acid to inactivate macromolecules involved in the production and breakdown of cAMP and cGMP. These agents must then be removed by ether extraction, base neutralization, or eliminated on alumina columns. Such procedures greatly complicate the assays and lead to significant loss of cyclic nucleotides. Dr. Hatch has found that a 2-sec heat treatment to boiling of cellular samples completely inactivates phosphodiesterases and other macromolecules which interfere with the radioimmunoassay. The sample can then be sonicated and micropore-filtered to remove cellular debris and used directly in the radioimmunoassay. Recovery of cyclic nucleotides after these procedures is high (95 ± 2%) and shows little variability. Moreover, small changes in cyclic nucleotide content are more readily detected. We have now used this assay to assess the effects of several chemoattractants and chemotactic modulators on PMN cGMP and cAMP levels (20). I shall summarize and give representative examples of his findings below.

EFFECTS OF CHEMOATTRACTANTS ON NEUTROPHIL CYCLIC NUCLEOTIDE LEVELS

Ignarro and George (33) have reported that zymosan-treated serum, which possesses complement-derived chemotactic activity, elevates cGMP levels in human PMNs. Recently, we have investigated the effects of other chemoattractants on the levels of cGMP and cAMP in human neutrophils (20). The bacterial factor derived from $E.$ $coli$ produced a dose-dependent increase in cGMP in PMNs (Table 5). Cyclic AMP levels following stimulation with BF could not be determined, since the filtrate contained significant amounts of cAMP (107 nM). Similar concentrations of cAMP in medium alone had no effect on PMN cGMP levels, however. Since the bacterial factor has not been completely characterized, we sought a more basic substance to use in additional studies. Schiffmann and co-workers (44) have indicated that the low-molecular-weight formyl methionyl peptides possess chemotactic activity. We have found that formyl methionyl alanine (FMA), in concentrations of 10^{-3} and 10^{-4} M, significantly increase (39 to 42%) cGMP levels in human PMNs. An elevation is detectable after 5

TABLE 5. *Dose-response of the* Escherichia coli *bacterial chemotactic factor (BF) on PMN levels of cGMP*

Concentration of BF (%)	Cyclic GMP fmoles/10^6 PMNs	Control (%)
0	21 ± 6	100
5	39 ± 8	186
10	54 ± 11	257
15	38 ± 7	181

Note: Cells preincubated at 37°C for 30 min. A 5-min incubation followed addition of the BF. Each value represents the mean ± SE of 3 incubations with 2 assay tubes per incubation.

min of incubation with the agent; this response peaks at 10 min and persists for at least 30 min. We have also confirmed that zymosan-treated serum and trypsinized human complement elevate cGMP levels in isolated preparations of human PMNs. The increase observed with these complement-derived chemotactic factors is usually significantly higher than that produced by the BF or FMA.

In agreement with Rivkin and co-workers (41), we have seen no effects of these chemoattractants on cellular levels of cAMP.

EFFECTS OF CHEMOTACTIC MODULATORS ON NEUTROPHIL CYCLIC NUCLEOTIDE CONCENTRATIONS

We next examined the effects of several *chemotactic modulators* on PMN cyclic nucleotide levels. As mentioned previously, these agents act to enhance or depress the chemotactic response but do not by themselves initiate chemotaxis.

TABLE 6. *Effect of chemotactic modulators on PMN cyclic-GMP levels*

Agent	Cyclic-GMP fmoles/10^6 PMNs	Control (%)	p
Control	39.2 ± 2.5		
PMA 10 ng/ml	48.6 ± 2.0	124	<0.05
PGF$_{2\alpha}$ 10^{-8} M	55.6 ± 2.0	142	<0.05
Phenylephrine 10^{-4} M	57.2 ± 2.5	146	<0.05

Note: Each value represents the mean ± SEM for 3 incubations with 2 assay tubes per incubation.

In multiple experiments, we have found that phorbol myristate acetate, prostaglandin F$_{2\alpha}$, and phenylephrine, in doses which enhance the chemotactic response, cause a significant increase in PMN cGMP levels (Table 6 shows a representative experiment). The elevation induced by these agents was generally small, however, averaging 25% of the initial level. The time course of the cGMP rise with the enhancing modulators was similar to that seen with the chemoattractants.

In similar studies, the inhibitory modulators isoproterenol and prostaglandin E$_1$ were found to increase PMN cAMP levels significantly (37 to 58% above control). Isoproterenol also acted to increase the level of cGMP in PMNs but the actual femtomole rise was not as great as that seen for cAMP (51 ± 9.1 vs 33 ± 7.8). A similar effect of this agent has been documented in rat heart tissue (1). The fact that isoproterenol depressed chemotaxis (1) while elevating both cAMP and cGMP suggests to us that cGMP effects may be masked when a simultaneous rise in cAMP occurs. Such a phenomenon might aid in explaining the biphasic dose-response curves observed with many of these agents.

EFFECTS OF COMBINATIONS OF CHEMOTACTIC MODULATORS AND CHEMOATTRACTANTS ON PMN cGMP LEVELS

If increases in cAMP and cGMP are important in modulating the chemotactic response, one might expect to see an additive or synergistic effect of chemoattractants and chemotactic modulators on cellular cyclic nucleotide levels. Using 5% BF and the chemotactic modulators listed above, we have found that the effects are less than additive. It is likely, however, that the concentration of BF present at the surface of the migrating PMNs is much less than 5% at the start of the chemotaxis assay. The modulator, which usually is added to the cell side of the chamber or preincubated with the cells, would be present at the cell surface in the predetermined concentration. For this reason, we have performed experiments with low concentrations of the BF (1%) alone and in combination with the chemotactic modulators. Under these conditions, the BF has only minimal effects on cellular cGMP levels. The modulators, however, continue to exert their full effects, and the resulting cGMP levels produced by the combination of modulator and attractant approximate those produced by the modulators alone. These results suggest to us, therefore, that an elevation of cGMP is inherent in the action of the enhancing chemotactic modulators. An increase in cAMP, with or without an increase in cGMP, results from stimulation with the inhibitory modulators. Since all the chemoattractants studied thus far also have an effect on PMN cGMP levels, it appears that the modulators exert their effects when the concentration of chemoattractant at the cell surface is minimal (i.e., has little effect on cellular cGMP). This may explain why other investigators have observed a more pronounced modulator effect when a less potent chemotactic stimulus is used (42). I might add that this is why we have routinely used the BF, which has an intermediate level of chemotactic activity, rather than the strong attractants produced by endotoxin or zymosan activation of serum.

MECHANISM OF CYCLIC NUCLEOTIDE MODULATION OF CHEMOTAXIS

Although there are a number of studies reported in the literature on the effects of cGMP and cAMP on leukocyte function, few have been designed to determine the mechanisms of action of these agents. In fact, the complete mechanism has been worked out for cAMP in only one system, that of glycogen metabolism. Adenylate cyclase catalyzes the synthesis of cAMP from ATP, and this substance, in turn, activates a family of similar enzymes termed *protein kinases*. Other enzymes, including phosphorylase kinase, are also phosphorylated. These activated enzymes are capable of phosphorylating a number of other proteins, including, perhaps, those in microtubular elements and contractile tissues. The mechanism of action of cGMP is even more poorly understood, but there is recent evidence of protein kinases which preferentially respond to this cyclic nucleotide rather than cAMP. Calcium, also, probably has a major role in the modulatory effects of cGMP and cAMP and in actually initiating cell movement. Becker and Showell (3) and we (12) have shown that chemotactic responsiveness is partially dependent upon the concentration of calcium and magnesium in the surrounding medium. Boucek and Snyderman (4) have reported that exposure of PMNs to chemotactic factors results in an influx of calcium. Gallin and Rosenthal (13) observed that exposure of PMNs to C5a results in an increase in pseudopod formation and appearance of microtubular structures when a gradient is present. Weissmann et al. (49) observed similar changes in PMNs exposed to zymosan-treated serum. In addition, they found that exposure of cells to cAMP depressed microtubular formation, while cGMP enhanced the appearance of these structures. The mechanism by which such agents cause these cellular morphologic and functional changes is unknown. The results above, combined with the fact that microtubular protein is a natural substrate for protein kinase, suggest that cyclic nucleotides exert their effect on the microtubular system. Cyclic GMP may, therefore, affect microtubular and/or microfilament function, enhancing both random and directed motility, while cAMP inhibits these same processes. Chemotactic factors, by increasing cGMP levels, may act to specifically stabilize certain microtubular elements, resulting in a net vector of motion, as suggested by Gallin and Rosenthal (13). Potent chemoattractants should, therefore, be capable of (a) initiating cell movement, perhaps through an effect on calcium flux, and (b) increasing cellular cGMP levels. Enhancing modulators should be capable of increasing cGMP levels but have no effect to initiate chemotaxis (i.e., have no effect on calcium flux), while inhibitory modulators should elevate cellular cAMP.

FUNCTIONAL GRANULOCYTE ABNORMALITIES SECONDARY TO ALTERED CYCLIC NUCLEOTIDE METABOLISM

A number of patients have recently been described with abnormalities of the cellular components of the inflammatory reaction. Enhanced PMN chemotactic responses have been found in otherwise healthy persons with cutaneous (25), pulmonary (30), and systemic bacterial infections (23). In contrast, depressed function has been observed in a number of patients including those with (a) diabetes mellitus (29,36,37); (b) hyperimmunoglobulinemia E associated with eczema (26,27,28); (c) allergic disease such as allergic rhinitis or urticaria without extreme hyperimmunoglobulinemia E (21,31); and (d) in patients with Chediak-Higashi syndrome (7,10). The mechanism of altered leukocyte function in these patients is unknown. There are, however, several observations which suggest that the absolute level or the relative proportions of cellular cAMP and cGMP are altered in these patients. Recently, we have studied the leukocytes in a patient with chronic cutaneous infection who had a hyperactive chemotactic response. The concentration of cGMP in the patient's PMNs was fourfold higher than that of controls. Circulatory factors produced by the patient's own immune

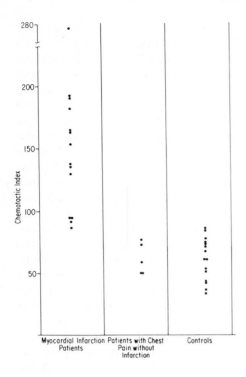

FIG. 1. Chemotactic responses of neutrophils from patients with myocardial infarction and controls.

system or the actively metabolizing, infecting bacteria may have altered this patient's cyclic nucleotide levels.

Chapman (9), working in my laboratory, has recently observed that the PMNs from 11 of 14 patients with myocardial infarction were hyperactive in their response to chemotactic stimulation (Fig. 1). The remaining patients with normal to depressed activity were suffering from shock or congestive heart failure at the time of chemotactic testing. The hyperactive response of the uncomplicated myocardial infarction patient's PMNs persisted for 14 days but had decreased to normal levels in 1- to 3-month follow-up specimens. A serum enhancer of chemotaxis could not be detected, suggesting a labile mediator of this response. Recently, George et al. (14) have shown in experimental animals that hypoxia and ischemia elevate myocardial levels of cGMP and increase lysosomal enzyme release. Such a mechanism might possibly explain the chemotactic enhancement observed. Additional studies are underway to determine cyclic nucleotide levels in the PMNs of such patients.

Patients with diabetes mellitus may also have depressed PMN chemotactic function as a result of an imbalance in the levels of cAMP and cGMP. Insulin is capable of enhancing the depressed response of diabetic PMNs (29,36,37). We have observed this effect even in the absence of glucose, suggesting a direct pharmacologic effect of insulin on the PMN. Insulin has been shown to raise

TABLE 7. *Effect of insulin and cyclic-GMP on a diabetic patient's (H.W.) PMN chemotactic responses to BF*

Cells	Agent tested[a]	Chemotactic index
H.W.	Medium 199	33
H.W.	Insulin 100µU	60
H.W.	cGMP 10^{-7} M	56

[a] Added to cell side of chamber during 3-hr assay.

cellular cGMP in lymphocytes (46). Moreover, we have found that incubation of diabetic PMNs with cGMP increases their directional movement toward a chemotactic stimulus in a manner similar to that of insulin (Table 7).

The mechanism of defective PMN chemotactic responses in patients with allergic disease with or without hyperimmunoglobulinemia E also remains obscure. Rivkin and Becker (40) and we (22) have found that histamine inhibits chemotaxis. Bourne et al. (6) have shown that histamine causes accumulation of cAMP in PMNs. Recently Busse and Sosman (8) have confirmed this finding and indicated that the response is mediated through a histamine H_2 receptor on the surface of the PMN. These authors also showed that histamine alters lysosomal enzyme release. These findings, along with the fact that burimamide, a H_2 histamine blocking agent, and levamisole, a drug which alters cellular cAMP and cGMP ratios, improve chemotactic function in some of these patients (2,21,32), suggest a role for cyclic nucleotides in the pathogenesis of this common chemotactic deficiency syndrome.

Recently, Oliver and Zurier (38) and Boxer and co-workers (7) have provided direct evidence for a role of cyclic nucleotides in the leukocyte abnormalities associated with Chediak-Higashi syndrome. Abnormal concanavallin A cap formation, as well as granule formation by the PMNs from both human subjects and an experimental animal model with this syndrome, was corrected by incubation with cGMP and cholinergic agonist. In addition, a patient with the disease was found to have abnormally high concentrations of cAMP in his PMNs (7). Neutrophil degranulation and chemotaxis in this patient dramatically improved after *in vivo* treatment with ascorbate. Clinical improvement was associated with a decrease in cAMP levels in the PMNs of this individual.

The patients reviewed above suggest the clinical importance of altered cyclic nucleotide metabolism in altered inflammatory states. More importantly, the limited investigations indicating that drugs such as ascorbate, burimamide, and levamisole may reverse functional abnormalities *in vitro* and *in vivo* suggest the possibility of pharmacologic modification of the inflammatory response.

ACKNOWLEDGMENTS

I wish to thank Drs. Paul G. Quie, Richard D. Estenson, and Nelson D. Goldberg, who participated in the initial studies on cyclic GMP and modulation of neutrophil chemotaxis, and Drs. Gary E. Hatch, William K. Nichols, and Hal Chapman who have worked on subsequent *in vitro* and clinical studies. I also thank Nancy A. Hogan and Mary R. Portas for technical assistance, and Oliva Hoyt and Patti Lorenz for secretarial aid.

This work was supported in part by United States Public Health Service grants AM 18354 and AI 13150.

Dr. Hill is an investigator of the Howard Hughes Medical Institute.

REFERENCES

1. Amer, M. S., and Byrne, J. E. (1975): Interchange of adenyl and guanyl cyclases as an explanation for transformation of beta to alpha adrenergic responses in the rat atrium. *Nature,* 256:421–424.
2. Anderson, R., Glover, A., Koornhof, H. S., and Rabson, A. R. (1976): In vitro stimulation of neutrophil motility by levamisole: Maintenance of cGMP levels in chemotactically stimulated levamisole-treated neutrophils. *J. Immunol.,* 117:428–432.
3. Becker, E. L., and Showell, H. J. (1972): The effect of Ca^{2+} and Mg^{2+} on the chemotactic responsiveness and spontaneous motility of rabbit polymorphonuclear leukocytes. *Z. Immunitaetsforsch.,* 143:466–476.
4. Boucek, M. M., and Snyderman, R. (1976): Calcium influx requirement for human neutrophil chemotaxis: Inhibition by lanthanum chloride. *Science,* 193:905–907.
5. Bourne, H. R., Lichtenstein, L. M., Melmon, K. L., Henney, C. S., Weinstein, Y., and Shearer, G. M. (1974): Modulation of inflammation and immunity by cyclic AMP. *Science,* 184:19–28.
6. Bourne, H. R., Melmon, K. L., and Lichtenstein, L. M. (1971): Histamine augments leukocyte adenosine 3'5'-monophosphate and blocks antigenic histamine release. *Science,* 173:743–745.
7. Boxer, L. A., Watanabe, A. M., Rister, M., Besch, H. R., Jr., Allen, J., and Bachner, R. L. (1976): Correction of leukocyte function in Chediak-Higashi syndrome by ascorbate. *N. Engl. J. Med.,* 295:1041–1045.
8. Busse, W. W., and Sosman, J. (1976): Histamine inhibition of neutrophil lysosomal enzyme release: An H_2 histamine receptor response. *Science,* 194:737–738.
9. Chapman, H. A., and Hill, H. R. (1976): Enhanced neutrophil chemotactic responses following myocardial infarction. *Clin. Res.,* 24:445A.
10. Clark, R. A., and Kimball, H. R. (1971): Defective granulocyte chemotaxis in the Chediak-Higashi syndrome. *J. Clin. Invest.* 50:2645–2652.
11. Estensen, R. D., Hill, H. R., Quie, P. G., Hogan, N. A., and Goldberg, N. D. (1973): Cyclic GMP and cell movement. *Nature,* 245:458–460.
12. Estensen, R. D., Reusch, M. E., Epstein, M. L., and Hill, H. R. (1976): Role of Ca^{++} and Mg^{++} in some human neutrophil functions as indicated by ionophore A23187. *Infect. Immun.,* 13:146–151.
13. Gallin, J. I., and Rosenthal, A. S. (1974): The regulatory role of divalent cations in human granulocyte chemotaxis: Evidence for an association between calcium exchanges and microtubule assembly. *J. Cell. Biol.,* 62:594–609.
14. George, W. J., Busuttil, R. W., and Ignarro, L. J. (1975): Reduction of myocardial cyclic GMP content as a possible mechanism for protection of the hypoxic heart by methylprednisolone. *Pharmacology,* 17:269.
15. Goetzl, E. J., Wasserman, S. I., Gigli, I., and Austen, K. F. (1974): Enhancement of random migration and chemotactic response of human leukocytes by ascorbic acid. *J. Clin. Invest.,* 53:813–818.
16. Goldberg, N. D. (1975): Cyclic nucleotides and cell function. In: *Cell Membranes, Biochemistry, Cell Biology and Pathology,* edited by G. Weissmann and R. Claiborne, pp. 185–201. H. P. Publishing Co., New York.
17. Goldberg, N. D., Haddox, M. K., Hartle, D. K., and Hadden, J. W. (1972): The biological role of cyclic 3'5'-guanosine monophosphate. *Proc. 5th Int. Congr. Pharm.,* 5:146–169.
18. Goldberg, N. D., Haddox, M. K., Nicol, S. E., Glass, D. B., Sanford, C. H., Kuehl, F. A.,

Jr., and Estensen, R. (1975): Biologic regulation through opposing influences of cyclic GMP and cyclic AMP: The Yin Yang hypothesis. In: *Advances in Cyclic Nucleotide Research,* edited by G. I. Drummond, P. Greengard, and G. A. Robison, pp. 307–330. Raven Press, New York.

19. Hatch, G. E., Nichols, W. K., and Hill, H. R. (1976): A simplified procedure for cyclic nucleotide radioimmunossay and its application to human blood leukocytes. Submitted for publication.

20. Hatch, G. E., Nichols, W. K., and Hill, H. R. (1976): Cyclic nucleotide changes in human neutrophils induced by chemoattractants and chemotactic modulators. *J. Immunol.,* 119:450–456, 1977.

21. Hill, H. R., Estensen, R. D., Hogan, N. A., and Quie, P. G. (1976): Severe staphylococcal disease associated with allergic manifestations, hyperimmunoglobulinemia E, and defective neutrophil chemotaxis. *J. Lab. Clin. Med.,* 88:796–806.

22. Hill, H. R., Estensen, R. D., Quie, P. G., Hogan, N. A., and Goldberg, N. D. (1975): Modulation of human neutrophil chemotactic responses by cyclic 3'5' guanosine monophosphate and cyclic 3'5' adenosine monophosphate. *Metabolism,* 24:447–456.

23. Hill, H. R., Gerrard, J., Hogan, N. A., and Quie, P. G. (1974): Hyperactivity of neutrophil leukotactic responses during active bacterial infection. *J. Clin. Invest.,* 53:996–1002.

24. Hill, H. R., Hogan, N. A., Mitchell, T. G., and Quie, P. G. (1975): Evaluation of a cytocentrifuge method for measuring neutrophil granulocyte chemotaxis. *J. Lab. Clin. Med.,* 86:703–710.

25. Hill, H. R., Kaplan, E. L., Dajani, A., Wannamaker, L. W., and Quie, P. G. (1974): Leukotactic activity and reduction of nitroblue tetrazolium by neutrophil granulocytes from patients with streptococcal skin infection. *J. Infect. Dis.,* 129:322–326.

26. Hill, H. R., and Quie, P. G. (1974): Raised serum-IgE levels and defective neutrophil chemotaxis in three children with eczema and recurrent bacterial infections. *Lancet,* 1:183–187.

27. Hill, H. R., and Quie, P. G. (1975): Defective neutrophil chemotaxis associated with hyperimmunoglobulinemia E. In: *The Phagocytic Cell in Host Resistance,* edited by J. A. Bellanti, and D. H. Dayton, pp. 249–266. Raven Press, New York.

28. Hill, H. R., Quie, P. G., Pabst, H. F., Ochs, H. D., Clark, R. A., Klebanoff, S. J., and Wedgwood, R. J. (1974): Defect in neutrophil granulocyte chemotaxis in Job's syndrome of recurrent "cold" staphylococcal abscesses. *Lancet,* 2:617–619.

29. Hill, H. R., Sauls, H. S., Dettloff, J. L., and Quie, P. G. (1974): Impaired leukotactic responsiveness in patients with juvenile diabetes mellitus. *Clin. Immunol. Immunopathol.,* 2:395–403.

30. Hill, H. R., Warwick, W. J., Dettloff, J., and Quie, P. G. (1974): Neutrophil granulocyte function in patients with pulmonary infections. *J. Pediatr.,* 84:55–58.

31. Hill, H. R., Williams, P. B., Krueger, G. G., and Janis, B. (1976): Recurrent staphylococcal abscesses associated with defective neutrophil chemotaxis and allergic rhinitis. *Ann. Intern. Med.,* 85:39–43.

32. Hogan, N. A., and Hill, H. R. (1977): Levamisole enhances PMN chemotaxis and elevates cellular cGMP. *Clin. Res.,* 25:181A.

33. Ignarro, L. J., and George, W. J. (1974): Hormonal control of lysosomal enzyme release from human neutrophils: Evaluation of cyclic nucleotide levels by autonomic neurohormones. *Proc. Natl. Acad. Sci. U.S.A.,* 71:2027–2031.

34. Ignarro, L. J., Lint, T. F., and George, W. J. (1974): Hormonal control of lysosomal enzyme release from human neutrophils: Effects of autonomic agents on enzyme release, phagocytosis, and cyclic nucleotides. *J. Exp. Med.,* 139:1395–1414.

35. McCall, C. E., Caves, J., Cooper, R., and DeChatelet, L. (1972): Functional characteristics of human toxic neutrophils. *J. Infect. Dis.,* 135:376–387.

36. Miller, M. E., and Baker, L. (1972): Leukocyte functions in juvenile diabetes mellitus: Humoral and cellular aspects. *J. Pediatr.,* 81:979–982.

37. Mowat, A. G., and Baum, J. (1971): Chemotaxis of polymorphonuclear leukocytes from patients with diabetes mellitus. *N. Engl. J. Med.,* 284:621–627.

38. Oliver, J. M., and Zurier, R. B. (1976): Correction of characteristic abnormalities of microtubule function and granule morphology in Chediak-Higashi syndrome with cholinergic agonists. *J. Clin. Invest.,* 1239–1247.

39. Parker, C. W., Sullivan, T. J., and Wedner, H. J. (1974): Cyclic AMP and the immune response. In: *Advances in Cyclic Nucleotides, Vol. 4,* edited by P. Greengard and G. A. Robison, pp. 1–79. Raven Press, New York.

40. Rivkin, I., and Becker, E. L. (1972): Possible implication of cyclic 3'5'-adenosine monophosphate in the chemotaxis of rabbit peritoneal polymorphonuclear leukocytes. *Fed. Proc.,* 31:657.

41. Rivkin, I., Rosenblatt, J., and Becker, E. L. (1975): The role of cyclic AMP in the chemotactic responsiveness and spontaneous motility of rabbit peritoneal neutrophils. *J. Immunol.,* 115:1126–1134.
42. Sandler, J. A., Gallin, J. I., and Vaughan, M. (1975): Effects of serotonin, carbamylcholine, and ascorbic acid on leukocyte cyclic GMP and chemotaxis. *J. Cell Biol.,* 67:480–484.
43. Sandoval, I. V., and Cuatrecasas, P. (1976): Opposing effects of cyclic AMP and cyclic GMP on protein phosphorylation in tubulin preparations. *Nature,* 262:511–513.
44. Schiffmann, E., Corcoran, B. A., and Wahl, S. M. (1975): N-formylmethionyl peptides as chemoattractants for leukocytes. *Proc. Natl. Acad. Sci. U.S.A.,* 72:1059–1062.
45. Schreiner, G. F., and Unanue, E. R. (1975): The modulation of spontaneous and anti-Ig-stimulated motility of lymphocytes by cyclic nucleotides and adrenergic and cholinergic agents. *J. Immunol.,* 114:803–808.
46. Strom, T. B., Bear, R. A., and Carpenter, C. B. (1975): Insulin-induced augmentation of lymphocyte-mediated cytotoxicity. *Science,* 187:1206–1208.
47. Tse, R. L., Phelps, P., and Urban, D. (1972): Polymorphonuclear leukocyte motility in vitro: VI. Effect of purine and pyrimidine analogues: Possible role of cyclic AMP. *J. Lab. Clin. Med.,* 80:264–274.
48. Ward, P. A., Lepow, I. H., and Newman, L. J. (1968): Bacterial factors chemotactic for polymorphonuclear leukocytes. *Am. J. Pathol.,* 52:725–736.
49. Weissman, G., Goldstein, I., Hoffstein, S., and Tsung, P. (1975): Reciprocal effects of cAMP and cGMP on microtubule-dependent release of lysosomal enzymes. *Ann. N.Y. Acad. Sci.,* 253:750–762.
50. Zurier, R. B., Weissmann, G., Hoffstein, S., Kammerman, S., and Hsiung Tai, H. (1974): Mechanism of lysosomal enzyme release from human leukocytes: II. Effects of cAMP and cGMP, autonomic agonists, and agents which affect microtubule function. *J. Clin. Invest.,* 53:297–309.

DISCUSSION

Dr. Becker: As you know, Dr. Hill, we have previously studied the effect of bacterial factor and C5 fragment on levels of cyclic-AMP in rabbit peritoneal neutrophils and found no effect. It is interesting that you were able to demonstrate changes in cyclic-AMP with isoproterenol. Were there changes in cyclic-GMP levels at those concentrations or at different concentrations?

Dr. Hill: I must admit that we have not looked at a number of different concentrations. We have just completed the development of this assay and have not had a chance to examine each one of the modulators at the various concentrations. We selected the concentrations that had the most profound effects on chemotaxis.

Dr. Ward: It is interesting that bacterial factor added to your phagocytosis system increases chemiluminescence. Was there an effect on rate or extent of phagocytosis?

Dr. Hill: The particle-phagocyte ratio was so high that it was difficult to evaluate phagocytosis. However, as you recall, bacterial factor brought about an increase in chemiluminescence even though phagocytosis is blocked. Chemotactic factor must act on an ectoenzyme system which stimulates chemotaxis and enhances chemiluminescence.

Dr. Gallin: From your time course of the effect of the chemotactic factor on elevation of cyclic-GMP, if I understood it correctly, it takes about 10 min until you see your maximum effects. Why do you think it takes so long to get that effect when we assume that locomotion starts very soon after interaction with the stimulus? Did you look at the ability of your cells to migrate after 10 min in the chemotactic factor? Also, if cyclic nucleotides are involved directly in the locomotion process, there might be local changes in cyclic nucleotides in the front and back sides of the cell. Is there any evidence for localized cyclic nucleotide changes within the cell?

Dr. Hill: Dr. Gallin, all I can say is that in most other tissues that have been examined, it has taken approximately 5 to 10 min for modulators to affect cyclic-GMP. The way we routinely perform chemotactic experiments is to add the modulator to the top of the chambers and incubate with chemotactic factor below. We have done some preincubation experiments in which we incubated the agent and the cell for 10 min, then washed them gently and put them into the assay system, and they were still markedly enhanced in chemotactic responsiveness.

Dr. Schiffmann: Dr. Hill, with respect to what Dr. Gallin said, did you include inhibitors of phosphodiesterase in one of your assays? This may permit detection of early, rapid increases in levels of cyclic nucleotides. It also may be important to see whether or not some of the modulators themselves may actually stimulate phosphodiesterase activity.

With respect to the biphasic effect of isoproterenol, you may be aware that Nirenberg and Klee have shown that opiates cause an immediate depression of adenylcyclase activity followed by a longer-term tolerance phenomenon during which intrinsic adenylcyclase is increased. It would be interesting to see if opiates could, in a sense, dissect the biphasic effect of isoproterenol and allow cyclic-GMP to be raised, thereby enhancing chemotaxis.

Dr. Hill: We tried opiates and morphine and have seen enhanced chemotactic responses and changes in cyclic nucleotide levels in preliminary experiments.

Dr. Wright: Dr. Hill, I was very interested to see your results with levamisole. Drs. Gallin, Charles Kirkpatrick, and I have had an opportunity to study a number of hyperimmunoglobulin E patients at the NIH, and to examine the chemotactic responses of both their mononuclear cells and neutrophils after treatment with levamisole. We found, as you did, that there were increased chemotactic responses by cells from these patients after the patients had taken levamisole (300 mg over 2 days). It was a consistent finding. In addition, we could show that those concentrations of levamisole which stimulate leukocyte migration *in vitro* also increased cyclic-GMP levels.

Dr. Nelson: I would like to return to your observation that addition of bacterial factor to the assay for measurement of neutrophil chemiluminescence augmented this leukocyte function. Bacterial factor may not influence leukocyte function. We have recently observed that addition of certain amino acids or soluble proteins can augment chemiluminescence by serving as a substrate for secondary light-producing reactions by activated forms of oxygen. Bacterial factor may be a similar substrate in your experiments.

Leukocyte Chemotaxis, edited by John I. Gallin
and Paul G. Quie. Raven Press, New York
© 1978.

The Nature of Histamine Control of Eosinophil Localization

*Richard A. F. Clark, John I. Gallin, and Allen P. Kaplan

Allergic Diseases Section, and Clinical Physiology Section, National Institute of Allergy and Infectious Diseases, National Institutes of Health, Bethesda, Maryland 20014

Both systemic and localized eosinophilia are initiated and modulated at several different levels including cell maturation, bone marrow release, endothelial adherence, and tissue translocation, of which only the last has been under intensive investigation (6). From the studies of *in vitro* eosinophil migration recently published, it appears that multiple factors initiate and modulate eosinophil movement; these mediators probably vary *in vivo*, depending on the initiating stimulus (Table 1). Parasitic infections, which are noted for their ability to stimulate massive local and systemic eosinophilia, ostensibly initiate this phenomenon through the activation of both immediate and delayed hypersensitivity reactions and the complement pathways (28). In the other disorders listed in Table 1, eosinophils are most likely mobilized by more limited mechanisms; that is, in allergic asthma and rhinitis, eosinophils are attracted by mediators released by basophils and mast cells through specific immediate hypersensitivity reactions, while in vesiculobullous diseases and atopic eczema, combinations of basophil and mast cell-associated mediators, complement pathway products, and/or lymphokines derived from cell-mediated immunity may each affect the eosinophil influx.

EOSINOPHIL LOCALIZATION

At least two lymphokines that effect eosinophil localization are released in cell-mediated immunity reactions induced by specific antigens. One factor called eosinophil stimulation promotor (ESP) (9) can be released from sensitized mouse T cells (17) by *Schistosoma mansoni* antigen, and it enhances the migration of mouse eosinophils out of an agarose microdroplet (4). The other lymphokine, when incubated with specific immune complexes, generates a potent eosinophil chemotactic factor (8). Products of complement activation, C5a and the $C\overline{567}$ complex, were shown initially to be chemotactic for neutrophils (37,38) but were subsequently shown to be chemotactic for eosinophils by Ward (36) and Kay (19). These studies suggested that the eosinophil responded to comple-

---

* Present Address: Massachusetts General Hospital, Department of Dermatology, Boston, Massachusetts 02114

TABLE 1. *Presumed mechanisms for eosinophil localization* in vivo

Representative disorders with tissue eosinophilia	Putative eosinophilia localization factors
Parasitic infections	ESP, histamine, ECF-A, C5a, and lymphokine-antigen complex
Allergic asthma and rhinitis	Histamine and ECF-A
Vesiculobullous diseases	C5a, histamine and ECF-A
Atopic dermatitis	?Lymphokine-antigen complex, histamine, and ECF-A

ment products in exactly the same way as the neutrophil. The products derived from cell-mediated immune reactions and complement activation are important in defining those factors that promote eosinophil localization but they do not explain the selective accumulation of eosinophils listed in Table 1 nor do they elucidate how eosinophil movement is modulated.

Kay, Stechschulte, and Austen (21), in 1971, showed that when actively or passively sensitized guinea pig lung was challenged with specific antigen, the lung diffusate was selectively chemotactic for guinea pig peritoneal eosinophils. This eosinophil chemotactic factor of anaphylaxis (ECF-A) had a molecular weight of approximately 500 daltons, as estimated by G25 Sephadex gel filtration, and was subsequently purified from human lung tissue and synthesized by Goetzl and Austen (16). The latter article demonstrated that ECF-A consists of two tetrapeptides which, although not selective for the eosinophil, do cause a preferential migration of eosinophils from a mixed leukocyte population, and, furthermore, effect a preferential deactivation of eosinophils. Additional studies have demonstrated that similar if not identical substances can be released as a result of the interaction of human IgE immunoglobulin and antigen utilizing sensitized human lung fragments (20), or nasal polyps (18); can be extracted from a human lung tumor associated with eosinophilia (39); can be liberated from human leukemic basophils by calcium ionophore (24); and, finally, can be released from human neutrophils by calcium ionophore (11) or during phagocytosis (23). Whether all these substances are identical to the two tetrapeptides delineated by Goetzl and Austen (17) must await further studies; however, the unique occurrence of eosinophil chemotactic factors (ECF) in immediate hypersensitivity reactions is no longer tenable, and it would seem that ECF might be released from neutrophils in a host of acute inflammatory reactions that are not characterized by eosinophilia. Thus, we return to the question of how selective tissue accumulation of eosinophils occurs. We have found that histamine is one factor that possesses selective eosinophil chemotactic activity and, furthermore, modulates eosinophil movement by three different means, as described below.

THE SELECTIVE EOSINOPHIL CHEMOTACTIC ACTIVITY OF HISTAMINE

Since Dale (12) first described histamine as a mediator of the immediate hypersensitivity reaction complex, there has been considerable interest in whether histamine produces eosinophilia, either locally or systemically. *In vivo* studies by several investigators demonstrated that histamine induces local eosinophilia (1,14,22,35); however, others had noted that histamine induces systemic eosinophilia but not local eosinophilia (29,33,34). Meanwhile, *in vitro* studies, until our recent report (4), had failed to demonstrate an effect of histamine upon eosinophil migration (10,21,30). Our finding that histamine was a *selective* eosinophil chemotactic factor happened quite fortuitously while we were looking for ECF-A activity in the supernatant from the incubation of human leukemic basophils and rabbit anti-human IgE. This supernatant demonstrated preferential eosinophil chemotactic activity; however, when increasing volumes of the mediator supernatant were assayed for histamine, slow-reacting substance of anaphylaxis (SRS-A), platelet-activating factor (PAF), and ECF-A activity in parallel, the eosinophil migration was diminished at higher concentrations of mediator supernatant, while histamine, SRS-A, and PAF activities showed no diminution at higher concentrations (5). Thus, it appeared that an inhibitor of eosinophil chemotaxis was interfering with the assay. Furthermore, upon fractionation of this material over G25 Sephadex gel filtration columns, a double peak of eosinophil chemotactic activity was observed (Fig. 1). The initial peak along the upstroke of the histamine activity was located at the approximate position of ECF-A, as previously reported (21), but the second peak along the downstroke of the histamine had not been reported previously (5). Since the nadir between the two peaks of chemotactic activity corresponded to the apex of the histamine peak, we considered the possibility that histamine, in high concentrations, was

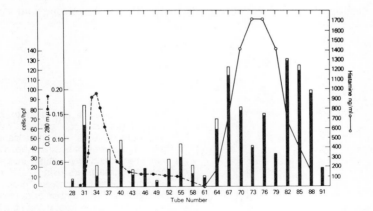

FIG. 1. Sephadex G25 gel filtration of the reaction supernatant from human leukemic basophils incubated with a 1/2,000 dilution of rabbit antihuman IgE antibody. The major protein (O.D. 280) peak occurred at the elution volume and therefore was excluded from the column (720,000 mol. wt.). The histograms represent chemotaxis (cells/hpf) of a mixed leukocyte population (60% eosinophils, 40% neutrophils). Eosinophils/hpf are represented by the height of the solid portion of the histogram and neutrophils per hpf are shown by the upper open portion of the histogram. (From Clark et al., ref. 5, with permission.)

the inhibitor of our chemotaxis assay. We therefore pooled the gel filtration fractions from the first chemotactic peak through the second chemotactic peak, concentrated the pool by lyophilization, and incubated the concentrate with diamine oxidase (histaminase) to destroy the histamine (5). Instead of abrogating the inhibition of chemotaxis, this enzymatic reaction destroyed virtually all the eosinophil chemotactic activity. Trypsin, chymotrypsin, and subtilisin had no effect on this chemotactic activity, while pronase effected a small reduction in activity (5). This set of experiments was our first evidence that histamine was not only an inhibitor of eosinophil chemotaxis but at the appropriate concentrations an eosinophil chemotactic factor itself.

To elucidate further the activity of histamine on eosinophil chemotaxis, we simplified our system by utilizing purified histamine diphosphate in our assays. In the first series of experiments, we delineated the selectivity of histamine for the eosinophil and the dose response on eosinophil migration (Fig. 2). The assay for these experiments was performed by visual inspection of polycarbonate filters using 2.3×10^6 granulocytes/ml with increasing proportions of eosinophils on the cell side of modified Boyden chambers and 10^{-8}, 10^{-7}, 10^{-6}, 10^{-5}, 10^{-4} M histamine or buffer on the stimulus side of the chamber (4).

As shown in Fig. 2, histamine was absolutely selective for the eosinophil; that is, the chemotactic response varied directly with the density of eosinophils used, and there was no migration of neutrophils to any dose of histamine. The striking dependence of eosinophil chemotaxis upon the percentage of eosinophils in the final preparation might be an inhibiting effect of the contaminating neutrophils upon eosinophil movement or might be merely a function of the absolute eosinophil count. Therefore, we assayed a cell preparation, containing 93% eosinophils and 7% neutrophils, with 10^{-6} M histamine and compared

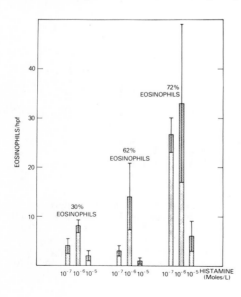

FIG. 2. Eosinophil migration to histamine using Hypaque-Ficoll purified eosinophil-neutrophil mixtures from three patients with differing degrees of eosinophilia. The assay was performed by visual inspection of polycarbonate filters using 2.3×10^6 granulocytes/ml with increasing proportions of eosinophils. The number of neutrophils migrating was never greater than background. (From Clark et al., ref. 4, with permission.)

the resultant eosinophil migration to the eosinophil migration obtained when these cells were mixed 1:1 with a cell preparation containing 95% neutrophils and 5% eosinophils which had no detectable eosinophil chemotaxis. The mixture, which had 49% eosinophils, had half the response of the preparation containing 93% eosinophils. Thus, no inhibitory effect of neutrophils upon eosinophils or upon eosinophil chemotaxis was observed, since the amount of migration was directly proportional to the absolute eosinophil count.

The dose response of histamine on eosinophil migration in these same experiments consistently showed maximal eosinophil migration in 10^{-6} M histamine with a diminution of migration to 10^{-5} M or higher concentrations of histamine (Fig. 2). A possible explanation for the diminution in response at higher concentrations of histamine was that the cells were falling off the filter. A modification of the ^{51}Cr radioassay for neutrophil chemotaxis, as described by Gallin et al. (15), was therefore utilized. A 5 μm pore 12 μm thick polycarbonate filter was inserted on top of a 3 μm pore, 145 μm thick cellulose nitrate filter in order to assess cell migration. Figure 3 demonstrates that the diminution of eosinophil migration to higher doses of histamine is apparent whether counting ^{51}Cr-labeled cells by counts per minute in the lower cellulose nitrate filter or morphologic inspection of the upper polycarbonate filter (4). Since the 1 hr incubation used in this modified technique does not allow the cells to migrate through the second filter, the decrease in eosinophil migration seen at higher doses cannot be attributable to cells falling off the filter. Figure 3 also demonstrates that when equal concentrations of histamine were placed on each side of the Boyden chamber, the eosinophil migration response was no greater than background, thus indicating that the increase in eosinophil migration seen with histamine on the stimulus side of the filter was a result of true chemotactic

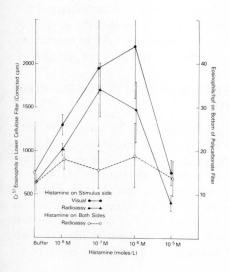

FIG. 3. Chemotactic dose-response curves of eosinophils to histamine expressed in counts per min (cpm) of ^{51}Cr-labeled cells in the lower cellulose intrate filters and in cells per hpf of eosinophils that had migrated through to the lower surface of the upper polycarbonate filter. A flat response by the ^{51}Cr radioassay was obtained when histamine was placed on both sides of the filters. Points at each concentration were shifted slightly to demonstrate the standard error more clearly. (From Clark et al., ref. 4, with permission.)

activity and not simply activated random migration. Final proof that histamine was the selective chemotactic factor for eosinophils came from the demonstration that histamine produced enzymatically from histidine possessed chemotactic activity (4).

THE NONHOMOGENEITY OF EOSINOPHILS

The specificity of histamine-stimulated chemotaxis for the eosinophil, the dose response of histamine chemotactic activity, and the minimal ability of histamine to increase eosinophil random migration were all confirmed by using the assay described by Zigmond and Hirsch (40). In this assay, 3 μm pore, 145 μm thick cellulose nitrate filters were used and incubated in Boyden chambers for 30 to 60 min so as not to allow the cells sufficient time to migrate across the entire filter thickness. Cells were counted at different levels in the filters by focusing with a microscope micrometer to the desired levels. Histamine 10^{-6} M on the stimulus side increased the number of eosinophils observed throughout the filter, while histamine 10^{-6} M placed on both sides of the filter yielded no increase in cell number over background, again indicating that histamine was a chemotactic factor; however, histamine caused no en masse movement into the filter (4), as expected for a chemotactic factor (40). This phenomenon, however, was a function of the eosinophils and not an attribute of histamine, as shown by the fact that when C5a was used as the chemotactic factor, eosinophil did *not* move en masse into the filter, while neutrophils did. Since the expectation that eosinophils move en masse into the filter under the influence of a chemotactic gradient comes from the assumption that they move as a homogeneous population (40), this hypothesis was tested by plotting $\log_e$ eosinophils/hpf against the square of the distance that the eosinophils had migrated using histamine or C5a as the chemotactic stimulus. The migration of a homogeneous population of cells would plot as a straight line (40); however, this was not obtained for the eosinophils. This is consistent with previous observations that the eosinophil is a long-lived recirculating cell (13) and, therefore, less likely to be homogeneous when compared to the neutrophil, which is short-lived and does not recirculate.

EFFECT OF H_1 AND H_2 RECEPTOR ANTAGONISTS ON EOSINOPHIL MIGRATION

Histamine exerts physiologic and pharmacologic effects by interaction with at least two different groups of receptors. The H_1 receptors mediate the action of histamine on the smooth muscle of the gastrointestinal tract and bronchi, and these effects are reversibly blocked by classic antihistamines (2) such as diphenhydramine, mepyramine, and their analogs. In contrast, the action of histamine on the gastric parietal cell, on the guinea pig atria, and on the rat uterus is not inhibited by the classic antihistamines, but it is reversibly blocked by the thiourea analogs of histamine, burimamide, and metiamide (3). This second series of histamine receptors have been designated the H_2 receptor. More

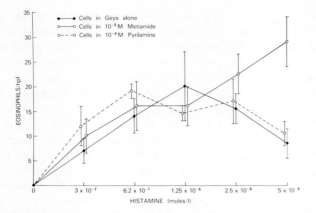

FIG. 4. Chemotactic dose-response curves of eosinophils to histamine in the presence and absence of 10^{-5} M metiamide and 10^{-5} M pyrilamine.

recently histamine has been shown to inhibit its own release (25), inhibit the cytotoxicity of T cells (31), decrease the number of antibody-forming cells (27), inhibit enzyme release from human polymorphonuclear leukocytes (41), and inhibit delayed hypersensitivity skin tests, including antigen-induced thymidine uptake and migration inhibitory factor (MIF) production (32). These inhibitory effects appear to be mediated through the H_2 receptor. As previously discussed, the dose response of histamine for eosinophil chemotaxis consistently showed a maximum response at 10^{-6} M histamine. As shown in Fig. 4, when the single polycarbonate filter chemotactic assay was used, a linear dose response was seen from 3×10^{-7} M to 1.25×10^{-6} M histamine; however, at higher histamine concentrations, the chemotactic response was markedly depressed. When 10^{-5} M mepyramine maleate, an H_1-receptor antagonist, was placed on the cell side of the chamber, the chemotactic activity was not significantly altered; however, when 10^{-5} M metiamide, an H_2-receptor antagonist, was added to the cells immediately before loading the chemotactic chambers, the dose response was linear from 3×10^{-7} M to 5×10^{-6} M histamine. These data strongly suggest that although the stimulation of cell motility by histamine was not dependent upon either H_1 or H_2 receptors, the diminution of cell migration observed at higher histamine doses was dependent upon the H_2 receptor. Deactivation obtained when histamine was preincubated with the cells could not be reversed by H_1 or H_2 antagonists (Clark, R. A. F., *unpublished observations*), suggesting that this interaction was mediated through some undefined site, as was observed with histamine chemotactic stimulation of eosinophils.

HISTAMINE MODULATION OF EOSINOPHIL MIGRATION

In the previous studies, the inhibitory effect of histamine upon eosinophil migration was examined by using histamine as the chemotactic agent. These observations lead to the question of whether concentrations of 10^{-5} M histamine or greater added to the cell side of the chemotactic chamber could inhibit eosinophil responsiveness to other chemotactic agents. Therefore, in all the following experiments, the eosinophils were preincubated with histamine for 5 to 10 min prior to the placement of the cells in modified Boyden chambers.

Using the 5 μm pore, 12 μm thick polycarbonate filters and determining eosinophil migration by visual inspection of the number of cells that had transversed the filter, we noted that preincubation of 10^{-5} M histamine with the eosinophils significantly reduced their migration to endotoxin-activated serum and to kallikrein (Fig. 5). Addition of 10^{-4} M metiamide to the preincubation of 10^{-5} M histamine with the eosinophils abrogated this diminution of migration, while preincubation of 10^{-4} M metiamide alone with the eosinophils did not significantly effect eosinophil migration. These data seemed to confirm the hypothesis that histamine, at sufficient concentrations, inhibited eosinophil migration through the H_2 receptor. However, we could not confirm this when we used the standard ^{51}Cr radioassay (15) in which two 3 μm pore, 145 μm thick cellulose nitrate filters are sandwiched in a modified Boyden chamber and the amounts of labeled cells reaching the *bottom* filter are measured as counts of radioactivity. Table 2 gives the results from three such experiments with the eosinophils preincubated in either buffer or 10^{-5} M histamine, and endotoxin-activated serum was used as the chemoattractant. No consistent effect of histamine is seen. Even more confusing were our results using the Zigmond and Hirsch assay (40) and measuring the migration fronts. As shown in Table 3, both 10^{-6} M and 10^{-5} M histamine affected a significant enhancement of the migration fronts to endotoxin-activated serum, and this enhancement was re-

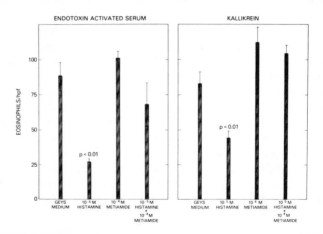

FIG. 5. Histamine-mediated inhibition of eosinophil migration to either endotoxin-activated serum or kallikrein and its abrogation by metiamide, an H_2-receptor antagonist. The bar represent the mean and SEM of four determinations after subtraction of the buffer control using visual inspection of 5 μm pore, 12 μm thick polycarbonate filters. p values are compared to a 10 min preincubation in Geys medium using the Student's t test.

TABLE 2. *Failure to detect inhibition on eosinophil chemotaxis using a ^{51}Cr radioassay*

^{51}Cr eosinophils preincubated in	Stimulus	^{51}Cr Eosinophil migration (corrected cpm)		
		Exp. no. 1	Exp. no. 2	Exp. no. 3
Buffer	Activated serum	392 ± 59	307 ± 15	175 ± 33
	None	65 ± 30	95 ± 14	44 ± 2.8
10^{-5} histamine	Activated serum	263 ± 22	348 ± 38	222 ± 33
	None	21 ± 8	98 ± 15	32 ± 7.2

TABLE 3. *Effect of histamine on eosinophil chemotaxis using the leading-front morphologic assay*

Eosinophils preincubated in	Migration fronts to endotoxin-activated serum	
	Exp. no. 1	Exp. no. 2
Buffer	92 ± 1.8	97 ± 4.0
10^{-7} M histamine	99 ± 2.6[a]	88 ± 3.5
10^{-6} M histamine	103 ± 1.8[b]	125 ± 2.3[b]
10^{-5} M histamine	98 ± 2.8	112 ± 2.5[c]
10^{-4} M pyrilamine	98 ± 4.1	97 ± 3.5
10^{-4} M pyrilamine + 10^{-5} M histamine	81 ± 2.1[b]	94 ± 3.4

[a] $p < 0.05$ Compared to eosinophils
[b] $p < 0.01$ preincubated in buffer
[c] $p < 0.001$

versed by the presence of pyrilamine. These data appeared to contradict our data from visual counts of thin filters in that here preincubation of histamine with eosinophils was presumably enhancing cell migration through the H_1 receptor.

This apparent paradox was resolved when we examined the entire population of migrating eosinophils by utilizing the Zigmond and Hirsch assay (40), but this time counting the cells/hpf at 10 μm intervals through the entire filter thickness (Fig. 6). All three doses of histamine used inhibited net eosinophil movement into the filter (267 ± 9.2 with 10^{-3} M histamine, 369 ± 6.3 with 10^{-4} M histamine, and 374 ± 17.7 with 10^{-5} M histamine)[1] compared to eosinophils preincubated in buffer alone (453 ± 19.5)[1]; however a significant increase in the number of eosinophils migrating further than 60 μm was observed with 10^{-4} M and 10^{-5} M histamine. These observations again demonstrated heterogeneity of the eosinophil response among eosinophils isolated from different patients as well as heterogeneity of the eosinophil response using cells isolated from a

---

[1] The mean ± SEM (six determinations) of the total number of eosinophils in a rectangular volume of filter measuring 50 X 50 X 150 mm.

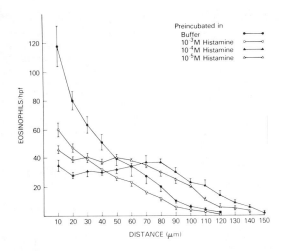

FIG. 6. Population curves of eosinophil migration through cellulose nitrate filters in response to endotoxin-activated serum after incubation for 30 min at 37°C in 100% humidity and 5% CO_2. The eosinophils were preincubated for 10 min at 37°C in buffer, 10^{-3} M histamine, 10^{-4} M histamine, or 10^{-5} M histamine. Each point represents the mean and SEM of six determinations.

single patient. To explore this observation further, the area under selected portions of the eosinophil population curves was integrated and shown in Fig. 7. The responding cells are represented as eosinophils/hpf/distance in that section of the filter. Such a manipulation allows simplified analysis of the effect of 10^{-5} M histamine on the responding eosinophil population to endotoxin-activated serum. In the 10 to 20 μm section, the number of eosinophils responding was significantly diminished when the cells were preincubated in 10^{-5} M histamine. Therefore, in these experiments, we observed a heterogeneity in the eosinophils' response to histamine which, for simplicity, can be divided into two different subpopulations of eosinophils: one in which 10^{-5} M histamine inhibited directed migration, and a second in which this concentration of histamine enhanced the chemotactic response. Metiamide, an H_2-receptor antagonist, abrogated the inhibition, while pyrilamine, H_1-receptor blockade, reversed the enhancement but had no effect upon the inhibition (Fig. 7).

The histamine inhibition of eosinophil migration has been further characterized, recently (7), to act through the H_2 receptor by increasing the intracellular levels of cyclic-AMP. This finding was not surprising, since stimulation of H_2 receptors by histamine has been shown to increase gastric secretion (3) and cardiac contractibility (26), and to inhibit cytotoxic T cells (31) and the release of histamine from human leukocytes (25), all of which are mediated through the increase of intracellular cyclic-AMP.

Thus far, histamine appears to be the only known *specific* chemoattractant for human eosinophils, and this activity is not influenced by H_1- or H_2-receptor

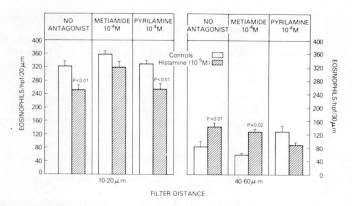

FIG. 7. The effect of the H_2-receptor antagonist, metiamide, and the H_1-receptor antagonist, pyrilamine, upon histamine inhibition and enhancement of eosinophil migration stimulated by endotoxin-activated serum. The eosinophils were preincubated in buffer or 10^{-5} M histamine with or without 10^{-4} M metiamide or 10^{-4} M pyrilamine for 10 min at 37°C. The eosinophils were then allowed to migrate into cellulose nitrate filters in response to endotoxin-activated serum for 30 min at 37°C in 100% humidity and 5% CO_2. Population curves were determined and the 10 to 20 μm and 40 to 60 μm filter section were integrated. Each histogram represents the mean and SEM of the integration of six population curve sections. p values are comparisons to controls with no antagonist using the Student's t test.

antagonists; however histamine-dependent inhibition of the eosinophil chemotactic response to other agents is mediated through the H_2 receptor and is associated with an intracellular cyclic-AMP increase. Histamine-dependent enhancement of the eosinophil chemotactic response to other agents is mediated through the H_1 receptor. Thus, the heterogeneous behavior of eosinophils may reflect differences in H_1- or H_2-receptor density and/or cell responsiveness to receptor stimulation. These data suggest that histamine may play a central role in the tissue localization of eosinophils as a result of its ability to stimulate eosinophil migration itself and modulate eosinophil responsiveness to other chemotactic factors.

REFERENCES

1. Archer, R. K. (1956): The eosinophil response in the horse to intramedullary and intradermal injections of histamine, ACTH and cortisone. *J. Pathol.,* 72:87–94.
2. Ash, A. S. F., and Schild, H. D. (1966): Receptors mediating some actions of histamine. *Br. J. Pharmacol.,* 27:427–439.
3. Black, J. W., Duncan, W. A. M., Durant, C. J., Canellin, C. R., and Parsons, E. M. (1972): Definition and antagonism of histamine H_2-receptors. *Nature (Lond.),* 236:385–390.
4. Clark, R. A. F., Gallin, J. I., and Kaplan, A. P. (1975): The selective eosinophil chemotactic activity of histamine. *J. Exp. Med.,* 142:1462–1476.
5. Clark, R. A. F., Gallin, J. I., and Kaplan, A. P. (1976): Mediator release from basophil granulocytes in chronic myelogenous leukemia: Demonstration of the eosinophil chemotactic activity of histamine. *J. Allergy Clin. Immunol.,* 58:623–634.
6. Clark, R. A. F., and Kaplan, A. P. (1975): Eosinophil leukocytes: Structure and function. *Clin. Haematol.,* 4:635–649.

7. Clark, R. A. F., Sandler, J. A., Gallin, J. I., and Kaplan, A. P. (1977): Histamine modulation of eosinophil migration. *J. Immunol.*, 118:137–145.
8. Cohen, S., and Ward, P. A. (1971): In vitro and in vivo activity of a lymphocyte and immune complex-dependent chemotactic factor for eosinophils. *J. Exp. Med.*, 113:133–146.
9. Colley, D. G. (1973): Eosinophils and immune mechanisms: I. Eosinophil stimulation promoter (ESP): A lymphokine induced by specific antigen or phytohemagglutinin. *J. Immunol.*, 110:1419–1423.
10. Czarnetzki, B. M., Konig, W., and Lichtenstein, L. M. (1976): Antigen-induced eosinophil chemotactic factor (ECF) release by human leukocytes. *Inflammation*, 1:201–215.
11. Czarnetzki, B. M., Konig, W., and Lichtenstein, L. M. (1976): Eosinophil chemotactic factor (ECF): I. Release from polymorphonuclear leukocytes by the calcium ionophore A23187. *J. Immunol.*, 117:229–234.
12. Dale, H. H. (1913): An anaphylactic reaction to plain muscle in the guinea pig. *J. Pharmacol. Exp. Ther.*, 4:167–223.
13. Dale, D. C., Hubert, R., and Fauci, A. S. (1976): Eosinophil kinetics in the hypereosinophil syndrome, *J. Lab. Clin. Med.*, 487–495.
14. Eidinger, D., Wilkinson, S. R., and Rose, D. A. (1964): A study of cellular responses in immune reactions utilizing the skin window technique. *J. Allergy Clin. Immunol.*, 35:77–85.
15. Gallin, J. I., Clark, R. A., and Kimball, H. R. (1973): Granulocyte chemotaxis: An improved in vitro assay employing ^{51}Cr-labeled granulocytes. *J. Immunol.*, 110:233–240.
16. Goetzl, E. J., and Austen, K. F. (1975): Purification and synthesis of eosinophilotactic tetrapeptides of human lung tissue: Identification as eosinophil chemotactic factor of anaphylaxis. *Proc. Natl. Acad. Sci. U.S.A.*, 72:4123–4127.
17. Greene, B. M., and Colley, D. G. (1976): Production of lymphokine eosinophil stimulation promotor by mouse T lymphocytes. *J. Immunol.*, 116:1078–1083.
18. Kaliner, M. A., Wasserman, S. I., and Austen, K. F. (1973): Immunologic release of chemical mediators from human nasal polyp tissue. *N. Engl. J. Med.*, 289:277–281.
19. Kay, A. B. (1970): Studies on eosinophil leukocyte migration: II. Factors specifically chemotactic for eosinophils and neutrophils generated from guinea-pig serum by antigen-antibody complexes. *Clin. Exp. Immunol.*, 8:723–737.
20. Kay, A. B., and Austen, K. F. (1971): The IgE-mediated release of an eosinophil leukocyte chemotactic factor from human lung. *J. Immunol.*, 107:899–902.
21. Kay, A. B., Stechschulte, D. J., and Austen, K. F. (1971): An eosinophil leukocyte chemotactic factor of anaphylaxis. *J. Exp. Med.*, 133:602–619.
22. Kline, B. S., Cohen, M. B., and Rudolph, J. A. (1932): Histologic changes in allergic and non-allergic wheals. *J. Allergy Clin. Immunol.*, 3:531–541.
23. Konig, W., Czarnetzki, B. M., and Lichtenstein, L. M. (1976): Eosinophil chemotactic factor (ECF): II. Release from human polymorphonuclear leukocytes during phagocytosis. *J. Immunol.*, 117:235–241.
24. Lewis, R. A., Goetzl, E. J., Wasserman, S. I., Valone, F. H., Rubin, R. H., and Austen, K. F. (1975): The release of four mediators of immediate hypersensitivity from human leukemic basophils. *J. Immunol.*, 114:87–92.
25. Lichtenstein, L. M., and Gillespie, E. (1973): Inhibition of histamine release by histamine, controlled by H_2-receptor. *Nature (Lond.)*, 244:287–288.
26. McNeil, J. H., and Verma, S. C. (1974): Blockade by burimamide of the effects of histamine and histamine analogs on cardiac contractility, phosphorylase activation and cyclic adenosine monophosphate. *J. Pharmacol. Exp. Ther.*, 188:180–188.
27. Melmon, K. L., Bourne, H. R., Weinstein, Y., Shearer, G. M., Kram, J., and Bauminger, S. (1974): Hemolytic plaque formation by leukocytes in vitro: Control by vasoactive hormones. *J. Clin. Invest.*, 53:13–21.
28. Ottesen, E. A., and Cohen, S. G. (1977): Eosinophils, eosinophilia and eosinophil-related disorders. In: *Allergy Principles and Practice*, edited by C. E. Reed, E. Middleton, and E. Ellis. C. V. Mosby Co., St. Louis *(In press)*.
29. Parish, W. E. (1970): Investigation on eosinophilia: The influence of histamine, antigen-antibody complexes containing gamma-1 or gamma-2 globulins, foreign bodies and disrupted mast cells. *Br. J. Dermatol.*, 82:42–64.
30. Parish, W. E. (1974): Substances that attract eosinophils in vitro and in vivo and that elicit blood eosinophilia. *Antibiot. Chemother.* 19:233–270.

31. Plaut, M., Lichtenstein, L. M., Gillespie, E., and Henney, C. S. (1973): Studies on the mechanism of lymphocyte-mediated cytolysis: IV. Specificity of the histamine receptor on effector T cells. *J. Immunol.,* 111:389–394.
32. Rocklin, R. E. (1976): Modulation of cellular immune response *in vivo* and *in vitro* by histamine receptor-bearing lymphocytes. *J. Clin. Invest.,* 57:1051–1058.
33. Spiers, R. S. (1955): Physiological approaches to an understanding of the function of eosinophils and basophils. *Ann. N.Y. Acad. Sci.,* 59:706–731.
34. Vaughn, J. (1953): The function of the eosinophil leukocyte. *Blood,* 8:1–15.
35. Vegad, J. L., and Lancaster, M. C. (1972): Eosinophil leukocyte-attracting effect of histamine in the sheep skin. *Indian J. Exp. Biol.,* 10:147–148.
36. Ward, P. A. (1969): Chemotaxis of human eosinophils. *Am. J. Pathol.,* 54:121–128.
37. Ward, P. A., Cochrane, C. G., and Müller-Eberhard, H. J. (1966): Further studies on the chemotactic factor of complement and its formation *in vivo. Immunology,* 11:141–153.
38. Ward, P. A., and Newman, L. J. (1969): A neutrophil chemotactic factor from human C-5. *J. Immunol.,* 102:93–99.
39. Wasserman, S. I., Goetzl, E. J., Ellman, L., and Austen, K. F. (1974): Tumor-associated eosinophilotactic factor. *New Engl. J. Med.,* 290:420–424.
40. Zigmond, S. A., and Hirsch, J. G. (1972): Leukocyte locomotion and chemotaxis: New methods for evaluation and demonstration of a cell-derived chemotactic factor. *J. Exp. Med.,* 137:387–410.
41. Zurier, R. B., Weissman, G., Hoffman, S., Kammerman, S., and Tai, H. H. (1974): Mechanisms of lysosomal enzyme release from human leukocytes: II. Effects of cAMP and cGMP, autonomic agonists and agents which effect microtubule function. *J. Clin. Invest.,* 53:297–309.

DISCUSSION

Dr. Snyderman: Is there any *in vivo* situation in which histamine has been demonstrated to cause eosinophil accumulation?

Dr. R. A. F. Clark: Yes, there were three articles in the literature. The first was in the 1930s (*J. Allergy,* 3:531–541, 1932) and this was confirmed later by two articles in the 1960s (*J. Allergy,* 35:77–85, 1964; *J. Allergy,* 40:73–87). These investigators showed that histamine injected intradermally in atopic patients who had eosinophilia, caused local influx of eosinophils. In patients who did not have eosinophilia, no influx was demonstrated.

Dr. Snyderman: In the guinea pig skin, it is virtually impossible to demonstrate eosinophil accumulation after histamine injection.

Dr. R. A. F. Clark: I am certainly well aware of the negative reports in the literature, and I do not really have an explanation for that; however, the work from our lab and that from Dr. Goetzl's, when taken together, show that eosinophil influx is mediated by a host of factors. I am prejudiced and think histamine plays a central role in the local accumulation of eosinophils in that it not only is a specific chemoattractant, but that it also modulates the response through H_1 and H_2 receptors. Nevertheless, the tetrapeptides, the lipid factors reported by Dr. Goetzl, and, in some reactions, C5a and lymphokines contribute to eosinophil influx.

Dr. Altman: Regarding the modulating effect of histamine on other chemotactic factors, since most chemotactic factors are not specific for eosinophils, and in most of your experiments you were not using pure populations of eosinophils, how did you know that the enhancement or inhibition of cell migration was specific for eosinophils? I could see how that distinction would be possible in a visual assay; it would seem to be impossible in a radiolabel assay.

Dr. R. A. F. Clark: Most of these experiments were done in a visual assay, that is, counting the cells migrating into the filter via the Zigmond-Hirsch technique.

Dr. Schiffmann: Do you know anything about the metabolism of histamine during the chemotactic response by eosinophils? Have you tried something like monamine oxidase inhibitors to see whether or not they affect chemotaxis?

Dr. R. A. F. Clark: No, we have not, and, as far as I know, no one has looked at the metabolism of histamine by eosinophils during chemotaxis. Certainly, the eosinophils have histaminase, as has been reported by Zeiger from Dr. Harvey Colten's laboratory. The histamase activity in eosinophils, however, is about the same as is found in neutrophils. Furthermore, monocytes, which do not have histaminase but do contain methyltransferase, metabolize histamine 10-fold faster than do either neutrophils or eosinophils. Therefore, it appears that the eosinophils do not have a potent mechanism for metabolizing histamine. That is a rather indirect answer but that is really all that is known.

Dr. Snyderman: I must say I am confused about eosinophil chemotaxis. If I understand your data and Dr. Goetzl's, you said that histamine causes eosinophil accumulation in atopic but not in normal tissues. In addition, it seems as though no dose of the tetrapeptides ever produces a maximum chemotactic response including the total number of eosinophils that can respond to other chemotactic factors. Histamine may be similar. Your data also show that you only see chemotactic responses when you get above a certain percentage of eosinophils in a mixture of granulocytes or in a patient. Is this suggesting that normally there are different populations of eosinophils circulating or that they must possess different states of activation before they will respond to these chemotactic agents? Could one separate the eosinophils on the basis of what chemotactic factors they respond to?

Dr. Williams: I was thinking about the same thing. The patients that you study, those from whose blood you can get 70% eosinophils, are very unusual. How do you know that that population of eosinophils that is in the peripheral blood of normal subjects is like the 80% eosinophils of your patients? In other words, how do you know you have not loaded the dice by the person that you actually study?

Dr. Goetzl: There is no question that many of these patients have abnormal eosinophils. Chris Spry has shown that they are degranulated, vacuolated, and have receptors for IgG that are not present on normal eosinophils and which disappear as the eosinophilia subsides. Other patients who have lesser eosinophilia do not have such profound defects but may exhibit qualitatively comparable alterations. Abnormal chemotactic responsiveness to C5a and ECF-A is not, however, a general characteristic of the cells of hypereosinophilic states.

Dr. R. A. F. Clark: We have studied eosinophils from a patient with schistosomiasis who had eosinophilia. These eosinophils showed the same response to histamine as did the eosinophils from patients with hypereosinophilia.

Dr. Williams: Have you ever done an experiment to try to quantitate the number of H_1 and H_2 sites on individual cells? Is there, for instance, a population that just has H_1 and a population of H_2 receptor eosinophils? It would be very interesting, for instance, if in an allergic family everybody in the family had more H_2 than H_1 receptors.

Dr. R. A. F. Clark: I agree. That needs to be done.

Dr. Ward: I share some of Dr. Snyderman's confusion about the fact that these so-called eosinophil-specific chemotactic factors do not incite the great intensity of response that the nonspecific ones, like the C5 fragment, will. And you have indicated that the accumulation of eosinophils in response to the injection of these materials is not particularly impressive unless there is a significant eosinophilia. But that has to be taken in the context of the basophil story. In the cutaneous basophil reaction, in spite of the fact that basophils represent an equally small or smaller numbers in the circulation, the cellular inflammatory reactions are almost completely selective for basophils, in spite of the fact that they represent maybe 1 or 2% of the circulating leukocytes. So if the eosinophil chemotactic factors represent the major selective chemotactic peptides for eosinophils, neither the *in vitro* nor the *in vivo* studies confirm this fact.

Dr. Becker: Yes, but Dr. Ward, one can get an eosinophil infiltration into a site at low levels of blood eosinophils, just as with the basophil. What that really suggests to me is that the 65% of the activity, for example, of the lung extracts, or whatever tissue that Dr. Goetzl mentioned, which has not been chemically characterized as yet, that 65% could well be extremely important in an *in vivo* situation.

Dr. Ward: But if you inject agents like histamine, the accumulation of eosinophils is really not terribly impressive on the basis of morphologic criteria. One sees a mixture of cells, a very small infiltrate, with about an equal percentage of neutrophils and eosinophils. Now that just may be a problem of the technique, but you know, it is not like some of the other mediators that, when injected, give an intense and localized infiltration.

Dr. Goetzl: A study by Dr. Kay recently published in *Immunology* showed that levels of 10^{-3} M to 10^{-4} M of either tetrapeptide injected alone or in combination subcutaneously in monkeys and humans without peripheral blood eosinophilia resulted in an eosinophil reaction in the skin. Thus, the methodology required for investigating cutaneous responses included a complete dose-response curve over a long time period.

Dr. Quie: I wonder if you have any evidence that histamine that is associated with cell surfaces or has been acted on by cells is more "attracting" than native histamine? Several years ago, while working with Ronald Walls in Dr. Beeson's laboratory, we noticed that basophils (mast cells) disappeared from the peritoneal cavity when guinea pigs which were sensitized to *Trichinella spiralis* were injected intraperitoneally with trichinella larvae. Eosinophils and neutrophils dominated and a particularly fascinating observation was the rosetting of eosinophils around large macrophages which may have contained antigen antibody complexes. There appeared to be specific attraction for eosinophils.

Dr. R. A. F. Clark: First, I would like to comment on the observation that mast cells disappear. A reasonable alternative would be that the mast cells have degranulated, thus being unrecognizable. Dr. Hal Dvorak has shown that mast cells can continue to synthesize and release histamine, even after they have degranulated. Hence, there can be a continued release of histamine. One of the problems with injecting histamine is that there is only a single bolus and no continuing release of histamine over hours or even days as in the *in vivo* processes.

Dr. Snyderman: Dr. Quie's point is very interesting, because Spiers from Downstate has extremely interesting phase-contrast photographs, of eosinophils responding chemotactically in the presence of macrophages interacting with antigen. His films demonstrate one of the most dramatic examples of chemotaxis that I have seen. Eosinophils will migrate to and around the areas of macrophage antigen interaction. They mass around there, walk away, and then come back again. I wonder if anybody has looked at the relationship between macrophage products and eosinophil chemotaxis?

Dr. Goetzl: The most critical point that has been raised is the persistent enigma of the mechanism(s) responsible for rapid and selective influx of eosinophils in immediate immunologic reactions. While the factors that have been described can produce eosinophilia under some circumstances, they do not account for the immunologic events that have been described.

Dr. R. A. F. Clark: One thing that has not been studied well, and may be important for that brisk response, is a factor that causes increased adherence of eosinophils to endothelial cells. Such adherence to endothelial cells may be a necessary initial prerequisite for local eosinophil accumulation.

Leukocyte Chemotaxis, edited by John I. Gallin
and Paul G. Quie. Raven Press, New York
© 1978.

Mechanisms for Modulation of the Inflammatory Response: Generation and Inactivation of C5a by Products Stored in the Granules of Human Neutrophils

Daniel G. Wright and John I. Gallin

Laboratory of Clinical Investigation, National Institute of Allergy and Infectious Diseases, National Institutes of Health, Bethesda, Maryland 20014

It is well recognized that the contents of neutrophil granules fulfill bactericidal and digestive functions within these cells once released into phagocytic vacuoles. It is increasingly evident, however, that neutrophil granules are not restricted to intracellular functions. Contents of both the azurophil and specific granules have been shown to be released extracellularly not only during phagocytosis (20,28,36) but under a variety of conditions *in vitro* (10,12,14,18,33,34,37). The specific (or secondary) granules are particularly accessible for extracellular release (19,34), and these granules have been shown to behave like the storage granules of secretory cells when neutrophils are exposed to certain chemical degranulating agents (phorbol myristate acetate and ionophore A23187) (30,34). In addition, granule contents, in particular those of specific granules, are released when neutrophils adhere to glass or nylon surfaces *in vitro* (18,33), and a comparable secretion of granule contents appears to occur when neutrophils marginate and enter inflammatory sites *in vivo* (33).

Our laboratory has had a special interest in the concept that neutrophils, on arriving at a site of inflammation, exert important modulating effects upon the evolution of inflammatory responses, regardless of the initial inflammatory stimulus. Recent studies have lent support to this concept by showing that products of neutrophil granules interact with complement not only to generate but to inactivate complement-derived chemotactic factors (24,25,27,32,35). These studies, summarized in this chapter, define mechanisms by which exudate neutrophils may not only amplify and localize an acute inflammatory response but may also limit this response, once sufficient numbers of cells have arrived at the site of inflammation.

GENERATION OF CHEMOTACTIC ACTIVITY FROM SERUM BY NEUTROPHIL GRANULE LYSATES AND BY POSTPHAGOCYTIC MEDIA

An involvement of neutrophils in the generation of chemotactic factors was first suggested by studies of the early 1960s, in which neutrophil extracts or

TABLE 1. *Generation of chemotactic activity from serum by lysates of neutrophils and by lysates of neutrophil granules*

Stimulus	Chemotactic activity (COR CPM LF)[a]
Buffer	166 ± 19
Neutrophil lysate[b]	150 ± 21
Neutrophil granule fraction[c]	181 ± 23
Serum alone	750 ± 78
Serum + neutrophil lysate[b]	1,619 ± 138
Serum + granule fraction[c]	1,843 ± 157

[a]Corrected counts per min in the lower filter: mean ± SEM, 6 determinations.
[b]Obtained by freeze/thaw of a suspension of 10^7 neutrophils/ml.
[c]Obtained by differential centrifugation of a lysate of 10^7 neutrophils/ml (36).

products of these cells in culture were found to cause or to magnify exudative inflammatory lesions in experimental animals (5,17,21). Subsequently, it was shown by Borel, Keller, and Sorkin that the lysosomal fraction of rabbit neutrophils could generate chemotactic activity from serum *in vitro* (4), and Ward and his associates demonstrated that this phenomenon could be explained in part by direct cleavage of C5 and the production of a chemotactic fragment (25). Ward showed further that rabbit neutrophils released a C5-cleaving enzyme during phagocytosis of immune complexes and that a comparable enzyme could be recovered from human inflammatory joint fluids (26,27).

Using human neutrophils, purified from blood by hypaque-ficoll/dextran sedimentation techniques, and a chemotaxis assay that employs ^{51}Cr-labeled leukocytes (7), we could readily confirm the observations of others that both neutrophil lysates and lysates of a granule-rich fraction of the cells could generate chemotactic activity from serum (32,35). As shown in Table 1, while both whole-cell and granule lysates lacked intrinsic chemotactic activity, these preparations more than doubled the chemotactic activity of fresh serum during 60-min incubations with the serum at 37°C. This effect was most apparent when 37°C incubations of lysates with serum were followed by 30-min incubations at 56°C.

When neutrophils were allowed to phagocytize latex particles *in vitro,* we found that postphagocytic incubation media also had the ability to generate chemotactic activity from serum, while it lacked intrinsic chemotactic activity in the absence of serum (32). Latex particles were particularly useful in these studies because they were readily ingested by the cells in the absence of serum or plasma proteins and because it could be shown that these particles lacked intrinsic chemotactic activity and did not themselves generate chemotactic activity from serum. As shown in Fig. 1, the media of phagocytizing neutrophils showed an increasing ability to generate chemotactic activity from serum as phagocytosis progressed, while lysates of neutrophils recovered at different times of phagocytosis showed a progressive loss of their ability to activate serum. The presence of a serum activator in postphagocytic media was detected after

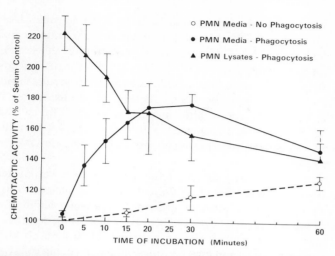

FIG. 1. Kinetics of serum-activator release from human neutrophils during phagocytosis. Neutrophil media and lysates obtained from 10^7 cells/ml incubated with and without latex particles (25 particles/cell) for 0 to 60 min. Postphagocytic media and cell lysates incubated with fresh serum for 60 min at 37°C and 30 min at 56°C before measurement of chemotactic activity. Results represent means ± SEM, 3 determinations. (From ref. 32, with permission.)

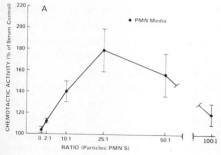

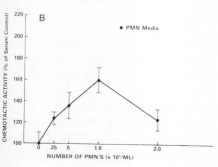

FIG. 2. A: Serum activator release from neutrophils with varying phagocytic challenges. Media obtained from 10^7 cells/ml incubated for 20 min with and without latex particles (0 to 100 particles/cell). **B:** Serum activator release from neutrophils with varying densities of phagocytizing cells. Media obtained from 0 to 2×10^7 cells/ml incubated for 20 min with latex particles (25 particles/cell). Media incubated with serum for 60 min at 37°C and 30 min at 56°C before measurement of chemotactic activity. Results are means ± SEM, 4 determinations. (From ref. 32, with permission.)

only 5 min of phagocytosis and was maximal by 20 to 30 min. Unexpectedly, this serum activator was found to be less apparent in 60 min postphagocytic media. This finding could not be explained by instability of the serum activator in solution, for postphagocytic media obtained at 20 min of phagocytosis did not lose its ability to generate chemotactic activity from serum during further incubation at 37°C in the absence of cells. Indeed, this media did not noticeably lose its ability to activate serum after incubation at 56°C for 30 min. Media from cells that had not been incubated with latex particles also showed the appearance of a serum activator but much less so than was observed with post-phagocytic media.

In other studies (32), we found that the recovery of a serum activator in postphagocytic media was related to the conditions of phagocytosis (Fig. 2). The ability of postphagocytic media to generate chemotactic activity from serum increased with increasing phagocytic challenges or increasing densities of phago-cytizing cells, but in both cases only up to a point. Both high phagocytic chal-lenges (>50 particles: 1 cell) and high densities of phagocytizing cells (>1.0 X 10^7 cells/ml) were associated with a diminished ability of the media to generate chemotactic activity from serum.

MECHANISMS OF SERUM ACTIVATION BY POSTPHAGOCYTIC MEDIA

Ward and his associates have reported that neutrophil granule lysates can cleave C5 directly to produce a chemotactic molecule related to C5a, and they have suggested that generation of chemotactic activity from serum by these lysates results from a direct effect on C5 (25). In an effort to identify the chemo-tactic molecules generated in serum by postphagocytic media, we incubated fresh serum with postphagocytic media and then chromatographed this serum on G-75 Sephadex. As shown in Fig. 3 (bottom panel), a distinct, new peak of chemotactic activity was found that had elution characteristics compatible with a molecular weight of about 17,000 daltons. The chemotactic activity re-covered from these elution fractions was stable at 56°C for 30 min and was inhibited by goat antiserum to human C5 but not by antiserum to human C3. Therefore, it was possible to conclude that the chemotactic activity generated in serum by postphagocytic media resulted in large part from C5a production (32).

When we incubated purified C5 for 30 min with postphagocytic media prepared with human neutrophils ingesting latex particles, some chemotactic activity was generated from the C5 preparation, confirming Ward's results; however, the increases in activity were small compared to those observed in whole serum, and we thought it possible that complement activation might contribute to the generation of C5a in serum by postphagocytic media. We were able to test this possibility with serum from a patient with congenital C3 deficiency, gener-ously provided to us by Dr. Arthur Rabson (South Africa). Although there

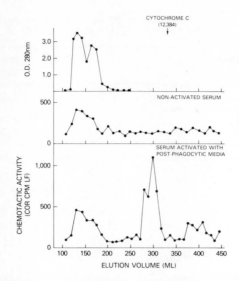

FIG. 3. G-75 Sephadex chromatography of fresh human serum after incubation with postphago-cytic media. Media prepared from 10^7 neutrophils/ml incubated with 25 latex particles per cell for 20 min. Media incubated with serum for 60 min at 37°C and 30 min at 56°C before chromatography of serum. Shown are optical densities of elution fractions at 280 nm from serum chromatography (top panel), chemotactic activity of elution fractions from chromatography of control serum (middle panel), and chemotactic activity of elution fractions from chromatography of serum incubated with postphagocytic media (bottom panel).

were normal amounts of C5 in this serum, it lacked detectable levels of C3 (1). As shown in Table 2, mimimal chemotactic activity was generated from this C3-deficient serum by postphagocytic media compared with that generated from normal serum. Addition of C3 to this deficient serum, however, resulted in normal generation of chemotactic activity by postphagocytic media. The media

TABLE 2. *Generation of chemotactic activity from C3-deficient serum by post-phagocytic media[a]*

Stimulus	Chemotactic activity (% of serum control)[b]
Normal serum	
+ postphagocytic media	172 ± 14
C3-deficient serum	
+ postphagocytic media	109 ± 6
+ postphagocytic media + 100 μ C3	163 ± 11

[a]Postphagocytic media obtained from 10^7 neutrophils/ml incubated for 20 min with latex particles (25 particles/cell).

[b]Mean ± SEM, 4 determinations. Chemotactic activity of 100 μ human C3 alone, postphagocytic media alone, and C3 + postphagocytic media were no different from buffer alone.

TABLE 3. *Generation of chemotactic activity from serum by postphagocytic media:* [a] *effects of EDTA and Mg-EGTA*

Stimulus	Chemotactic activity (% of serum control) [b]
Serum and postphagocytic media	223 ± 15
Serum and postphagocytic media	
+ EDTA (5 mM)	104 ± 16
+ Mg-EGTA (5 mM Mg, 10 mM EGTA)	202 ± 16

[a] Postphagocytic media obtained from 10^7 neutrophils/ml incubated for 20 min with latex particles (25 particles/cell).
[b] Mean ± SEM; 4 determinations.

did not generate chemotactic activity from C3 alone, nor did the addition of C3 to normal serum enhance its ability to be activated by postphagocytic media. These experiments indicated that most of the C5a produced in serum by postphagocytic media results from complement activation through C3 rather than from direct cleavage of C5.

In related experiments, it was found that activation of normal serum by postphagocytic media was completely inhibited by EDTA (5 mM) but not by Mg-EGTA (5 mM Mg, 10 mM EGTA), as shown in Table 3. This result indicated that complement activation by postphagocytic media proceeds at least in part through the alternate pathway, which has been shown to be magnesium-dependent but not calcium-dependent (6,13). In agreement with our findings, Goldstein and his associates have reported independently that lysates of human neutrophil granules induce complement activation in whole serum, thereby generating C5a-related lysosomal enzyme-releasing activity in the serum. Their studies, by demonstrating an effect of granule lysates on C3 proactivator, have also implicated the alternate pathway (11).

ADDITIONAL RELEASE OF A C5a INACTIVATOR BY PHAGOCYTIZING NEUTROPHILS

In the experiments shown in Figs. 1 and 2, prolonged phagocytosis (>30 min), high phagocytic challenges, and high densities of phagocytizing cells resulted in diminished activation of serum by postphagocytic media, and, as stated previously, these findings could not be explained by instability of the serum activator in solution. Rather, these findings suggested that under conditions of relatively intense phagocytosis an inactivator of C5a chemotactic activity is released by neutrophils in addition to the serum activator. To explore this possibility, postphagocytic medium was obtained from a high density of phagocytizing cells and was incubated both with serum previously activated by *Escherichia coli* endotoxin and with partially purified C5a (8). As shown in Figure 4, the chemotactic activity of both the endotoxin-activated serum and the C5a preparation was significantly inhibited by the postphagocytic media (32).

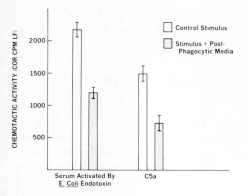

FIG. 4. Inactivator of C5a-associated chemotactic activity in postphagocytic media. Media obtained from 3×10^7 neutrophils/ml incubated with latex particles (25 particles/ml) for 45 min. *Escherichia coli* endotoxin-activated serum and partially purified C5a were incubated for 30 min at 37°C with and without the media before measurement of chemotactic activity. Results are means ± SEM, 6 determinations. (From ref. 32, with permission.)

Goetzl has reported that a heat-stable "neutrophil-immobilizing factor" is released from phagocytizing neutrophils and has an effect of rendering leukocytes unresponsive to chemotactic stimuli (9). It was quite possible, therefore, that the results shown in Fig. 4 reflected an effect of postphagocytic media upon the leukoytes in the chemotactic assays rather than upon the stimuli; however, the effects of postphagocytic media shown in Fig. 4 were almost completely eliminated by heating the media at 56°C for 30 min. Furthermore, as illustrated in Fig. 5, the inhibitory effects of postphagocytic media on the chemotactic activity of endotoxin-activated serum or of C5a increased with the time of incubation of these stimuli with the media, indicating a direct effect by the media on the stimuli (35). Neutral and acid proteases of diverse substrate specificities have been isolated from neutrophil granules (16), and it appeared likely from our results that one or more of these enzymes is released during phagocytosis and is able to degrade chemotactically active complement fragments. In agreement with this conclusion are reports by Venge and Olsson that chymotrypsin-

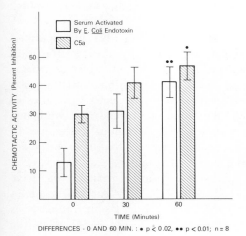

FIG. 5. Progressive inactivation of C5a chemotactic activity with time of exposure to postphagocytic media. Media obtained from 3×10^7 neutrophils/ml incubated with latex particles (25 particles/cell) for 45 min. Media incubated with chemotactic stimuli for 0 to 60 min before measurement of chemotactic activity. Results are expressed as percent inhibition of stimuli by incubation with the media and represent means ± SEM, 4 determinations.

like cationic proteins prepared from human neutrophil granules can interact with multiple-complement components and can abolish the chemotactic activity of porcine C5a or activated human C5 (24).

DIFFERENTIATION OF THE SERUM ACTIVATOR AND C5a INACTIVATOR IN POSTPHAGOCYTIC MEDIA

It seemed possible that the effects of postphagocytic media, both to generate chemotactic activity from serum by complement activation and to inactivate C5a, could result from the same molecule or molecules, and that the domination of one effect or the other depended upon incubation conditions and the relative concentrations of reactants. It was possible, however, to show that these effects are mediated by separate neutrophil products released from the cells (35). As stated before, the capacity of postphagocytic media to activate serum was found to be heat-stable, unlike its ability to inactivate C5a. Furthermore, the kinetics with which the serum activator and C5a inactivator appeared in the media during phagocytosis clearly differed. While it could be shown that the serum activator appeared rapidly in the media and was evident maximally by 20 to 30 min of phagocytosis, the serum inactivator appeared more slowly and was not maximal until 45 to 60 min (35). This result, by itself, suggested that the effects of postphagocytic media on serum and on C5a were mediated by neutrophil products contained in separate granule populations. In studies using the same conditions of phagocytosis illustrated in Fig. 1, it was found that lysozyme, contained to a large extent in the specific granules (23,29,34), was released rapidly by neutrophils, like the serum activator, while β-glucuronidase, contained only in the azurophil granules (23,29,34), was released more slowly, like the C5a inactivator. From work by Bainton (2), by Leffell and Spitznagel (19), and by others (12,30), as well as from work in our own laboratory (33,34), it is now known that the specific and azurophil granules not only degranulate at different rates but are quite different in terms of their availability for extracellular release.

Using an adaptation of a technique described by West (29), we separated specific and azurophil granules from human neutrophils by ultracentrifugation of cell lysates on continuous sucrose gradients. An example of the granule separation achieved by this method is shown in Fig. 6. Ultracentrifugation of a lysate of 10^8 neutrophils on a sucrose gradient, with a range of sucrose densities as is indicated, resulted in separation of three granule-rich bands. The two bands of greatest density, A and B, have been shown by cytochemical techniques to contain relatively large, round, peroxidase-positive granules that have been identified as primary or azurophil granules (23,29). The lighter band, C, has been found to contain small, pleomorphic, peroxidase-negative granules that have been identified as secondary or specific granules (23,29). Azurophil granules separated by this method contain acid hydrolases such as β-glucuronidase, as well as acid and neutral proteases, and myeloperoxidase (23,29,34), while the

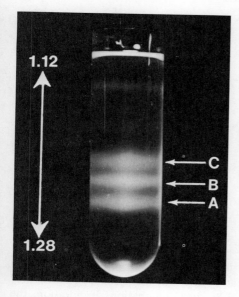

FIG. 6. Neutrophil granule separation by sucrose density centrifugation, prepared from a lysate of 10^8 neutrophils. The range of sucrose density (expressed as specific gravity) is shown.

specific granules contain two-thirds of the neutrophil lysozyme and most of the cell-associated lactoferrin (23,29,34). After selectively pumping out these different granule bands, we examined lysates of these preparations both for serum-activating and C5a-inactivating capacity. As is indicated by the representative study summarized in Table 4, the serum activator was found to be stored in the specific granules, C, while the C5a inactivator was found in the azurophil granules, B (35).

TABLE 4. *Localization of the neutrophil serum activator and C5a inactivator in different granule populations*

Granule type[a]	Generation of chemotactic activity from serum[b] (% of control)	Inactivation of C5a[c] (% inhibition of control)
A	136 ± 12	9 ± 7
B	116 ± 14	37 ± 6
C	258 ± 22	5 ± 5

[a]Granule-rich bands from 5×10^7 neutrophils, selectively aspirated from sucrose gradient (as in Fig. 6), washed in 0.34 M sucrose, pelleted, resuspended in sterile normal saline, and lysed by freeze/thaw.

[b]Granule lysates were incubated with serum (60 min at 37°C and 30 min at 56°C) before measurement of chemotactic activity. Results are expressed as the percent of chemotactic activity in control, untreated serum, and represent means ± SEM, 6 determinations.

[c]Granule lysates incubated with partially purified C5a (60 min at 37°C). Results are expressed as the percent inhibition of chemotactic activity in control, untreated C5a, and represent means ± SEM, 4 determinations.

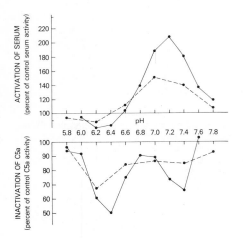

FIG. 7. pH optima of serum activation and C5a inactivation by postphagocytic media *(dashed lines)* and by granule lysates *(solid lines)*.

Top panel: Generation of chemotactic activity from serum by postphagocytic media (10^7 neutrophils/ml incubated with 25 latex particles/cell for 30 min) and by C granule lysates prepared from 5×10^7 cells.

Bottom panel: Inactivation of C5a by incubation at 37°C for 30 min with postphagocytic media (prepared as indicated above) and with B granule lysates prepared from 5×10^7 cells. Results are expressed as the percent of chemotactic activity found in control untreated serum or in untreated C5a.

As is the case with postphagocytic media, the serum activator located in the specific granules was resistant to heating at 56°C, while the C5a inactivator in the azurophil granules was destroyed by 56°C incubation. In addition, the optimal pH ranges for serum activation and for C5a inactivation by specific granule or azurophil granule lysates matched those identified with postphagocytic media (35). As shown in Fig. 7, generation of chemotactic activity from serum, both by postphagocytic media and by C granule lysates, was optimal at pH 7.2 to 7.4; inactivation of C5a by the same postphagocytic media and by B granule lysates was observed both at neutral pH and at a more acid pH, 6.2 to 6.3.

FURTHER CHARACTERIZATION OF THE SERUM ACTIVATOR AND C5a INACTIVATOR

The identification of two pH optima for C5a inactivation by azurophil granule lysates suggested that both these granules and postphagocytic media contained at least two separate C5a inactivators. Chromatography of B granule lysates on G-75 Sephadex also indicated the existence of several different C5a inactivators (31,35). Fractions eluted from Sephadex were incubated (60 min at 37°C) with aliquots of endotoxin-activated serum, which were then assayed for chemotactic activity. Inactivation of this chemotactic stimulus occurred with fractions at two distinct elution volumes, indicating inactivators with molecular weights of about 65,000 and 30,000 daltons (31,35). The smaller of these inactivators is similar in size to the neutrophil cationic proteins reported by Venge and Olsson to degrade C5 and C5a (24). Chemotactic factor inactivation also occurred with elution fractions that were consistent with a molecule of 10,000 to 12,000 daltons but this was not a consistent finding in the replicate studies that we have done (35). In related studies, isoelectric focusing of B granule lysates was done, and fractions after focusing were evaluated for their ability to destroy the chemotactic activity of endotoxin-activated serum. While some inactivator activity was consistently located at an isoelectric point of pH 8.0, most of the activity was found at an isoelectric point in the acid range, pH 5.0 to 5.5 (35). In separate studies, it was found that inactivation of C5a by B granule lysates was prevented when lysates were exposed to the enzyme inhibitors EDTA (ethylenediaminetetraacetic acid) and EACA (ϵ-aminocaproic acid), but unchanged after exposure of the lysates to DFP (diisopropyl fluorophosphate) (31,35).

Chromatography of C (specific) granule lysates on both G-75 and G-200 Sephadex and evaluation of elution fractions for the ability to generate chemotactic activity from serum have shown that the serum activator recovered from these granules is a large molecule in excess of 150,000 daltons. This material maintains its activity after heating for 30 min at 56°C and after exposure to trypsin (35).

SUMMARY AND CONCLUSIONS

Work from several laboratories has indicated that materials stored in human neutrophil granules can interact with individual complement components, with the intact complement system in serum, and with the chemotactic fragment C5a. It has been shown in particular that separate neutrophil granule products can (a) activate the complement system via the alternate pathway (11,32), (b) generate a chemotactic fragment from isolated C5 (23,25,32), and (c) destroy the chemotactic activity of preformed C5a (24,32).

In addition, we have found that these neutrophil products, with apparently counteracting effects, are located in different granule populations, and we believe that this finding is important for an understanding of how these cell products may act together to modulate an inflammatory response. The location of the serum activator in the specific (or secondary) granules and C5a inactivators in the azurophil (or primary) granules is significant, for there is evidence that specific granules are not only mobilized more rapidly (2) but are more accessible for extracellular release than are azurophil granules (5,12,19,30,33,34). In addition, we have recently presented evidence that the process of margination and exudation by itself is a stimulus for some degree of specific granule secretion by neutrophils *in vivo* (33). Granule separation studies that compared exudate neutrophils with neutrophils from peripheral blood have shown a preferential if not selective loss of specific granules from exudate cells (33). Also, measurement of granule-associated enzymes in sterile exudate fluids has indicated an early extracellular release of the contents of neutrophil-specific granules. These studies indicate that extracellular release of the neutrophil-derived serum activator located in the specific granules may occur during acute inflammation generally and that, regardless of the initial inflammatory stimulus, once neutrophils begin to arrive at a site of inflammation, they may amplify and localize the response by mediating complement activation. In this regard, it is of interest that exudation of leukocytes, as measured by the Rebuck skin window technique, was markedly delayed in a patient with C3 deficiency, whose serum did not support complement activation and C5a production (3). This observation supports the concept that an intact complement system is necessary for an early amplification phase of leukocyte exudation even in nonimmune injury, as is the case with the superficial abrasion used as an inflammatory stimulus in the skin window assay.

Extracellular release of azurophil granule contents by neutrophils would appear to become quantitatively more significant at a site of inflammation as the inflammatory response develops and the density of exudate cells increases. In addition, difference in the pH optima of the neutrophil serum activator and C5a inactivators suggest that as pH decreases in an evolving inflammatory lesion, C5a inactivation would be favored over complement activation, thus limiting the effect of C5a as an inflammatory mediator.

There is evidence that secretory products of neutrophils may influence the accumulation of neutrophils at inflammatory sites by mechanisms other than those summarized here. It is reported that, after phagocytosis of crystals, neutrophils synthesize and secrete a small molecule with serum-independent chemotactic activity (22). Also, under certain conditions, neutrophils are reported to release a factor that renders leukocytes unresponsive to chemotactic stimuli (9). Nonetheless, the studies reviewed in this chapter suggest that neutrophils may have an important role in modulating acute inflammatory responses through the release of granule products that interact with the complement system.

REFERENCES

1. Alper, C. A., Colten, H. R., Rosen, F. S., Rabson, A. R., McNab, G. M., and Gear, J. S. S. (1972): Homozygous deficiency of C3 in a patient with repeated infections. *Lancet,* 2:1179–1181.
2. Bainton, D. F. (1973): Sequential degranulation of the two types of polymorphonuclear leukocyte granules during phagocytosis of microorganisms. *J. Cell Biol.,* 58:249–264.
3. Ballow, M., Shira, J. E., Harden, L., Yang, S. Y., and Day, N. K. (1975): Complete absence of the third component of complement in man. *J. Clin. Invest.,* 56:703–710.
4. Borel, J. F., Keller, H. V., and Sorkin, E. (1969): Chemotaxis: XI. Effect on neutrophils of lysosomal and other subcellular fractions from leukocytes. *Int. Arch. Allergy Appl. Immunol.,* 35:194–205.
5. Estensen, R. D., White, J. G., and Holmes, B. (1974): Specific degranulation of human polymorphonuclear leukocytes. *Nature,* 248:347–350.
6. Fine, D. P., Marney, S. R., Colley, D. G., Sergent, J. S., and Des Prez, R. M. (1972): C3 shunt activation in human serum chelated with EGTA. *J. Immunol.,* 109:807–809.
7. Gallin, J. I., Clark, R. A., and Kimball, H. R. (1973): Granulocyte chemotaxis: An improved in vitro assay employing ^{51}Cr-labeled granulocytes. *J. Immunol.,* 110:233–240.
8. Gallin, J. I., and Rosenthal, A. S. (1974): The regulatory role of divalent cations in human granulocyte chemotaxis. Evidence for an association between calcium exchanges and microtubule assembly. *J. Cell Biol.,* 62:594–609.
9. Goetzl, E. J., and Austen, K. F. (1972): A neutrophil-immobilizing factor derived from human leukocytes: I. Generation and partial characterization. *J. Exp. Med.,* 136:1564–1580.
10. Goldstein, I. M., Hoffstein, S. T., and Weissmann, G. (1975): Mechanisms of lysosomal enzyme release from human polymorphonuclear leukocytes: Effects of phorbol myristate acetate. *J. Cell Biol.,* 66:647–652.
11. Goldstein, I. M., and Weissmann, G. (1974): Generation of C5-derived lysosomal enzyme releasing activity (C5a) by lysates of leukocyte lysosomes. *J. Immunol.,* 113:1583–1588.

12. Goldstein, I. M., Weissmann, G., Dunham, P. B., and Soberman, R. (1975): The role of calcium in secretion of enzymes by human polymorphonuclear leukocytes. In: *Calcium Transport in Contraction and Secretion,* edited by E. Carafoli, pp. 185–193. North Holland Publishing Co., Amsterdam.

13. Goodkofsky, I., and Lepow, I. (1971): Functional relationship of factor B in the properdin system to C3 proactivator of human serum. *J. Immunol.,* 107:1200–1204.

14. Henson, P. M. (1971): Interactions of cells with immune complexes: Adherence, release of constituents, and tissue injury. *J. Exp. Med.* 134 (Suppl.):114–135.

15. Hurley, J. V. (1964): Substances promoting leukocytic emigration. *Ann. N.Y. Acad. Sci.,* 116:918–935.

16. Janoff, A., ed. (1972): Symposium: Neutrophil proteases as mediators of tissue injury. *Am. J. Pathol.,* 68:537–623.

17. Janoff, A., and Zweifach, B. W. (1964): Adhesion and emigration of leukocytes produced by cationic proteins of lysosomes. *Science,* 144:1456–1458.

18. Klock, J. C., and Bainton, D. F. (1976): Degranulation and abnormal bactericidal function of granulocytes procured by reversible adhesion to nylon wool. *Blood,* 48:149–161.

19. Leffell, M. S., and Spitznagel, J. K. (1974): Intracellular and extracellular degranulation of human polymorphonuclear azurophil and specific granules induced by immune complexes. *Infect. Immun.,* 10:1241–1249.

20. May, C. D., Levine, B. B., and Weissmann, G. (1970): The effects of compounds that inhibit antigenic release of histamine and phagocytic release of lysosomal enzymes on glucose utilization by leukocytes in humans. *Proc. Soc. Exp. Biol. Med.,* 133:758–763.

21. Moses, J. M., Ebert, R. M. O., Graham, R. C., and Brine, K. L. (1964): Pathogenesis of inflammation: I. The production of an inflammatory substance from rabbit granulocytes *in vitro* and its relationship to leukocytic pyrogen. *J. Exp. Med.,* 120:57–82.

22. Spilberg, I., Gallacher, A., Mehta, J. M., and Mandel, B. (1976): Urate crystal induced chemotactic factor. *J. Clin. Invest.,* 58:815–819.

23. Spitznagel, J. K., Dalldorf, F. G., Leffell, M. S., Folds, J. D., Welsh, I. R. H., Cooney, M. H., and Martin, L. E. (1974): Character of azurophil and specific granules purified from human polymorphonuclear leukocytes. *Lab. Invest.,* 30:774–785.

24. Venge, P., and Olsson, I. (1975): Cationic proteins of human granulocytes: VI. Effects on the complement system and mediation of chemotactic activity. *J. Immunol.,* 115:1505–1508.

25. Ward, P. A., and Hill, J. H. (1970): C5 chemotactic fragments produced by an enzyme in lysosomal granules of neutrophils. *J. Immunol.,* 104:535–543.

26. Ward, P. A., and Zvaifler, N. J. (1971): Complement derived leukotactic factors in inflammatory synovial fluids of humans. *J. Clin. Invest.,* 50:606–616.

27. Ward, P. A., and Zvaifler, N. J. (1973): Quantitative phagocytosis by neutrophils: II. Release of the C5-cleaving enzyme and inhibition of phagocytosis by rheumatoid factor. *J. Immunol.,* 111:1777–1782.

28. Weissmann, G., Zurier, R. B., and Hoffstein, S. (1972): Leukocyte proteases and the immunological release of lysosomal enzymes. *Am. J. Pathol.,* 68:539–559.

29. West, B. C., Rosenthal, A. S., Gelb, N. A., and Kimball, H. R. (1974): Separation and characterization of human neutrophil granules. *Am. J. Pathol.,* 77:41–62.

30. White, J. G., and Estensen, R. D. (1974): Selective labilization of specific granules in polymorphonuclear leukocytes by phorbol myristate acetate. *Am. J. Pathol.,* 75:45–60.

31. Wright, D. G., and Gallin, J. I. (1975): Inactivation of the chemotactic molecule C5a by products contained in human polymorphonuclear leukocytes and released during phagocytosis. *Fed. Proc.,* 34:1019.

32. Wright, D. G., and Gallin, J. I. (1975). Modulation of the inflammatory response by products released from human polymorphonuclear leukocytes during phagocytosis: Generation and inactivation of the chemotactic factor C5a. *Inflammation,* 1:23–39.

33. Wright, D. G., and Gallin, J. I. (1976): The selective mobilization of specific granules by human neutrophils during adherence *in vitro* and during exudation *in vivo. Clin. Res.,* 24:355A.

34. Wright, D. G., and Gallin, J. I. (1977): The differential release of human neutrophil granules: Effects of phorbol myristate acetate and ionophore A23187. *Am. J. Pathol.,* 87:273–284.

35. Wright, D. G., and Gallin, J. I. (1977): Functional differentiation of human neutrophil granules: Generation of C5a by a specific (secondary) granule product and inactivation of C5a by azurophil (primary) granule products. *J. Immunol. (in press).*

36. Wright, D. G., and Malawista, S. E. (1972): The mobilization and extracellular release of granular enzymes from human leukocytes during phagocytosis. *J. Cell Biol.*, 53:788–797.
37. Zurier, R. B., Hoffstein, S., and Weissmann, G. (1973): Cytochalasin B: Effect on lysosomal enzyme release from human leukocytes. *Proc. Natl. Acad. Sci. U.S.A.*, 70:844–848.

DISCUSSION

Dr. Ward: These are very nice studies. I wonder if you have evidence that the chemotactic factor generator is in fact operating as an enzyme? Could it be a lipid or other heat-stable factor?

Dr. Wright: That question has been of particular interest to us and, in fact, my suspicion is that it may not be an enzyme and perhaps not a protein, but we do not have much data on that. It is resistant to heating at 56°C. Also, we have been unable to show that the active large molecule that we obtain by chromatography is particularly sensitive to various concentrations of trypsin. But that is about the extent of what we have done with it. We are intrigued with the possibility that this material could be a polysaccharide.

Dr. Ward: In the experiments in which you added the extracts from the granules to serum and showed that they would generate chemotactic activity, what is the effect of these extracts on chemotactic activity present in activated serum? Also, what sort of cell equivalents or concentrations were you using?

Dr. Wright: First, we were not looking at activated serum; we were looking at partially purified C5a. Our activated serum was heated at 56°C for 30 min prior to chromatography on G-75, which should have eliminated much of the enzyme activity you are concerned with. Also, separation of the granules permits one to obtain a large amount of active material from the cells and provides an opportunity to begin to characterize these molecules. Working with post-phagocytic media has been less useful in efforts to characterize the various neutrophil products biochemically.

Dr. Robert Clark: One of the inactivators you mentioned was similar in size to the antimicrobial cationic proteins. These cationic proteins have chymotrypsin-like protease activity. Certain properties of the cationic proteins, such as bactericidal activity and cytotoxic activity, are independent of the enzymatic activity, but are blocked by heparin, presumably through modifying the strong positive charge of the molecules. Have you looked to see which of these properties of cationic proteins, that is, charge or enzymatic activity, might be responsible for the inactivation of chemotactic factors?

Dr. Wright: No, we were looking simply for degradation of chemotactic factors. It really is not terribly surprising that one or more of the proteases, of which many have already been described in neutrophil granules, could act upon a complement fragment to alter its activity; however, the mechanisms of chemotactic inactivation by the granule-derived molecules have not been worked out.

Dr. Altman: Have you looked at leukemic or otherwise diseased polymorphonuclear leukocytes or immature cells to see if you can isolate either a serum activator or C5a inactivator? These types of cells might serve as valuable probes for further investigation.

Dr. Wright: We have only studied normal neutrophils.

Dr. Schiffmann: Does there appear to be any involvement of contractile elements of the cell in the export of granules during the phagocytosis stimulus, and does colchicine inhibit this release?

Dr. Wright: It can be shown that colchicine both *in vivo* and *in vitro* will inhibit the extracellular release of specific granule products when the cells are exposed to several different kinds of stimuli. Phagocytosis is one such stimulus and there has been a controversy over whether the effect of colchicine on inhibiting either extracellular or intracellular release of granular enzymes during phagocytosis represents more an effect on the ingestion process, or the adherence of particles to the cell, than it does on some internal event. But with other degranulating stimuli, such as the chemical agents phorbol myristate acetate and ionophore A23187, or adherence to surfaces like nylon wool, it can again be shown that degranulation is inhibited by colchicine.

Dr. Quie: Dr. Wright, have you studied the phenomenon of neutropenia that occurs when patients are dialyzed? Is the C5 fragment or a reaction product of complement produced first, which brings about a change in neutrophils? Is it possible that neutrophils release something that leads to the formation of C5 fragments?

Dr. Wright: We have been very interested in the problem, not so much from the point of view of dialysis, but in terms of filtration leukapheresis. As you know, Drs. Phillip Craddock and Harry Jacobs and their associates at Minnesota have been very interested in the finding that cells exposed to nylon wool, as used in filtration leukapheresis, pick up complement on their surfaces, and their feeling is that the nylon surfaces cause complement activation. We feel that this is not the case, but that the cells are induced to degranulate when they adhere to nylon wool, and that complement activation occurs as a consequence of the release of a complement activator by the cells.

Dr. Williams: In doing those elegant types of granule studies, have you examined people who have been leukapheresed? It is conceivable they are only losing the specific granules.

Dr. Wright: We have compared the granulation of neutrophils obtained by filtration leukapheresis with that of neutrophils obtained from peripheral blood of the leukapheresis donors. We have found that the cells exposed to nylon wool have lost a proportion of their specific granules.

Dr. Williams: How about doing it on people just after dialysis?

Dr. Wright: I do not think you would see any change under those conditions. What you would like to do is to compare cells that had adhered with those still circulating. I do not believe that the circulating cells are changed in terms of their granule content. Rather, the cells that have interacted with either the dialysis tubing or the nylon wool are changed.

Dr. Leddy: At Rochester, Drs. Jacob Nusbacher, Stephen Rosenfeld, and I are studying the neutropenia in donors during nylon fiber filtration leukapheresis and the rebound leukocytosis they have later. Dr. Nusbacher at the Red Cross Transfusion Service in Rochester has published an article dealing with the leukocyte kinetics of the donors. Recently Dr. Rosenfeld and I have looked at the associated complement changes. I am very attracted to what you said about complement activation somehow being an effect of something released from leukocytes. We find that if patient's plasma is put through the nylon filters, there is little or no demonstrable complement consumption. But if whole blood is used, there is remarkable complement consumption. It appears to be via the classical pathway in our hands, not the alternative pathway. C1, C4, and C2 are markedly depressed, and there is only a modest reduction in C3. We are not sure yet just what the ultimate neutropenia-producing factor is, and we are not even sure that the complement activation is the cause of the neutropenia. They just go hand in hand. It is very attractive to think that C5a or something like this is being produced, and we are aware of the other observation from Dr. Craddock in Minnesota that C5a can produce neutrophil aggregation in an aggregometer *(J. Clin. Invest.,* 60:260–264, 1977).

Dr. Wright: Perhaps I can elaborate on that. We have looked at this question in a similar way, comparing either plasma alone or plasma enriched with cells that can be diverted simultaneously from a cell separator, both of which were then run through filters. With plasma alone, we found neither complement consumption nor generation of chemotactic activity in the plasma. Only when cells are available did these events occur. Our studies, i.e., with Mg-EGTA, do not eliminate the possibility of classical pathway complement activation by granule products.

Dr. Ward: Dr. J. O'Flaherty in my laboratory, having previously worked with Drs. Jacobs and Craddock, has been able to show that the purified chemotactic factors (C5 fragment, bacterial factor, and the synthetic peptides) induce neutropenia after infusion. This almost exactly parallels the dose response of the peptides in chemotactic chambers. The dose that will cause attraction of the leukocytes is the dose which, when infused *in vivo,* will cause the sudden leukopenia, with about 50 to 60% reduction in the leukocyte count across the pulmonary vascular flow. So, this is direct evidence that at least some chemotactic factors can induce neutropenia *in vivo.*

Dr. Wright: That result invokes the issue that has been discussed informally that *in vivo* chemotactic factors may have a major effect simply on the adherence of cells to endothelial walls, rather than on the induction of directed migration.

Dr. Ward: It has also been shown, however, that the direct treatment of leukocytes with these factors not only causes a volume change, which itself might interfere with their passage through the pulmonary capillaries, but also causes cell aggregation. (O'Flaherty, J. and Ward, P. A. *J. Immunol.,* 119:232–239, 1977. Therefore, it may be a physical trapping and not necessarily increased margination of cells that causes the neutropenia.

Dr. Williams: This issue is important. We also have been very interested in people before and after dialysis. We now have three patients with lupus and rapidly progressive glomerulonephritis in whom we looked at circulating immune complexes in the serum in the solid phase (Clq assay). We could show that

24 hr after dialysis there are no more circulating complexes. They were detectable in the serum from the patient, yet we can not find them on the dialysis membrane. We think that the mechanisms are exactly what you described. The leukocytes are being activated and sucking up complexes in the lung. The patient thus may be using his lung as a splint.

Dr. Ward: The pulmonary capillary tree is not unique, because, if you do these experiments across any arteriovenous network, such as the femoral artery and vein, the same results obtain; however, the pulmonary tree would seem to be one of the most important capillary beds involved in leukocyte-trapping.

Dr. Williams: According to Craddock and Jacobs, most of the leukocytes adhere in the lung.

Dr. Stossel: Of course, that is the only place they looked.

Dr. Ward: That is probably because, in shunted patients, the pulmonary capillary bed is the first capillary bed the manipulated leukocytes are delivered to.

Dr. Stossel: Another factor, aside from aggregation, that probably accounts for some of the sequestration is recognition of damaged cells by mononuclear cells. We think that the final common pathway for this damage is oxygen. John Klock and I have shown that the adherent cells are induced to generate metabolites of oxygen. You can protect cells that are interacting with nylon by letting them adhere in the presence of mannitol, sodium benzoate, superoxide dismutase, or ascorbate, all free radical scavengers. The assay for "damage" is to feed the eluted cells to other phagocytes (polymorphonuclear leukocytes) and then measure the metabolic response of the responding cells. And, interestingly, chronic granulomatous diseased cells can be put on nylon wool, then eluted, and they are not recognized by the other cells. The idea being the cell immolates itself with its own toxic oxygen products.

Dr. Quie: My interpretation of the evidence is that nylon wool or dialysis membrane brings about neutropenia by a process requiring both leukocytes and plasma.

Dr. Wright: This is also our interpretation. In the setting of nylon wool adherence, as with adherence to glass, adherence is a stimulus for the cells to degranulate partially, and this event results not only in complement activation if complement is present but also perhaps in hydrogen peroxide and superoxide production at the surface of the cell.

Dr. Jensen: I wonder what role this might play *in vivo*. With the very potent anaphylatoxin inactivators that are circulating, a small amount of C5a produced would be very rapidly degraded.

Dr. Wright: The same issue could be raised with the Arthus reaction, in which the role of complement has been clearly demonstrated. Certainly, one would expect that complement activation locally might have effects that are restricted to a specific site because of circulating inactivators.

Dr. Snyderman: In an *in vivo* model using the peritoneal cavity, we showed that if endotoxin or other substances that activate an inflammatory response are injected, the first thing seen kinetically is the production of chemotactic activity before cellular influx. This occurs within the first hour or two. Then, the accumulation of neutrophils starts to become visible. By the time that neutrophil accumulation is increasing rapidly, the amount of free chemotactic activity falls down markedly. By the time the number of neutrophils are at their peak, there is no detectable free chemotactic activity. I think that indicates that the initial event is the generation of C5a by the classical and alternative complement pathways. Following this, the neutrophils migrate in and ingest the inflammatory stimulant. Depending on the amount and digestibility of the inflammatory stimulus they find when they get there, they may release additional enzymes which cleave more C5 to produce more cellular influx. But if there is no strong phagocytic stimulus, the generation of more C5a ceases. Free C5a may dissipate by absorption of the chemotactic factors to the PMNs, or perhaps, because of chemotactic factor inactivators which break down chemotactic activity.

Dr. Wright: The model of endotoxin injected into the peritoneal cavity is very different from a sterile inflammatory lesion, such as the skin window. As was noted, in a C3-deficient patient, the kinetics of the skin window response has been found to be quite abnormal, suggesting that complement activation early in the inflammatory response, mediated perhaps by a secreted neutrophil product, is important in the normal development of the response. But, at the same time, we agree that the release of chemotactic factor inactivators may be important in shutting off an inflammatory response once it has developed.

Dr. Leddy: I would like to return to Dr. Jensen's question for just a moment, because this problem of why C5 fragment can survive to produce chemotactic activity, in the presence of the peptide inactivator (s), is a very puzzling one. The extremely rapid inactivation of C5a that has been recorded in the literature pertains to the anaphylatoxin activity. And here, the inactivation is so efficient that you cannot generate anaphylatoxin in human serum, unless you have EACA added at high molar concentration. Yet, we are all generating complement-dependent chemotactic activity in our chambers. Almost everyone's work seems to indicate that the major chemotactic factor is some fragment related to C5. So there must be a mechanism for a chemotactically active C5 fragment to survive, at least in some measure.

Leukocyte Chemotaxis, edited by John I. Gallin
and Paul G. Quie. Raven Press, New York
© 1978.

Chemotactic Factor Inhibitory Activity in Rabbit Neutrophils

John P. Bronza and Peter A. Ward

*Department of Pathology, University of Connecticut Health Center,
Farmington, Connecticut 06032*

Regulation of the inflammatory response is an essential feature of an acute insult to tissue that brings about a wave of infiltrating neutrophilic granulocytes (neutrophils). The reversed passive Arthus reaction has been used as a convenient model to study mediation of the injury which occurs as a consequence of the formation of immune complexes in tissues (3). It is now known that the complement system is an essential requirement for the developing inflammatory reaction and that the production of leukotactic factors generated by activation of the complement system is necessary for the accumulation of neutrophils (10,13). Subsequently, phagocytic ingestion of the complexes and release of proteolytic enzymes are responsible for the tissue injury (3,12). It has been shown that the accumulation of neutrophils in these reactions has two paradoxical effects. The first is tissue injury (referred to above), while the second is a termination of the inflammatory reaction (4). The latter has been assumed to be a result of phagocytic removal of the immune complexes. The results to be described will document the fact that neutrophils phagocytizing zymosan particles release a factor(s) that brings about inactivation of leukotactic mediators. This may represent an important mechanism for control of inflammatory responses that are mediated by leukotactic factors.

MATERIALS AND METHODS

Chemotaxis

Modified Boyden chambers were used to quantitate the migratory responses of rabbit neutrophils derived from glycogen-induced peritoneal exudates. Cells were suspended in Hank's medium containing 0.1% bovine serum albumin. Details of the technique are given elsewhere (2).Chemotactic factors employed consisted of the bacterial chemotactic factor present in a culture filtrate of *Escherichia coli*, the C3 fragment generated in human serum (containing 1M ε-amino caproic acid (EACA) and treated with inulin at 37°C for 1 hr), and the C5 fragment generated by zymosan activation of EACA-treated human serum. Deatails of these reagents are given elsewhere (9,11). The C3 and the

C5 fragments were isolated in crude form by elution of activated serum from a Sephadex G100 column and pooling of the post-albumin fractions. Amounts of the chemotactic preparations corresponded to 50 μl culture filtrate in the case of the bacterial chemotactic factor, and the equivalent of 20 μl of activated serum. Chemotactic factor inactivator activity was determined by the amount of reduction in chemotactic activity after a given factor was incubated for 30 min at 37° C with an appropriate test sample (2). When supernatant fluids of phagocytizing neutrophils were tested for inactivator activity, 50 μl of supernatant fluid was used. This would be the equivalent of culture fluid from 1×10^5 phagocytizing neutrophils.

Phagocytosis

Zymosan particles (2 mg) were first incubated with 1.0-ml fresh rabbit serum for purposes of opsonization. After the yeast suspension was incubated at 37°C for 1/2 hr, the zymosan particles were washed twice by diluting 10-fold with Hanks' medium (pH 7.4) and centrifuging ($1,000 \times g$). The yeast particles were then resuspended in Hanks' medium and added to rabbit neutrophils such that there were 2×10^7 neutrophils/2 mg zymosan in 1.0 ml. After incubation of cells and zymosan particles, with constant shaking at 37°C for 1/2 hr, the cells and particles were removed by centrifugation (see above) and the supernatant fluids assayed for the various contents.

Enzyme assays for the lysosomal enzyme β-glucuronidase and the cytosol enzyme lactic dehydrogenase (LDH) were done as described recently (14).

Subcellular Fractionation

These were accomplished by hypoosmotic means to disrupt neutrophils (in 0.34 M sucrose with 500 units heparin/ml) followed by differential sedimentation using sucrose gradients (5).

Density Gradient Ultracentrifugation

Continuous sucrose density gradients were made up from 5 to 35% sucrose in phosphate buffer (ionic strength, 0.2, pH 7.4) and ultracentrifugation carried out in a swinging bucket rotor, as previously described (2).

RESULTS

Release of Inactivator Activities from Phagocytizing Rabbit Neutrophils

When rabbit neutrophils were allowed to phagocytize opsonized zymosan particles, over a 60-min interval of time, approximately 25% of the lysosomal enzyme β-glucuronidase was released into the phagocytic (supernatant) fluid.

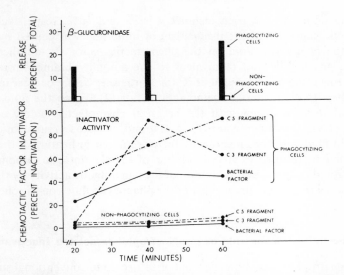

FIG. 1. Release from rabbit neutrophils of inactivator activity for the bacterial chemotactic factor and the C3 and C5 leukotactic fragments, in parallel with the release of β-glucuronidase.

In contrast, virtually none was released from nonphagocytizing cells (Fig. 1). When inactivator activities were measured for the three chemotactic factors (the bacterial factor, the C3, and the C5 fragments), significant amounts of inactivator activity were found during the hour-long period of incubation. The amounts of inactivator activities increased for the first 40 min and then either continued to increase in the case of the inactivator for the C5 fragment, to plateau with the bacterial factor inactivator, or to diminish after the 40-min interval in the case of the inactivator for the C3 fragment. Reasons for these differences are not known; they could relate either to different inactivators for each fragment, or to varying susceptibilities of each chemotactic factor to a common inactivator.

Mechanism of Inactivation Action

It seemed important to determine the nature by which the chemotactic factor activities were being suppressed. This could be caused either by an effect of the phagocytic fluids on the chemotactic factors, or by an inhibitory effect of the phagocytic fluids on the neutrophils per se (6). Two different experiments indicated that the suppressive effect was directed against the chemotactic factors and not against the indicator cells in the assay system. First, 50 μl of culture fluid from phagocytizing cells (equivalent of 1×10^5 neutrophils phagocytizing 100 μg zymosan) was added either to the 1.0-ml cell suspension in the upper compartment of the modified Boyden chamber, or into the lower compartment, which contained 50 μl bacterial chemotactic factor (in 1.0 ml). The inhibition of chemotactic activity in each instance was 92 and 16%, respectively. These data strongly suggest that the mechanism of inhibition was caused by a direct effect of the phagocytic fluid on the chemotactic factor. In another type of study, the phagocytic fluid (equivalent to the amount obtained from 1×10^5 phagocytizing cells) was heated at 56°C for 1 hr, either before or after incubation with the heat-stable bacterial chemotactic factor (2). When the fluid was *first* heated and *then* incubated with the bacterial chemotactic factor, only 35% inhibition of the chemotactic activity was found, whereas preincubation of the supernatant fluid with the chemotactic factor *followed by* heating of the mixture at 56°C for 1 hr resulted in 90% inhibition of the chemotactic response. These findings strongly suggest that inhibition of the chemotactic activity by the phagocytic fluids is a result of a direct effect of the phagocytic fluids on the chemotactic factors.

Subcellular Localization of the Neutrophil-associated Inactivator

Rabbit neutrophils were homogenized or subjected to conventional subcellular fractionation procedures and the equivalent of 1×10^5 leukocytes tested for inactivation of 50 µl of the bacterial chemotactic factor. The results are given in Table I. The whole-cell homogenate (which had been obtained by freeze-thawing five times of 1×10^5 neutrophils) inactivated 94% of the bacterial chemotactic factor, whereas no such effect was found with the nuclear fraction. The lysosomal fraction (which was obtained by differential centrifugation and then subjected to five cycles of freeze-thawing) was highly inhibitory (83% inactivation of the chemotactic activity), whereas the microsomal fraction reduced the chemotactic activity by only 26%. The cytosol fraction was halfway between the lysosomal and the microsomal fractions in terms of inactivation activity. The finding of an intermediate level (43%) of inactivation activity in the cytosol fraction could be a result of contamination by lysosomal enzymes (not suggested by the β-glucuronidase assays) or a result of the presence in the cytosol of an unrelated and independent inactivator activity. The results of β-glucuronidase assays were expected. The cell homogenates and the lysosomal

TABLE 1. *Localization of chemotactic factor inactivator activity in rabbit neutrophils*

Cellular or subcellular fraction[a]	Inactivation of bacterial fraction (%)	Enzyme content	
		Glucuronidase	LDH
Whole-cell fragments	94	100[b]	100[b]
Nuclear	0	5	0
Lysosomal	83	88	0
Microsomal	26	9	0
Cytosol	43	4	90

[a] From 2×10^7 peritoneal exudate neutrophils.
[b] Reference (100%) values for enzyme determinations.

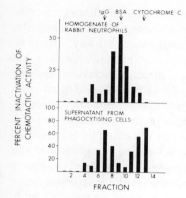

FIG. 2. Ultracentrifugal analysis in sucrose density gradients of the inactivator for the bacterial chemotactic factor. The homogenate of rabbit neutrophils is compared with the phagocytic supernatant fluid from phagocytizing leukocytes.

fractions contained high amounts of β-glucuronidase activity, whereas the other fractions had very low levels of enzyme. LDH assays confirmed the expected fractionation results: activity was predominantly in the whole-cell homogenate and in the cytosol fraction.

Ultracentrifugal Features of Leukocyte-derived Inhibitor

A homogenate from 1×10^7 rabbit neutrophils was obtained by five cycles of freeze-thawing, followed by removal of the particulate material by centrifugation ($15,000 \times g$ for 15 min). The cell lysate (0.25 ml) was applied to sucrose density gradient and then subjected to ultracentrifugation. Samples from the gradient were subsequently tested for ability to inactivate the bacterial chemotactic factor. Comparisons were made with similarly obtained samples that were derived from the phagocytic supernatant fluid after 2×10^7 neutrophils had ingested 2 mg opsonized zymosan over a 30-min period at 37°C.

The ultracentrifugal profiles of the inhibitor activity from the cell homogenate and from the phagocytic fluid are shown in Fig. 2. Although the cell homogenate contained a single peak of inhibitor activity in the position of the albumin (BSA) marker (Fig. 2, upper frame), the phagocytic fluid yielded a bimodal peak of inhibitor activity with a faster sedimenting peak coincident with the IgG marker, and a second zone of activity in the upper region of the gradient. Reasons for the differences in the sedimentation profiles for the two samples are unknown.

COMMENTS

The data reported in this chapter appear to confirm, at least in part, a recent report in which it is concluded that human neutrophils phagocytizing latex particles release into the phagocytic supernatant fluid a material that inactivates the C5-related leukotactic factor (15). This phenomenon was found under conditions in which maximal phagocytosis was occurring. Under conditions in which the intensity of the phagocytic stimulus was diminished, the authors reported the release of a material that had the net effect of generating chemotactic activity, at least in part, by activation of the alternative complement pathway. The presence in leukocytes of an activator of the alternative complement pathway has been previously described, as has the presence of a direct, C5-cleaving enzyme that generates C5 chemotactic fragments (7,12). Thus, products released from neutrophils during phagocytosis have complex effects that are difficult to predict.

The nature of the chemotactic factor inactivator activity described in this chapter is unknown. It seems likely that the inactivator is derived from lysosomal granules, that it is one of many substances released during phagocytosis, and that it may well be one of the many neutral proteases contained within in neutrophils (8). In unpublished data, we have found that the inactivator has a neutral pH optimum. There is, however, no information regarding the susceptibility of the inactivator to various inhibitors. No statements can be made regarding the relationship of the inactivator(s) to any of the traditional proteases in lysosomal granules of rabbit neutrophils or the possible physical-chemical relationship to the chemotactic factor inactivator present in normal human serum in low concentrations (1).

SUMMARY

Rabbit neutrophils release during phagocytosis of opsonized zymosan particles an inactivator(s) of the complement-derived C3 and C5 leukotactic factors and the bacterial chemotactic factor from *E. coli*. The release of this inactivator is time-dependent and occurs in parallel with the release of the lysosomal enzyme β-glucuronidase. By subcellular fractionation techniques, the inactivator occurs in high concentration in the lysosomal fraction. Analysis of the inactivator in sucrose density gradient ultracentrifugation reveals different patterns for the inactivator present in phagocytic supernatant fluids and that present in the leukocytic homogenate. The release from phagocytizing neutrophils of the chemotactic factor inactivator may represent an important regulatory mechanism in the inflammatory response.

REFERENCES

1. Berenberg, J. L., and Ward, P. A. (1973): The chemotactic factor inactivator in normal human serum. *J. Clin. Invest.*, 52:1200–1206.
2. Brozna, J. P., and Ward, P. A. (1975): Antileukotactic properties of tumor cells. *J. Clin. Invest.*, 56:616–623.
3. Cochrane, C. G. (1968): Immunologic tissue injury mediated by neutrophilic leukocytes. *Adv. Immunol.*, 9:97–214.
4. Cochrane, C. G., Weigle, W. G., and Dixon, F. J. (1959): The role of polymorphonuclear leukocytes in the initiation and cessation of Arthus vasculitis. *J. Exp. Med.*, 110:481.
5. deDuve, C. (1971): Tissue fractionation, past and present. *J. Cell. Biol.*, 50:20d–55d.
6. Goetzl, E., and Austen, K. F. (1972): A neutrophil-immobilizing factor derived from human leukocytes: I. Generation and partial characterization. *J. Exp. Med.*, 136:1564–1580.

7. Goldstein, I. M., and Weissmann, G. (1974): Generation of C5a activity in human serum by leucocyte lysosomal lysates. *Fed. Proc.*, 33:798 (abstract).
8. Janoff, A., Blondin, J., Sandhaus, R. A., Mosser, A., and Malenude, C. (1975): Human neutrophil elastase: In vitro effects on natural substrates suggest important physiological and pathological actions. In: *Proteases and Biological Control*, edited by E. Reich, D. B. Rifkin, and E. Shaw, pp. 603–620. Cold Spring Harbor Laboratory, New York.
9. Till, G., and Ward, P. A. (1975): Two distinct chemotactic factor inactivators in normal human serum. *J. Immunol.*, 114:843–847.
10. Ward, P. A., and Cochrane, C. G. (1965): Bound complement and immunologic vasculitis. *J. Exp. Med.*, 121:215.
11. Ward, P. A., Data, R., and Till, G. (1974): Regulatory control of complement derived chemotactic and anaphylatoxin mediators. In: *Progress in Immunology II*, Vol. 1, edited by L. Brent and J. Holborow, pp. 209–215. North-Holland Publishing Co., Amsterdam.
12. Ward, P. A., and Hill, J. H. (1970): C5 chemotactic fragments produced by an enzyme in lysomal granules of neutrophils. *J. Immunol.*, 104:535–543.
13. Ward, P. A., and Hill, J. H. (1972): Biologic role of complement products: Complement-derived leukotactic activity extractable from lesions of immunologic vasculitis. *J. Immunol.*, 108:1137–1145.
14. Ward, P. A., and Zvaifler, N. J. (1973): Quantitative phagocytosis by neutrophils: I. A new method with immune complexes. *J. Immunol.*, 111:1771–1775.
15. Wright, D. G., and Gallin, J. I. (1975): Modulation of the inflammatory response by products released from human polymorphonuclear leukocytes during phagocytosis: Generation and inactivation of the chemotactic factor C5a. *Inflammation*, 1:23–40.

DISCUSSION

Dr. Leddy: Dr. Ward, is the α-globulin chemotactic factor inhibitor elevated in Hodgkin's disease or are both serum inhibitors elevated?

Dr. Ward: In Hodgkin's disease the α-inhibitor is elevated. In sarcoidosis patients, cirrhosis patients, and a variety of others, both inhibitors are seen to be elevated.

Dr. Leddy: What does the β-inhibitor specifically inhibit?

Dr. Ward: The β-globulin inhibitor specifically inhibits the C3 chemotactic fragment. Both the α- and β-globulin inhibitors inactivate the bacterial chemotactic factor.

Dr. Van Epps: From this, could one conclude that C3 fragments have very little part in the inflammatory response?

Dr. Ward: Yes, that implication is correct. Early in our studies of inflammatory reaction, we searched for but could not find C3 fragments in developing Arthus lesions. There may be many C3 fragments floating around, but not with chemotactic activity.

Dr. Lynn: Are these fragments inhibitors?

Dr. Ward: We have to hedge on this. There is hydrolysis of chemotactic peptides and an associated aminopeptidase activity but there is no direct evidence of how CFI interacts with naturally occurring chemotactic factors.

Dr. Jensen: Dr. Ward, do you have any information about inhibitors in other animal species?

Dr. Ward: Our experiments have primarily involved CFI and chemotactic factors isolated from human serum, but we know that CFI will inactivate the chemotactic activity in the activated rat and guinea pig serums. The serum carboxypeptidase-*N*, which we isolate in the process of purifying the CFI from serum, has no inhibitory activity for the C5 fragment.

Dr. Jensen: Would you then say that C5 anaphylatoxin is not chemotactic?

Dr. Ward: No, I do not think that is correct. All the preparations of C5a that we have tested are chemotactically active, so whatever is in those preparations is chemotactically active. I believe C5 anaphylatoxin is chemotactically active, but it does not represent the bulk of the chemotactic activity in activated serum.

Dr. Quie: Dr. Ward, do you have any idea about the source of the inhibitor that is increased in inflammatory diseases? For example, what cells may be releasing the inhibitor?

Dr. Ward: We do not have any direct information.

Dr. Schiffmann: Does the inhibitor inactivate formylated peptides?

Dr. Ward: The most recent, highly purified preparations of CFI will totally block chemotactic activity in bacterial culture supernatants but will not touch the synthetic peptides.

Dr. Van Epps: Dr. Ward, will these inhibitors act on chemotactic factors released from stimulated lymphocytes?

Dr. Ward: Yes, at least the "unpurified" material does inactivate the chemotactic activity produced by activated lymphocytes. It also blocks MIF.

Dr. Van Epps: Did you notice any correlation between serum CFI in your patients and skin test anergy? In our experience, only about 50% of patients with liver disease will have a suppressed inflammatory response, and I noticed that the serum inhibitor was present in nearly 90% of your patients.

Dr. Ward: There is a correlation in leprosy patients. About 18 patients had high levels of inactivator and 17 of the 18 were anergic.

Leukocyte Chemotaxis, edited by John I. Gallin
and Paul G. Quie. Raven Press, New York
© 1978.

Serum Inhibitors of Leukocyte Chemotaxis and Their Relationship to Skin Test Anergy

Dennis E. Van Epps and Ralph C. Williams, Jr.

School of Medicine, University of New Mexico, Albuquerque, New Mexico 87131

Multiple humoral factors have been described which are capable of suppressing polymorphonuclear leukocyte (PMN) and monocyte chemotaxis. These circulating inhibitors are most prominent during states of severe systemic disease including liver disease (5,15,30), pulmonary disease (28,29), sepsis (28), Hodgkin's disease (34), leprosy (35), renal disease (3,6), neoplasms (21,23,32,33), in certain children who experience recurrent bacterial infections (22,37), and in some patients following bone marrow transplants (16). These inhibitors can be classified into two basic types: (a) those which inactivate chemotactic factors (4), and (b) those which exhibit a direct inhibitory effect on the responding cell (23,31, 32,33). Two chemotactic inhibitors which irreversibly inactivate chemotactic factors are found in low concentrations in normal serum (31) and in much higher concentrations in patients with cirrhosis (15), Hodgkin's disease (34), and leprosy (35). These inhibitors are heat-labile at 56°C and can be separated into a 4S inhibitor which irreversibly inactivates the chemotactic activity of C5a and a 7S inhibitor which irreversibly inactivates C3a (26), and have been characterized as amino peptidases (36). The second type of serum chemotactic inhibitors, the cell-directed inhibitors, are present in sera from patients with liver disease (30), IgA myeloma (32), other neoplastic diseases (21,23,33), children with recurrent infections (22,37), and normal serum (33). These cell-directed inhibitors are also apparent in the sera of most patients with suppressed delayed-type skin test responses (28,31). It is speculated in most instances that these various serum inhibitors of chemotaxis may either regulate the inflammatory response, or be at least partially responsible for *in vivo* suppression of inflammation and increased susceptibility to infection.

STUDIES ON ANERGIC PATIENTS

A total of 182 patients with various systemic diseases were studied with respect to serum chemotactic inhibitory activity. In each case, normal human polymorphonuclear leukocytes were used as indicator cells (28), and fresh normal serum, C5a, casein, kallikrein or *Escherichia coli*-derived chemotactic factor was used as chemotactic attractants (5,28,32). Serum chemotactic inhibitory activity was declared present if the addition of 10% patient serum to the lower compartment

TABLE 1. *Summary of patients with serum chemotactic inhibitory activity*

Disease	Number of patients with serum chemotactic inhibitory activity per total tested[a]
Liver disease	36/72
Pulmonary disease	13/29
Sepsis	5/6
Fractures	0/4
Burns	1/2
Malignancy (other than myeloma)	1/3
SLE	4/34
Viral infection	0/3
Congestive heart failure	0/2
Rheumatoid arthritis	1/5
Chronic inflammatory bowel disease	3/6
Children with recurrent infections	0/7
Hodgkin's disease	0/8
Cellulitis	1/1
Controls	0/37

[a] All tests shown utilized 10% fresh normal serum as a control chemotactic stimulus and normal human PMNs as indicator cells.

of the Boyden-type chamber resulted in a 30% reduction in the chemotactic response of normal human PMNs. Table 1 shows a summary of the studies we have performed on 182 patients and 37 normal adults. Sixty-five of the patients studied showed serum chemotactic inhibitory activity. The categories of patients where chemotactic inhibitors were most frequently encountered were those patients with liver disease, pulmonary disease, sepsis, and chronic inflammatory bowel disease.

Of the 182 patients shown in Table 1, 142 were skin-tested with six common skin test antigens including streptokinase-streptodornase, candida, mumps, coccidiodin, PPD, and trichophytin (28). Patients were considered to be anergic if less than 5 mm of induration was noted to all skin test antigens. In our original studies on 61 patients, we observed a highly significant association between skin test anergy and serum chemotactic inhibitory activity. In the larger series presented here, the association was still apparent and highly significant ($p < 0.001$), as shown in Table 2. It is of interest to note that of the 36 patients not conforming to the pattern of anergy with inhibitor or skin reactivity without inhibitor, more individuals were anergic without inhibitor than were skin test-positive with chemotactic inhibitory activity. This would imply that although serum inhibitors of chemotaxis are closely associated with skin test anergy, they are clearly not solely responsible for anergy itself. Both anergy and serum chemotactic inhibitory activity are transient conditions in most of these patients, and in several experiments performed on patients who regained their skin reactivity there was a direct parallel between anergy and chemotactic inhibitory activity (28,30). In these patients, chemotactic inhibitors were demonstrated concurrently

TABLE 2. *Summary of patients tested with respect to the presence or absence of anergy and serum chemotactic inhibitory activity*

	Number of patients	
Patients	With serum chemotactic inhibitory activity	Without serum chemotactic inhibitory activity
Anergic patients	55	26
Skin test-positive patients	10	51

$p < 0.001$ for the association of anergy and chemotactic inhibitory activity.

with skin test anergy, and when skin reactivity was regained, no chemotactic inhibitory activity was demonstrable.

It is apparent from more recent studies (20) that chemotactic inhibitors are not the only suppressive factors which became apparent in anergic patients. In these studies, when mouse femur cells were cultured in the presence of serum from patients with various systemic diseases, serum from anergic patients significantly suppressed mouse bone marrow colony formation when compared with either normal control serum or serum from patients with positive skin test responses. Similarly, patients with serum chemotactic inhibitory activity significantly suppressed mouse bone marrow colony formation when compared to normal control sera or sera from patients with positive skin test responses. This inhibition of bone marrow colony formation was caused by multiple factors (20). Whether some of these inhibitors are the same as those responsible for chemotactic inhibition remains to be seen. Further studies are warranted in order to determine the function of these factors *in vivo* and their relationship to host defense mechanisms.

STUDIES WITH WHOLE SERA CONTAINING CHEMOTACTIC INHIBITORS

Sera containing chemotactic inhibitory activity effectively suppressed PMN chemotaxis toward fresh normal serum, C5a, C3a, casein, kallikrein, and bacterial chemotactic factor (28,29). This broad spectrum of activity implied that the inhibitory effect on chemotaxis was cell-directed. This hypothesis was confirmed by the preincubation of PMNs with inhibitory serum, which resulted in a suppressed chemotactic response, and by the failure of these sera to inactivate the chemotactic activity of casein irreversibly (31). Although many of the sera were derived from patients similar to those in whom chemotactic factor inactivator activity has been detected and probably contain these factors (15), we have been unable, so far, to detect an irreversible inactivation of chemotactic factor by these sera or an adsorption of chemotactic inhibitor to insolubilized casein-adsorbent columns (31). In addition, the chemotactic inhibitory activity observed in the anergic patient sera studied here was heat-stable at 56°C for over 2 hr and, in fact, this treatment enhanced the inhibitory activity of these sera significantly—implying that either heat-labile antagonists of this system are present in serum or that 56°C heat treatment resulted in the aggregation of inhibitors to form a more effective suppressor substance (31). The presence of inhibitor antagonists was also implied by the neutralization of inhibitory activity which occurred with the addition of increasing concentrations of normal serum (29). The inhibition of chemotaxis by these sera from anergic patients was not restricted to PMN, but was also observed with monocytes. The suppression of monocyte chemotaxis is consistent with a function for these factors in anergy, since these cells are predominant in a normal delayed cutaneous response to antigen.

FRACTIONATION OF INHIBITORY SERA

Patient sera were separated by 5 to 20% sucrose density gradient centrifugation and fractions tested for the suppression of PMN chemotaxis (29,30). The representative patterns of inhibition shown in Fig. 1 indicate various levels of three major inhibitors in patients with liver disease, cellulitis, disseminated atypical mycobacterium, pulmonary edema, or IgA myeloma. These inhibitors have sedi-

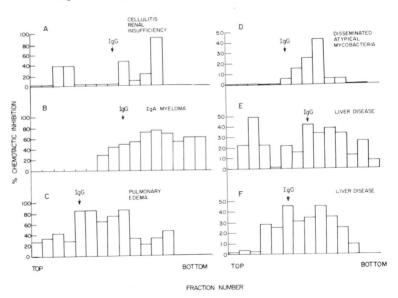

FIG. 1. Representative patterns of chemotactic inhibition observed when sera from patients with different systemic diseases were separated by 5 to 20% sucrose density gradient centrifugation. Samples were centrifuged for 12 to 16 hours at 100,000 × g. The position of the 7S IgG marker is shown for each sample. Sample A, C, D, E, and F were obtained from anergic patients; sample B from a patient with IgA myeloma who was not skin-tested. Fractions were used in the lower compartment of the Boyden chamber with 10% fresh normal serum as a chemotactic attractant.

mentation coefficients of approximately 4S, 7S, and 11 to 14S. In our studies of 10 anergic patients with chemotactic inhibitory activity, 7 of 10 showed 4S inhibitors, 9 of 10 showed 7S inhibitors, and 10 of 10 showed 11 to 14S inhibitors. These data indicate that a closer association exists between 7S and 11 to 14S inhibitors and anergy than between 4S inhibitors and anergy. Furthermore, in our system, the degree of inhibition resulting from 7S and 11 to 14S inhibitors was generally greater than that observed with the 4S inhibitors.

Our efforts have been directed at characterizing the inhibitors in the 7 to 14S range. Current evidence indicates that these factors are cell-directed inhibitors, since preincubation of normal PMN with sucrose density gradient fractions resulted in the suppression of PMN chemotaxis by both the 7S and 11 to 14S components. Further characterization of these larger inhibitors showed that these factors were precipitated from serum with 50% ammonium sulfate, had β-electrophoretic mobility as determined by starch block electrophoresis, they elute from Sephadex G-200 in the void volume and 7S regions, are heat-stable (28,29,30), and elute from DEAE with 0.01 M pH 6.0 buffer in fractions containing IgA and albumin. The apparent association of chemotactic inhibitory activity with fractions containing IgA indicated a possible involvement of this immunoglobulin in chemotactic inhibition. This was also implied by studies on patients with liver disease, which showed that IgA was significantly higher in patients with serum chemotactic inhibitory activity than in those without chemotactic inhibitory activity (30). Additional experiments showed that the 50% ammonium sulfate precipitable inhibitory activity from patients with liver disease could be specifically removed from the samples with insolubilized anti-IgA and anti-light chain-specific immunoadsorbent columns (30). Furthermore, inhibitory activity could be eluted from these columns with an acid buffer, and the absorption of inhibitory substances by these IgA-specific columns blocked by prior incubation of the immunoadsorbent column with human colostral IgA (30). All these data support the involvement of IgA in the inhibition of PMN chemotaxis.

STUDIES ON MYELOMA SERA

Confirmation of IgA involvement in chemotactic inhibition comes from data on 48 patients with IgA myeloma of which 28 showed serum chemotactic inhibitory activity (Fig. 2). This inhibition was not observed with sera from patients with Waldenströms' macroglobulinemia of IgG myeloma. Inhibition of chemotaxis by IgA myeloma sera occurred in chemotaxis systems mediated by C5a, fresh normal serum, casein, and bacterial-derived chemotactic factors. Treatment of IgA myeloma sera at 56°C for 30 min enhanced their chemotactic inhibitory activity (Fig. 2) in a manner similar to that previously shown with sera from anergic patients with chemotactic inhibitory activity (31). These same characteristics were observed with isolated IgA-M components and human colostral IgA (32).

The suppression of PMN chemotaxis by IgA M-components was not restricted

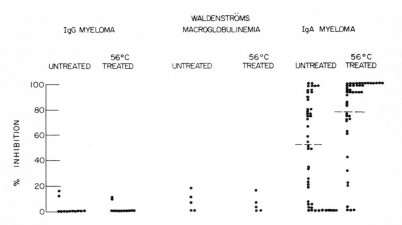

FIG. 2. Studies of the chemotactic inhibitory activity of patients with IgA and IgG myeloma, and patients with Waldenström's macroglobulinemia. Each point indicates a different patient serum tested both before and after a 56°C heat treatment for its effect on normal PMN chemotaxis toward fresh normal serum.

to neutrophils but also included monocytes, although IgA M-components generally were not as effective in suppressing monocyte chemotaxis as they were neutrophil chemotaxis (32). More recent experiments indicate that IgA M-components also exhibit a similar suppressive effect on human eosinophil chemotaxis (19). The effect of IgA on the PMN was predominantly on chemotaxis, since random mobility was either unaffected or only slightly reduced by the presence of IgA (32). These results contradict a possible inhibition of chemotaxis by α_1 antitrypsin of α_2 macroglobulin, which may be bound to IgA M-component (27), since these factors have been shown to enhance random mobility (7). The action of IgA was cell-directed, as demonstrated by preincubation of PMN with IgA M-components (32). This cell-directed inhibition of chemotaxis was partially reversible if PMN were cultured in medium supplemented with fetal calf serum (32).

Separation of whole IgA myeloma sera and isolated M-components showed chemotactic inhibitory activity in the 7 to 14S regions with the majority of inhibition falling in the 11 to 14S region where polymeric IgA would be found (Fig. 1). The role of polymeric IgA was investigated by dithiotreitol reduction and alkylation of isolated IgA M-components, which results in the conversion of polymeric IgA to its monomeric counterpart (10). This conversion of polymeric IgA to monomeric IgA resulted in a substantial loss of chemotactic inhibitory activity, as did removal of the Fc portion of the IgA M-component by pepsin digestion (32). These data indicate, first, that polymeric IgA is a more effective inhibitor than monomeric IgA, and second, that the suppressive effect of IgA is dependent upon the Fc portion of the molecule. This Fc-dependent inhibition of neutrophil chemotaxis also occurs with eosinophil chemotaxis (19). These data parallel previous work on the PMN IgA receptor showing Fc dependence and enhanced binding of IgA polymers (13,25). Furthermore, it is of interest to note that the percent of IgA myeloma patients exhibiting chemotactic inhibitory activity in their sera prior to heat treatment (58%) is similar to the percent of IgA myeloma patients showing over 10% polymeric IgA in their sera, 65% (18).

Two possible mechanisms of IgA-mediated chemotactic inhibition have been proposed. First, the interaction of IgA with the PMN IgA receptor may result in steric or functional interference of the PMN-chemotactic factor interaction and thus suppress a chemotactic response. If this is the mechanism of chemotactic inhibition, these data imply that human eosinophils may also have a receptor for IgA, since their chemotaxis is also inhibited by IgA M-components (19). Second, it is feasible that inhibition may be caused by a factor bound to IgA. This factor could then inhibit chemotaxis by steric or functional interference. The binding of various serum components to IgA has been well documented (14,17,27), and certain of these components that may bind to IgA (α_1 antitrypsin and α_2 macroglobulin) have also been shown to suppress PMN chemotaxis reversibly while enhancing random mobility (7). Although it is conceivable that these factors may be involved in chemotactic suppression, no enhancement of random migration was observed with IgA M-components (32). These data indicate that polymeric IgA or IgA with an associated component may account for chemotactic inhibition in the 11 to 14S regions of sucrose density gradient preparations.

EFFECT OF IGA M-COMPONENTS ON PMN PHAGOCYTOSIS AND CHEMILUMINESCENCE

The functional specificity of IgA for inhibition of chemotaxis was further tested by incorporating IgA M-components into assays designed to measure PMN bactericidal activity (12). As shown in Fig. 3, the addition of IgA to cultures of PMN plus normal serum opsonized *E. Coli.* resulted in a concentration-dependent decrease in bactericidal activity. It should be noted that although some IgA M-components tested, including the one shown in Fig. 3, totally inhibited chemotaxis at 0.5 mg/ml, they did not suppress PMN bactericidal activity to the same degree, even at final concentrations of 2 mg/ml. This observation was consistent with seven different IgA M-components with potent chemotactic inhibitory activity. Thus, IgA M-components were more effective inhibitors of chemotaxis than of phagocytosis. The partial inhibition of bactericidal activity by IgA M-components, like the suppression of chemotaxis, was also dependent on the Fc portion of IgA. Although data indicate that some suppression of bactericidal activity by IgA M-components occurs, substantial bacterial killing was still observed, indicating that much of the cellular machinery responsible for bactericidal activity was still intact. In an effort to define the mechanism of IgA-mediated chemotactic inhibition further, IgA M-components were tested for their effect on PMN chemiluminescence (11). Zymosan, which had been

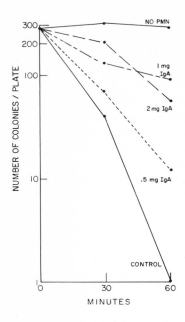

FIG. 3. The effect of increasing concentrations of IgA M-component on PMN bactericidal activity. The IgA M-component shown gave 100% inhibition of chemotaxis at a concentration of 1 mg per milliliter. Results are reported as the $\log_{10}$ of the number of *Escherichia coli* colonies per pour plate observed when sampling 0.001 ml of a 1-ml mixture of opsonized *E. coli*, PMNs, and IgA after various times of 37°C incubation.

opsonized with fresh human serum, was used to stimulate normal human PMN chemiluminescence in the presence or absence of IgA M-components. Results showed that the addition of isolated IgA M-components with potent chemotactic inhibitory activity had little or no effect on chemiluminescence. When concentrations as high as 2 mg/ml were used, less than a 10% reduction in chemiluminescence was observed. Experiments also showed that IgA M-components themselves did not stimulate chemiluminescence. These data, in addition to the lack of an effect on PMN random mobility, indicate that IgA-mediated suppression of PMN chemotaxis was not a result of a generalized inhibition of cell function or metabolic pathways such as hexose monophosphate shunt activation, which is common to all the cell functions examined. These data imply that inhibition of chemotaxis by polymeric IgA may be the result of interference with cell systems or receptors specific for chemotaxis.

COMMENTS

Many serum inhibitors of leukocyte chemotaxis have been described in normal serum and in association with a variety of systemic illnesses (Table 3). These inhibitors may be directed toward chemotactic factors (2,15,16,34,35,36), multiple effector cells (21,30,32,33), or exert a more specific cellular inhibition restricted to one particular cell type (23,24). From the data presented here and in previous studies, we can define several chemotactic inhibitors: First, are a 4S inhibitor and a 7S inhibitor known as chemotactic factor inactivators (CFI), which irreversibly inactivate chemotactic factors. These inhibitors are apparent in patients with cirrhosis (15), sarcoid (16), lepromatous leprosy (35), Hodgkin's disease (34), and can be found in low concentrations in normal serum (2). Similar factor-directed inhibitors have also been described in renal disease (3,6), although these have not been characterized. Second, there is a group of 7S cell-directed chemotactic inhibitors which are found in anergic patients (28, 29,30,31), patients with liver disease (30), sarcoma (21,33), carcinoma (33), and in low concentrations in normal sera (33). In normal serum, sarcoma, and carcinoma, these factors have also been shown to inhibit PMN phagocytosis. Whether all these 7S cell-directed inhibitors represent a single factor remains to be seen. Third, both α_1 antitrypsin and α_2 macroglobulin have been shown to suppress chemotaxis while enhancing random mobility (7). Fourth, IgA M-components have been shown to inhibit PMN, monocyte, and eosinophil chemotaxis. This suppression was cell-directed, dependent on the Fc portion of the IgA and associated with polymeric forms of this immunoglobulin (32), and, finally, low-molecular-weight chemotactic inhibitors derived from neoplasms which effect only macrophage chemotaxis (23,24). The relationship of each of these factors to the overall host inflammatory response remains to be defined. It is possible that the observed inhibition of leukocyte chemotaxis by serum from patients with various systemic diseases may be an important means of regulating the host inflammatory response. The consequence of this regulation could be an enhanced susceptibility to infections, as has been previously noted in many of the patient categories referred to here. In our studies, the appearance of chemotactic inhibitors in association with anergy (28,29,31) implies that *in vivo* these factors may function, as they do *in vitro,* by suppressing various aspects of the inflammatory response. Three alternatives exist: first, these factors may be the result of a suppressed inflammatory response; second, these factors may appear simultaneously with anergy in patients with severe systemic disease, but not function *in vivo* to suppress delayed cutaneous hypersensitivity; or third, that these inhibitors function as they do *in vivo* to inhibit various aspects of the inflammatory response, thus causing anergy. If the latter is true, it is likely that either the 7S or high-molecular-weight chemotactic inhibitors shown in Fig. 1 are responsible for anergy, since in our studies on anergic patients these inhibitors were most frequently encountered in multiple types of disease.

One of the major problems involved in relating our findings to the clinical course of disease in various anergic patients is the precise source of such inhibitory materials. It is not yet clear whether the factors which are apparently cell-directed, such as polymeric IgA, or those 7S factors initially described (28,29,30,31) in a wide variety of patients with acute systemic illness, are derived directly from the inflammatory process—possibly the inflammatory cells themselves much like the neutrophil-immobilizing factor released from neutrophils during phagocytosis (8)—or whether they arise somehow as a distant consequence of the acute systemic illness. Several recent studies have characterized chemotactic factors liberated by lymphocytes after various types of mitogenic challenge (1,38). Very little evidence is yet available concerning the possibility

TABLE 3. *Summary of current studies on serum chemotactic inhibitors*

Source of serum chemotactic inhibitor	Characteristics	Site of action	Other effects on phagocytic cells	References
Normal serum	a. 4S aminopeptidase (CFI); Heat-labile, α-globulin	Chemotactic factor (C5a, kallikrein, bacterial factor)	—	2, 17, 36
	b. 7S aminopeptidase (CFI); Heat-labile, β-globulin	Chemotactic factor (C3a, kallikrein, bacterial factor)	—	2, 17, 36
	c. 7S heat-stable inhibitor	Cell-directed (PMN, monocytes)	Inhibits phagocytosis	33
	d. α₁-antitrypsin, α₂-macroglobulin	Cell-directed (PMN)	Enhance random mobility	7
Patients with liver disease	a. Elevated 4S and 7S CFI	Chemotactic factor	—	15
	b. Inhibitor of casein and activated serum-mediated chemotaxis	—		5
	c. 4S, 7S, and 11S inhibitors; 7S and 11S heat-stable with β electrophoretic mobility	7S and 11S cell-directed; sera inhibit both monocyte and PMN chemotaxis	—	30
Hodgkin's disease	Elevated levels of CFI	Chemotactic factor	—	34
Lapromatous leprosy	Elevated levels of CFI	Chemotactic factor	—	35
Sarcoid	Elevated levels of CFI	Chemotactic factor	—	11
Anergic patients	4S, 7S, and 11S inhibitors; 7S and 11S dominant; heat-stable with β mobility	7S and 11S cell-directed.	—	28, 29, 30, and 32
IgA myeloma	11S to 14S; heat-stable; associated with polymeric IgA	Cell-directed (PMN, eosinophils, monocytes)	Partial inhibition of bactericidal activity	19, 31
Sarcoma and carcinoma	a. 7S heat-stable	Cell-directed PMN, monocytes	Inhibits phagocytosis	33
	b. Heat-stable, elutes with IgG from Sephadex	—	Inhibits phagocytosis	21

Neoplastic disease in mouse	Low-molecular-weight inhibitor (6,000 to 12,000 daltons) derived from tumor cells	Cell-directed (macrophages)	—	16, 23
Renal disease	a. Heat-labile	Chemotactic factor	—	6
	b. Found in rabbits w/drug-induced renal failure	Chemotactic factor	—	3
Bone marrow transplant patients	Inhibits PMN chemotaxis	—	—	4
Children with recurrent infections	a. Heat-stable, reversible	Cell-directed (PMN)	—	22
	b. Reversible inhibition	Cell-directed (PMN)	—	37

that lymphocytes, monocytes or possibly other inflammatory cells actually liberate chemotactic inhibitors themselves in the course of an acute systemic illness or disease associated with clinical anergy. A recent report by Greene et al. (9) bears directly on this point. These latter investigators were able to show a dramatic decrease in chemotactic effectiveness of polymorphonuclear leukocytes after conventional hemodialysis procedures. No evidence was derived in this particular study for a circulating inhibitor of PMN chemotaxis in these patients. It is conceivable that various metabolic events occur or may be induced by various disease processes within such cells as PMNs which partially turn off their metabolic machinery necessary for chemotaxis or other forms of cellular interaction. Studies directed at such intracellular processes as chemiluminescence or effective intracellular killing of ingested bacteria are certainly now in order in this regard.

Considerable interest has recently evolved in the relationship of chemotactic inhibitors to cancer. Studies by Snyderman et al. (23,24) have described production by various experimental tumors of a 6000 to 10,000 molecular weight factor which appears to inhibit accumulation of macrophages but was inactive against polymorphonuclear chemotaxis. These findings suggest that tissue cells themselves are indeed capable of producing chemotactic inhibitors; however, it is not clear what the cellular source for such chemotactic inhibitors is when one considers the wide variety of systemic illnesses clearly associated with relative skin test anergy and presence of chemotactic inhibition. Studies must now be directed at the precise cellular origin of these inhibitors associated with various anergic states.

ACKNOWLEDGMENTS

Supported by U.S.P.H.S. Grant numbers HL17179 from the National Heart and Lung Institute, and CA30819 from the National Cancer Institute, and the Arthritis Foundation.

REFERENCES

1. Altman, L. C., Snyderman, R., Oppenheim, J. J., and Mergenhagen, S. E. (1973): A human mononuclear leukocyte chemotactic factor: Characterization, specificity and kinetics of production by homologous leukocytes. *J. Immunol.*, 110:801–810.
2. Berenberg, J. L., and Ward, P. A. (1973): Chemotactic factor inactivator in normal human serum. *J. Clin. Invest.*, 52:1200–1206.
3. Clark, R. A., Hamory, B. H., Ford, G. H., and Kimbal, H. R. (1972): Chemotaxis in acute renal failure. *J. Infect. Dis.*, 126:460–463.
4. Clark, R. A., Johnson, F. L., Klebanoff, S. J., and Thomas, E. D. (1976): Defective neutrophil chemotaxis in bone marrow transplant patients. *J. Clin. Invest.*, 58:22–31.
5. Demeo, A. N., and Andersen, B. R. (1972): Defective chemotaxis associated with a serum inhibitor in cirrhotic patients. *N. Engl. J. Med.*, 286:735–745.
6. Gewurz, H., Page, A. R., Pickering, R. J., and Good, R. A. (1967): Complement activity and inflammatory neutrophil exudation in man. *Int. Arch. Allergy Appl. Immun.*, 32:64–90.
7. Goetzl, E. J. (1975): Modulation of human neutrophil polymorphonuclear leukocyte migration

by human plasma alpha-globulin inhibitors and synthetic esterase inhibitors. *Immunology,* 29:163–174.

8. Goetzl, E. J., Gigli, I., Wasserman, S., and Austen, K. F. (1973): A neutrophil immobilizing factor derived from human leukocytes. *J. Immunol.,* 111:938–945.

9. Greene, W. H., Cassan, R. S., Mauer, S. M., and Quie, P. G. (1976): The effect of hemodialysis on neutrophil chemotactic responsiveness. *J. Lab. Clin. Med.,* 88:971–974.

10. Hauptman, S., and Tomasi, T. B. (1975): Mechanism of immunoglobulin A polymerization. *J. Biol. Chem.,* 250:3891–3896.

11. Hill, H. R., Hogan, N. A., Bale, J. F., and Hemning, V. G. (1976): Evaluation of nonspecific (alternative pathway) opsonic activity by neutrophil chemiluminescence. *Int. Arch. Allergy Appl. Immun. (in press).*

12. Holley, T. R., Van Epps, D. E., Harvey, R. L., Anderson, R. E., and Williams, R. C., Jr. (1974): Effect of high doses of radiation on human neutrophil chemotaxis, phagocytosis, and morphology. *Am. J. Pathol.,* 75:61–72.

13. Lawrence, D. A., Weigle, W., and Spiegelberg, H. (1975): Immunoglobulins cytophilic for human lymphocytes, monocytes, and neutrophils. *J. Clin. Invest.,* 55:368–376.

14. Lewis, L. A., and Page, I. H. (1965): An unusual serum lipoprotein-globulin complex in a patient with hyperlipemia. *Am. J. Med.,* 38:286–297.

15. Maderazo, E., Ward, P. A., and Quintiliani, R. (1975): Defective regulation of chemotaxis in cirrhosis. *J. Lab. Clin. Med.,* 85:621–630.

16. Maderazo, E. G., Ward, P. A., Woronick, C. L., Kubik, J., and DeGraff, A. C. (1976): Leukotactic dysfunction in sarcoidosis. *Ann. Intern. Med.,* 84:414–419.

17. Mannik, M. (1967): Binding of albumin to gamma A myeloma proteins and Waldenström macroglobulins by disulfide bonds. *J. Immunol.,* 99:899–906.

18. Radl, J., Schutl, H. R., Mestecky, J., and Hijmans, W. (1974): The origin of monomeric and polymeric forms of IgA in man: The immunoglobulin A system, edited by J. Mestecky and A. R. Lanton. Plenum, New York.

19. Reed, K., Van Epps, D. E., and Williams, R. C., Jr. (1977): Supression of eosinophil chemotaxis by IgA paraproteins. *Fed. Proc.* 36:A4996.

20. Rhyne, R. L., Jr., Van Epps, D. E., and Williams, R. C., Jr. (1977): Serum inhibitors of mouse bone marrow colony formation in patients with systemic disease: Increased activity in anergic patients with chemotactic inhibitory activity. *J. Lab. Clin. Med.,* 90:195–203.

21. Ruutu, T., Ruutu, P., Vuopio, P., Franssila, K., Linder, E. (1975): An inhibitor of chemotaxis and phagocytosis in reticulum cell sarcoma. *Scand. J. Haematol.,* 15:27–34.

22. Smith, C. W., Hollers, J. C., Dupree, E., Goldman, A. S., and Cord, R. A. (1973): A serum inhibitor of leukotaxis in a child with recurrent infections. *J. Lab. Clin. Med.,* 89:878–885.

23. Snyderman, R., Pike, M. C. (1976): An inhibitor of macrophage chemotaxis produced by neoplasms. *Science,* 192:370–372.

24. Snyderman, R., Pike, M., Blaylock, B. L., and Weinstein, P. (1974): Effect of neoplasm on inflammation: Depression of macrophage accumulation after tumor implantation. *J. Immunol.,* 116:585–589.

25. Spiegelberg, H. L., Lawrence, D. A., and Henson, P. (1974): Cytophilic properties of IgA to human neutrophils. *Adv. Exp. Med. Biol.,* 45:67–74.

26. Till, G., and Ward, P. A. (1975): Two distinct chemotactic factor inactivators in human serum. *J. Immunol.,* 114:843–847.

27. Tomasi, T. B., and Hauptman, S. P. (1974): The binding of α_1 antitrypsin to human IgA. *J. Immunol.,* 112:2274–2277.

28. Van Epps, D. E., Frierson, J. A., and Williams, R. C., Jr. (1974): Immunological studies of anergic patients. *Infect. Immun.,* 10:1003–1009.

29. Van Epps, D. E., Palmer, D. L., and Williams, R. C., Jr. (1974): Characterization of serum inhibitors of neutrophil chemotaxis associated with anergy. *J. Immunol.,* 113:189–200.

30. Van Epps, D. E., Strickland, R. G., and Williams, R. C., Jr. (1975): Inhibitors of leukocyte chemotaxis in alcoholic liver disease. *Am. J. Med.,* 59:200–207.

31. Van Epps, D. E., and Williams, R. C., Jr. (1976): Serum chemotactic inhibitory activity: Heat activation of chemotactic inhibition. *Infect. Immun.,* 13:741–749.

32. Van Epps, D. E., and Williams, R. C., Jr. (1976): Suppression of leukocyte chemotaxis by human IgA myeloma components. *J. Exp. Med.,* 144:1227–1242.

33. Ward, P. A., Anton, T., and Maderazo, E. (1976): Defective leukotaxis in cancer patients. *Clin. Res.,* 24:463A.

34. Ward, P. A., and Berenberg, J. L. (1974): Defective regulation of inflammatory mediators in Hodgkin's disease: Supernormal levels of chemotactic-factor inactivator. *N. Engl. J. Med.,* 290:76–80.
35. Ward, P. A., Goralnick, S., and Bullock, W. E. (1976): Defective leukotaxis in patients with lepromatous leprosy. *J. Lab. Clin. Med.,* 87:1025–1032.
36. Ward, P. A., and Ozols, J. (1969): Characterization of the protease activity in the chemotactic factor inactivator. *J. Clin. Invest.,* 58:123–129.
37. Ward, P. A., and Schlegel, R. J. (1969): Impaired leukotactic responsiveness in a child with recurrent infections. *Lancet,* 2:344–347.
38. Ward, P. A., and Volkman, A. (1975): The elaboration of leukotactic mediators during the interaction between parental-type lymphocytes and F_1 hybrid cells. *J. Immunol.,* 115:1394–1399.

DISCUSSION

Dr. Ward: Your observations on IgA suggest that they may be a unique property of this material. If you take aggregated IgG, can you find similar effects in your system?

Dr. Van Epps: If we use isolated IgG, heat-treat it, and incubate with cells in the upper chamber at a 1 mg per ml concentration, we get some suppression of chemotaxis, although we have never found the same degree of inhibition with IgG as with polymeric IgA, which seems to be a much more effective inhibitor of the neutrophil chemotactic response.

Dr. Ward: Evidence in the literature suggests that if leukocytes first phagocytize, they are preempted for chemotactic responsiveness. Do you think this is what is going on in your system?

Dr. Van Epps: That is possible, but so far we have not been able to show any release of enzymes from the cells in the presence of soluble preparations containing polymeric IgA.

Dr. Jenson: Do you have any direct evidence that the IgA combines with the cell surface?

Dr. Van Epps: The data I have shown are indirect, but in addition we have obtained five IgA myeloma samples from Dr. Hans Spiegelberg. These were five of the samples utilized in the initial studies to show that there was an IgA receptor on the polymorphonuclear leukocyte. These same five IgA M-components suppressed the chemotactic response. As of now, this is the only direct evidence we have. Furthermore, in light of the evidence presented here for a chemotactic receptor, it should now be possible to determine if the interaction of polymeric IgA with the polymorphonuclear leukocyte will result in a direct interference with chemotactic factor-binding.

Dr. Snyderman: In your screening for chemotactic inactivators in serum, is it correct that you use either unheated or heated serum and dilute it 10% and add it to the top of the chamber? We found that there is a very large variation in serum in terms of its intrinsic chemotactic activity. Theoretically, the system that you use is extremely complex in that you would appear to have inhibitory activity if there is chemotactic activity in the serum tested for cell-directed inhibitors of chemotaxis. I wonder if you would discuss this.

Also, if I have interpreted your data correctly, you found that individuals with infections, mainly pulmonary infections, showed the increased serum chemotactic inhibitory activity. I think Dr. Hill has shown that such individuals frequently have supernormal chemotactic responsiveness of their cells. We have found similar results. How does this fit in with your data?

Dr. Van Epps: When we screened patients for chemotactic inhibitor, serum was used only in the lower compartment, so as not to reverse the chemotactic gradient. So, in our screening assays, we are actually looking only at the patients who have a tremendous amount of inhibitory activity, since, generally, as you increase the concentration of serum in the lower compartment of the chemotactic chamber, you will enhance the chemotactic response resulting from an increase in chemotactic factor. Whereas, what we are looking at in these studies is a reduction in chemotaxis by greater than 30% of what you would expect with only 10% normal serum in the lower chamber.

Dr. Snyderman: The individuals with pulmonary infection have increased inhibitory activity. I wonder if this is a different finding from Dr. Hill's studies and from the phenomenon that people with bronchial pneumonia in general have an increase in neutrophil chemotactic responses?

Dr. Van Epps: In answer to your second question, we have looked at cellular responses in some of these individuals. Generally, we do not screen for cellular defects, but in those on whom we have done this, we find individuals who show chemotactic inhibitory activity in their serum and have totally normal neutrophil responses when the cells are isolated and washed before testing. On the other hand, some individuals in the same disease category, with serum inhibitors, will have a suppressed neutrophil response.

Dr. Hill: In several patients, we studied serum inhibitors by incubating cells and serum on the cell side of the chamber. When the cells were allowed to settle onto the filters, a profound defect was noted. If we cytocentrifuged the cells onto the filter, however, the chemotactic defect disappeared.

Dr. Quie: Dr. Hill, are you suggesting inhibition of adherence?

Dr. Hill: Either adherence or settling of the cells.

Dr. Van Epps: We have not tried spinning the cells down on the filter as you do, but we have utilized M-components on both sides of the membrane. The suppressive effect is much greater when the patient's serum or isolated IgA component is in the upper compartment versus the lower compartment.

Dr. Altman: Dr. Van Epps, do patients with IgA myeloma have more infections or other complications than patients with IgG or IgM myeloma? This might be expected if your *in vitro* findings are representative of actual *in vivo* events. In other words, the fact that IgA myeloma proteins suppress polymorph chemotaxis while immunoglobulins of other classes do not suggests that PMN function in IgA myeloma patients might be more abnormal than in other myeloma patients. This would be very interesting, since the nature of the malignant disease process is presumably similar in all myeloma patients, except that the class of abnormal protein produced is different.

Dr. Van Epps: I can not answer that question right now. We have obtained samples from a variety of different sources, and we have not been able to review the clinical course of each of these individuals. I do not know if anybody has observed more infections in IgA myeloma patients than in IgG myeloma patients. Does anyone here have information on this point?

Dr. Stossel: It is said that patients with IgA myeloma do worse.

Dr. Robert Clark: We saw a patient with recurrent staphylococcal skin infections and advanced peridontal lesions who had a high concentration of an IgA M component in his serum, but he did not have myeloma. His serum was strongly inhibitory in assays similar to those which Dr. Van Epps described.

Dr. Leddy: Dr. Van Epps, did IgA inhibit chemotactic responsiveness to all the attractants you studied: i.e., kallikrein, C5 fragment.

Dr. Van Epps: Yes, everything that we tested including casein, bacterial-derived chemotactic factor, normal serum, and C5 fragment.

Dr. Wilkinson: Dr. Van Epps, do you also get inhibition of rosetting and FC-binding?

Dr. Van Epps: We have looked at these receptors because we assumed this might be a possible explanation for the inhibition of bactericidal activity as the result of interference with the opsonic receptor on the surface of the polymorphonuclear leukocyte. We did this by the classic rosetting technique, using complement-coated erythrocytes (EAC) and antibody-coated erythrocytes (EA). Neutrophil EA and EAC controls in the absence of IgA ranged from 72 to 96% and 87 to 92%, respectively. The addition of 1 mg/ml of five different IgA M-components resulted in a mean inhibition of 17% for EAC rosettes and 14% for EA rosettes. Whether this is enough inhibition to suppress bactericidal activity, I do not know. It is also possible that polymorphonuclear leukocyte ingestion is suppressed in the presence of IgA. This is all the evidence that we have right now but we are continuing these studies to determine if IgA M-components effect surface receptors or PMN ingestion.

Dr. Schiffmann: Have you tried to see whether or not you could change the activity of polymeric IgA by dialysis?

Dr. Van Epps: We have not done that. We are still attempting to dissociate a possible IgA-associated component but we have not succeeded in demonstrating any component that is common to all the IgA paraproteins that could account for chemotactic inhibition.

Dr. Schiffmann: Do you have a rough idea of what the effective molar concentration is of IgA? You mentioned 1 or 2 mg per assay but do you have more information?

Dr. Van Epps: No, and I think this may be a little difficult to determine because we are dealing with polymeric forms of IgA, which are more effective inhibitors than monomeric IgA and vary in concentration from sample to sample.

Dr. Snyderman: Have you looked at any serum of people with IgA deficiency to see if they have any inhibitory activity?

Dr. Van Epps: No, so far I have not tested any IgA-deficient serum. One of our initial suspicions was that we might be looking at an effect of alpha$_1$ antitrypsin or alpha$_2$ macroglobulin, and indeed in some of our preparations IgA was bound to alpha$_1$ antitrypsin; however, we found suppression in IgA preparations with alpha$_1$ antitrypsin and those without.

Dr. Goetzl: Does IgE inhibit leukocyte migration at concentrations comparable to the effective range for IgA?

Dr. Van Epps: We have tested serum from one patient with IgE myeloma and it showed virtually no suppression.

Dr. Maderazo: Dr. Van Epps, in those cases in which you showed chemotactic inhibitory activity in the serum, did you determine a dose response?

Dr. Van Epps: No.

Dr. Snyderman: We have been impressed that individuals with chronic granulomatous disease hardly ever have serum inhibitory activity and, if anything, their serum sometimes stimulates migration of polymorphonuclear leukocytes.

We have also looked at the pleural fluid from patients with a malignant condition, and find inhibitory activity for monocyte chemotaxis. These fluids have a predominance of what looks like a 4S inhibitor. This material elutes just behind albumin on Sephadex G-200. We were very interested in whether or not this was going to be a low-molecular-weight inhibitor that may be dissociating from serum protein.

Leukocyte Chemotaxis, edited by John I. Gallin
and Paul G. Quie. Raven Press, New York
© 1978.

Antigen-dependent Chemotaxis

Joerg A. Jensen, Violet Esquenazi, and George Cianciolo

*Department of Microbiology, School of Medicine, University of Miami,
Miami, Florida 33152*

I shall discuss chemotaxis initiated by antigen-antibody reactions involving the surface of the chemotactically responding cell. Thus, if the antigen is associated with the cell surface or is part of it, the specific antibody can chemoattract the cell, while the antigen becomes chemotactic if the cell carries the antibody. This kind of antigen-dependent chemotactic stimulus is quite different from the more familiar one, where antigen-antibody-complement interactions result in the generation of chemotactic factors. In this latter case, the immune reaction takes place independent of, and at a distance from, the chemotactically responding cell, which is not at all involved in the immune reaction itself.

We have shown previously that heterologous and homologous leukocytotoxic sera could chemoattract polymorphonuclear neutrophils (PMNs); that antibody against cell surface antigens mediated this chemoattraction; and that the participation of the complement system was essential (3,5).

We could also demonstrate that peritoneal PMNs obtained from guinea pigs immunized with ovalbumin were chemoattracted by ovalbumin but not by unrelated antigens (3,4). The serum of such immunized animals could be used to passively "arm" PMNs from nonimmunized guinea pigs which then were also specifically attracted by the antigen (3). We assumed that under these circumstances cytophilic antibodies were responsible for the specific recognition of the antigen and for the chemotactic response to it.

We proceeded to further investigate this phenomenon of antigen-induced chemotaxis mediated by cytophilic antibodies. This chapter deals with two aspects of these studies: one concerns the question of complement involvement and the other the characteristics of the mediating antibodies.

IS COMPLEMENT NECESSARY?

Guinea pig peritoneal PMNs (quite in contrast to human peripheral PMNs) required protein-supplemented Gey's medium in order to show any chemotactic responses (3). Initially we used crystallized bovine serum alubmin (BSA) as supplement; however, the results were very difficult to interpret because the concentration of BSA influenced strikingly the random mobility of the cells in the absence of any specific chemotactic agent. We could indeed simulate typical dose responses (in the absence of chemotactic materials) by setting up a series of chambers with increasing BSA concentrations from 0.0075% to 1.0%, where in each chamber the concentrations in the lower and upper compartment were identical. Since it was not known how BSA influenced cell migration, it seemed impossible to determine to what extent this nonspecific effect would be altered by the addition of antigen to the lower compartment.

Abandoning BSA as a protein supplement, we decided to try autologous, preimmune guinea pig serum. At concentrations of 0.5%, the cells responded well to chemotactic agents and the negative controls were acceptable. The same was true if the serum was added with the cells to the upper compartment only. This had two advantages: (a) chemotactic factors that might be generated or present in the serum would form a negative concentration gradient for the cells, and (b) possible interactions of the test antigens with the serum in the lower compartment were avoided.

Since the presence of 0.5% guinea pig serum in the upper chamber compartment effectively supported antigen-induced chemotaxis of immune PMNs and passively "armed" PMNs, it seemed important to obtain some information as to the specificity of this serum requirement and, especially, whether it represented complement participation.

Using partially purified porcine C5a at a concentration of 3.0 μg/ml in Gey's medium as chemoattractant in the lower compartment, we measured chemotaxis of peritoneal PMNs obtained from either immunized guinea pigs (immune PMNs) or from normal animals whose cells were treated (a) with immune serum or partially purified immunoglobulin fractions ("armed PMNs"), or (b) with normal autologous preimmune serum or the corresponding serum fractions (control PMNs). For each series of experiments, the cells were suspended either in Gey's medium alone or in Gey's medium containing one of the following supplements: (a) 0.5% autologous normal or preimmune guinea pig serum; (b) (a), heated for 45 min at 56°C; (c) (a), containing 0.02M EDTA; (d) 0.5% guinea pig pseudoglobulin fraction; (e) 0.5% guinea pig albumin; or (f) 0.5% bovine serum albumin. The supplemented media were placed in the upper compartments together with the cells, and the chemotaxis assays were run as described in Table 1.

The results were as follows: Neither C5a nor antigen was chemotactic for any of the cell preparations if Gey's medium was used without supplements. The response to C5a was strong in all supplemented media. It varied in 15 independent experiments between 150 and 400 cells per high-power field; but none of the supplements was clearly superior or inferior to any of the others. There was also no significant difference in the C5a-induced chemotactic responses of normal PMNs as compared with immune or "armed" PMNs.

In contrast, antigen-induced chemotaxis required whole guinea pig serum, either untreated or heat-treated or containing EDTA. The other three supplements did not support directional migration. Overall, the response to antigen was clearly less than that to C5a, varying at the most effective antigen concentra-

TABLE 1. *Antigen-induced chemotaxis[a] of guinea pig peritoneal PMNs*

Treatment[b] of PMNs (no)	CHP[c] at antigen concentrations (ovalbumin, $\mu g/ml$)								
	0	3.75	7.5	15	30	60	120	240	C5a[d]
A γ1	0	4	6	16	70	44	68		100
γ2	0	0	63	54	86	91	49		144
B γ1	4				18	65	100	86	145
γ2	0				36	35	88	23	373
C γ1	17			90	58	71	65		171
γ2	0.3			45	73	17	21		149
D γ1	24				53	121	94	67	153
γ2	14				84	68	75	106	106
E γ1	23				84	78	70	107	126
γ2	5				75	49	58	61	135
Specific Ig (γ2 & γ2)	5			67	41	40			117
Immune serum[e]	25			128	150	41	41	80	80
Immune PMNs	18				34	45	102	102	142

[a] *In vitro* chemotaxis was carried out and quantitated as described by Snyderman et al. (9). Modified Boyden chambers were set up in duplicate. Results are expressed as average number of PMNs per high-power field on the lower surface of the Millipore filters (5 μm pore size) separating the upper from the lower compartments of the chambers. Gey's medium was used throughout. Incubation: time, 3 hr; temperature, 37°C; in water-saturated 5% CO_2 in air.

[b] Arming of cells: Usually 2.5×10^7 peritoneal guinea pig PMNs were washed twice in Gey's medium, pelleted, and resuspended in 0.5 ml of (a) γ1 immune Ig pool or (b) γ2 immune Ig pool or (c) 1 : 5 diluted immune serum. The cell suspension was kept for 1 hr in an ice bath, and was then sedimented and washed twice with 2.5 ml of Gey's medium. Finally, the cell batches were resuspended at $2.2 \times 10^6/ml$ in Gey's medium containing 0.5% autologous normal guinea pig serum and added to the upper compartments of the chemotaxis chambers. Each compartment received 2×10^6 PMNs. The control cells were treated in exactly the same manner but with nonimmune γ1 and γ2 pools or preimmune serum.

[c] CHP = cells per high-power field.

[d] Partially purified porcine C5a was used at a concentration of 3.0 $\mu g/ml$ in the lower compartment to assess the chemotactic responsiveness of the various cell preparations.

[e] Immune serum which served as starting material for the preparation of the γ1 and γ2 pools.

tions between 60 and 180 cells per high-power field (CHP). Normal untreated cells or cells treated with preimmune serum never responded chemotactically to antigen. While untreated and heat-treated serum supported chemotaxis equally well, in the presence of EDTA higher antigen concentrations were required for optimal responses.

We concluded from these studies that antigen-induced chemotaxis of guinea pig PMNs required the presence of heat-stable serum factor(s), unrelated to the complement system. Wilkinson (10), studying antigen-induced chemotaxis of guinea pig macrophages treated ("armed") with guinea pig antihuman serum albumin, arrived at similar conclusions.

CHARACTERIZATION OF THE CYTOPHILIC ANTIBODIES MEDIATING CHEMOTAXIS

Pooled antiovalbumin immune serum raised in english short hair female guinea pigs, as described previously (3), was dialyzed against 0.005M potassium phosphate buffer pH 8.0 and applied to a DE-52 column equilibrated with the same buffer. After collecting the effluent and exhaustive washing of the column, it was stepwise-eluted with increasing salt concentrations of decreasing pH, as described by Osler et al. (7). Ovalbumin-reactive antibody of electrophoretic γ_2 mobility appeared in the effluent while the fractions eluting with 0.04 M phosphate buffer of pH 6.0 contained specific antibody of γ_1 mobility. Neither of the peak antibody-reactive fractions showed cross-contamination as judged by immunoelectrophoresis using antigen or goat anti-guinea pig 7S immunoglobulin. The antiovalbumin containing γ_1 and γ_2 immunoglobulin fractions were pooled, dialyzed against phosphate-buffered saline, and used for passive arming of guinea pig PMNs to be used for *in vitro* chemotaxis.

Table 1 contains typical data obtained with PMNs armed with the γ_1 and γ_2 antiovalbumin preparations responding to various antigen concentrations; it also shows, in comparison, cells armed with whole unfractionated immune serum, cells armed with specifically isolated antiovalbumin antibodies,[1] and immune PMNs obtained from an immunized guinea pig.

The following control cells were used: (a) normal PMNs as controls for immune PMNs, harvested and processed in the same manner; (b) cells treated with autologous preimmune serum as controls for cells armed with immune serum; (c) cells treated with γ_1 and γ_2 fractions obtained by DE-52 fractionation of normal pooled guinea pig serum, as controls for the corresponding specifically armed cells. None of these control cells showed directional, concentration-dependent migration toward ovalbumin but all were chemoattracted by C5a. The control data are not included in Table 1.

Our data show that both γ_1 and γ_2 antibodies can effectively arm PMNs for antigen-induced chemotaxis. Apparently very little is known about guinea pig antibodies cytophilic for PMNs. Boyden (1), working with antisheep erythrocyte antibodies, claimed that only macrophages carried cytophilic antibody. Current studies in our laboratory using fluorescein-conjugated ovalbumin and rabbit anti-guinea pig 7S Ig show that the arming procedure results in the cytophilic attachment of specific γ_1 and γ_2 antibody to the PMNs; however, there seem to be quantitative differences. While more than 90% of the cells show cytophilic γ_2 antibody, only about 10% have demonstrable γ_1 antibody on their surface. We know that these cells are not macrophages, but they might constitute a subpopulation of PMNs. It is interesting and puzzling that the arming with normal, nonimmune serum is very inefficient as judged by the fluorescence with anti-7S Ig antibody, though the normal serum contains large

---

[1] Prepared by immune absorption chromatography with ovalbumin conjugated to Sepharose 4B, as described by Grov (2).

amounts of γ_1 and γ_2 immunoglobulins. It appears as if the immune antibodies had strikingly different cytophilic properties as compared with the "natural" or uncommitted immunoglobulins. This would also explain the significant difference we observed between the fluorescence (after anti-7S treatment) of peritoneal PMNs from immunized as compared with nonimmunized guinea pigs.

Though we are reasonably sure that our γ_2 preparations do not contain γ_1, we cannot be certain that the reverse is also true. Quantitative considerations, based on Ouchterlony and immunoelectrophoretic studies using specific antigen and anti-guinea pig Ig antibodies, make it quite unlikely that the γ_1 fractions are contaminated with more than 5 to 10% γ_2 antibody. Where 10% contamination is assumed, a 1:10 dilution of the γ_2 fraction used for arming the cells should give the same results as the undiluted γ_1 fraction. This is not the case: cells armed with the 1:10 diluted γ_2 fraction were consistently less (about 25%) reactive with the same antigen concentration than cells armed with undiluted γ_1 fractions.

We have previously proposed that one of the most exciting aspects of the concept of chemotactic stimulation by cell surface immune reactions would be the chemoattraction of lymphocytes by antigen to which the cell carries recognition molecules (3,4). To establish whether lymphocytes respond chemotactically at all to the stimulus resulting from a cell surface immune reaction, we recently tested the chemoattraction of human peripheral lymphocytes by cytotoxic sera. We reasoned that the very effective chemoattraction of PMNs and macrophages by heterologous and homologous leukocytotoxic sera (13) might also be observed with lymphocytes as target cells.

Lymphocytes were separated from normal, heparinized human blood by the Ficoll-Hypaque method (6). The cells were freed from platelet and macrophage contamination by standard procedures, were washed several times in medium RPM1-1640 (GIBCO), and adjusted to 2.5 to 3.0 X 10^6/ml. The lower compartments of the chemotaxis chambers were filled with the same medium containing the cytotoxic sera at different concentrations. The upper compartments received 0.1 ml of the cell suspension and 0.2 ml of medium or control materials; the total lymphocyte number per chamber was 2.5 to 3.0 X 10^5. Nucleopore membrane filters (5 μm pore size) separated the compartments. The chambers were incubated for 2 hr under the same conditions as described in Table 1. After the incubation, the contents of the lower compartments were separately harvested; the cells contained in the fluid were sedimented, resuspended in 0.1 ml, and counted. The harvesting of the lower compartments was done in two steps: first, about 1/3 of the fluid was withdrawn with a Pasteur pipette. The resulting air bubble facilitated gentle washing of the lower filter surface by rocking the chambers back and forth 10 times. Then the rest of the fluid was collected.

The results of a typical experiment are given in Table 2. Though these studies must still be considered preliminary, results such as those listed in the table were rather consistently found, allowing the following statements to be made: (a) Not more than 10% to 15% of the cells migrated through the filter. (b) McCoy's medium did not allow migration. (c) No significant migration occurred

TABLE 2. *Chemoattraction of peripheral human lympocytes by nurse shark serum (NSS)*

NSS in medium (%)		Total number of lymphocytes	
Lower compartment	Upper compartment	Lower compartment	Upper compartment[a]
20	0	1.6×10^4	2×10^5
10	0	1.9×10^4	2×10^5
10	10	0	2×10^5
20(H)[b]	0	1.4×10^4	2×10^5
10(H)	0	1.5×10^4	2×10^5
10(H)	10(H)	0.4×10^4	2×10^5
0	0	0	2×10^5

[a] Initial number of lymphocytes per upper compartment.
[b] Heat-inactivated (40 min, 56°C)

with less than 2×10^5 cells per chamber. (d) In contrast to the earlier results obtained with PMNs, heat-inactivated serum was consistently almost as active as fresh serum. (e) The cells harvested at 2 hr from the lower compartments containing unheated shark serum were invariably dead (they truly committed suicide), which is not surprising, since the serum had a lymphocytotoxic titer of 1:64 to 1:128. (f) Controls, containing medium only in both compartments, were consistently negative; that is, not a single cell could be found in the lower compartment.

We considered the chemotactic responses observed by Russel et al. (8) of human B-lymphocyte cell lines and by Wilkinson et al. (11,12) of activated human peripheral lymphocytes, and we wondered whether an earlier state of cell activation (occurring within 2 hr) could be observed under our experimental conditions. Since blastogenesis, as measured by the uptake of tritiated thymidine, could certainly not be expected to occur, we decided to use tritiated L-leucine.

At the time this chapter is written, we have the results of one such experiment. Using the same medium, cells, shark serum, and incubation conditions as for the chemotaxis studies, we exposed 3×10^5 cells to various concentrations of fresh and heat-inactivated serum in the presence of ^{3}H-L-leucine. Compared with the uptake of cells incubated in the absence of shark serum, all fresh serum dilutions (1:30, 1:60, 1:90) were inhibitory by 30 to 40%; however, the heat-inactivated serum enhanced the uptake: the 1:30 dilutions by 10% and the 1:90 dilutions by 45%.

If these observations can be confirmed, they could indicate that the cell surface immune reaction may result in cell activation permitting directional migration.

SUMMARY AND CONCLUSIONS

We have no doubt that chemotaxis of PMNs and of macrophages induced by antigen and mediated by cytophilic antibodies is a real phenomenon. We hope that other laboratories besides Wilkinson's and our own will confirm our findings and help to elucidate the mechanisms involved. In contrast to chemoattraction of leukocytes by chemotactic factors, "antigen-dependent" chemotaxis exhibits a built-in immunologic specificity residing in the specificity of the cell surface immune reaction. Translated into *in vivo* conditions, this specificity has considerable potential, especially regarding the early encounter between leukocytes and antigenic materials. The chemotactic response to antigens (shed by grafted tissues or tumor cells or produced by microorganisms) could even precede a humoral immune response resulting in formation of cytophilic antibodies, if one assumes the existence of "natural" cytophilic or of Cohn's "associative" antibodies. Furthermore, if noncomplement-fixing cytophilic antibodies can mediate antigen-induced chemotaxis in humans (as they do in the guinea pig), such antibodies could be responsible for the accumulation of PMNs and/or macrophages under various conditions in which complement-dependent reactions are not demonstrable as, e.g., in early renal allograft rejections. Obviously, the demonstration of antigen-dependent chemotaxis of lymphocytes, though more elusive, would be of even greater significance. The recent results obtained in Wilkinson's laboratory with human B-cell lines and with mitogen-activated human T-cells show clearly that lymphocytes can be chemoattracted by chemotactic factors after they have been activated.

The question remains whether activation must precede chemotactic responsiveness or whether the activating event, that is, the interaction of the antigen with the recognition molecule, can serve as the chemotactic stimulus. Our preliminary results, using as chemoattractant antibody directed against lymphocyte cell surface antigens, would support a positive answer to this question, especially since the cell surface immune reaction appears to be the primary event causing chemotactic stimulation without the participation of complement.

ACKNOWLEDGMENTS

This work was supported by United States Public Health Service Grant Al 10726 from the National Institute of Allergy and Infectious Diseases and by institutional funds of the Veterans Administration Hospital, Miami, Florida. We should like to thank the Miami Seaquarium for holding nurse sharks for us, and Ms. Cynthia Chaddock for her technical assistance.

REFERENCES

1. Boyden, S. V. (1964): Cytophilic antibody in guinea pigs with delayed-type hypersensitivity. *Immunology,* 7:474–483.
2. Grov, A. (1973): Studies on the interaction between staphylococcal protein A and the Fc region of immunoglobulin G. *Acta Pathol Microbiol. Scand.,* A (Suppl.) 236:77–83.
3. Jensen, J. A., and Esquenazi, V. (1975): Chemotactic stimulation by cell surface immune reactions. *Nature,* 256:213–215.
4. Jensen, J. A., Esquenazi, V., Williams, D., and Cirocco, R. (1976): Chemotaxis of leucocytes induced by cell surface immune reactions. *Agents Actions,* 5:282.

5. Jensen, J. A., and Williams, D. (1973): Chemotaxis of human neutrophils induced by lymphocytotoxic sera. *Nouv. Rev. Fr. Hematol.,* 13:889–891.
6. Mittal, K. K., Singer, D. P., and Terasaki, P. I. (1968): Serotyping for homotransplantation: XVIII. Refinement of microdroplet lymphocyte cytotoxicity test. *Transplantation,* 6:913.
7. Osler, A., Oliveira, B., Shin, H. S., and Sandberg, A. (1969): The fixation of guinea pig complement by γ1 and γ2 immunoglobulins. *J. Immunol.,* 102:269–271.
8. Russel, R. J., Wilkinson, P. C., Sless, F., and Parrott, D. M. V. (1975): Chemotaxis of lymphoblasts. *Nature,* 256:646.
9. Snyderman, R., Shin, H. S., Phillips, J. K., Gewurz, H., and Mergenhagen, S. E. (1969): A neutrophil chemotactic factor derived from C5 upon interaction of guinea pig serum with endotoxins. *J. Immunol.,* 103:413–422.
10. Wilkinson, P. C. (1976): Cellular and molecular aspects of chemotaxis of macrophages and monocytes. In: *Immunobiology of the Macrophage,* edited by D. S. Nelson, pp. 349–365. Academic Press, New York.
11. Wilkinson, P. C. (1976): Recognition and response in mononuclear and granular phagocytes. *Clin. Exp. Immunol.,* 25:355–366.
12. Wilkinson, P. C., Roberts, J. A., Russell, R. J., and McLoughlin, M. (1976): Chemotaxis of mitogen-activated human lymphocytes and the effects of membrane-active enzymes. *Clin. Exp. Immunol.,* 25:280–287.
13. Williams, D., Esquenazi, V., Cirocco, R., and Jensen, J. A. (1976): The chemoattraction of neutrophils by heterologous and homologous cytotoxic sera. *J. Immunol.,* 116:554–561.

DISCUSSION

Dr. Snyderman: The polycarbonate filter can be used to study lymphocyte migration very easily, especially with the blind-well chamber. Dr. Jensen uses the U-shaped chamber. A given number of lymphocytes are put in the top compartment and one can quantitate the actual number of lymphocytes that migrate through. These cells do not stick to the filter and are found in the fluid in the lower compartment of the chamber. I have never analyzed lymphocyte migration the way Dr. Gallin has looked at PMN migration, but the appearance of lymphocytes going through a pore of a polycarbonate filter is completely different from that of a macrophage or a monocyte. One never sees any direct contact of the lymphocyte membrane with the polycarbonate filter. With a macrophage, however, one can not see any space whatsoever between the cell and the filter. Similar to PMNs and macrophages, lymphocyte migration is an active process. It occurs best at 37°C and is time-dependent; it could be inhibited by azide.

Dr. Wilkinson: We have talked for some time of lymphocyte locomotion and the appearance of these cells in movement is rather different from that of phagocytes. Moving lymphocytes seem to have a more stable oriented morphology with the nucleus well forward and, when moving, they nearly always have easily visible tails. The front edge is not as extensive as in phagocytes.

What I actually wanted to talk about was to go on from what Dr. Jensen was saying on the influences of antigen and to discuss how antigen affects the migration of primed lymphocytes. This work was based on the checkerboard assay. If one analyzes the locomotion of lymphocytes from unprimed mice in varying concentrations of serum albumin, one finds that serum albumin has a pronounced chemokinetic effect and there is little evidence of a chemotactic effect (Wilkinson, Parrott, Russell, and Sless, *J. Exp. Med.* 1977, *in press*).

If, in contrast, you have mice that have been immunized with serum albumin and lymphocytes are harvested from the draining lymph nodes between 3 and 10 days following challenge with the same antigen, the serum albumin again causes a chemokinetic reaction, but, as judged by the checkerboard assay, we also have good evidence for a response to the gradient of albumin as well, suggesting chemotaxis.

Ovalbumin proved not to be chemokinetic, so we primed mice with ovalbumin and took cells under the same regime. If there was no protein other than ovalbumin in the system, one saw really nothing at all. The cells hardly moved into the filter; however, if the lymphocytes were in serum albumin and their migration was then tested in various gradients of ovalbumin, a chemotactic response to the ovalbumin could be demonstrated. I think this suggests that cells do respond to an antigen gradient. Antigen is probably eliciting the same response from primed lymphocytes as from Dr. Jensen's cytophilic-antibody-coated neutrophils.

Dr. Williams: Dr. Jensen, in your system are the shark antibodies for the lymphocytes a 19S or IgM antibody?

Dr. Jensen: A 19S IgM antibody which is a very strong complement-fixing antibody. We have shown that the PMN reaction is complement-dependent.

Dr. Williams: You get the same effect with anti-HL-A serum of lymphocytotoxic antibody in human HL-A sera?

Dr. Jensen: Yes, we can get it for PMNs with anti-HL-A sera from multiparous women or from patients who rejected transplants, provided the PMNs are from people with the corresponding HL-A antigens.

Dr. Williams: What about lymphocytes?

Dr. Jensen: For lymphocytes we have done a few experiments. It looks as if the same is true but that it is not complement-dependent. Dr. Wilkinson has shown that lymphoblasts migrate very strongly and can be attracted after they have been primed by PHA or CON-A and then migrate toward PHA or chemotactic factors. So one of the questions was, must the lymphocyte be primed or activated first to migrate, or, can it migrate and get activated at the same time? We have done one single experiment. This was a 2-hr incubation. We figured if we could see any lymphocyte activation, it had to occur in 2 hr, and it had to occur in practically the same system. So we could not use tritiated thymidine; we used tritiated leucine and used heat-inactivated shark serum and approximately the same cell numbers. Actually during these 2 hr, during which in the parallel experiment the cells migrate through the membrane, leucine uptake can be demonstrated. So it could be that activation and chemotactic response are going on at the same time. But you do not have to start with primed lymphocytes to get them to migrate. Biologically, it would be most important to attract nonprimed lymphocytes to the vicinity of the corresponding antigen.

Dr. Becker: Dr. Jensen, I thought that γ_1 was not cytophilic, whereas γ_2 was.

Dr. Jensen: There is practically nothing known about guinea pig cytophilic antibodies for PMNs. Boyden is one of the last ones who did anything about it in the guinea pig. And he said there is no such thing. We have looked at these cells with fluorescent antigen as well as fluorescent goat and rabbit anti-guinea pig 7S immunoglobulin. Something very interesting comes out of that. First of all, if one treats the cells with normal guinea pig γ_1 and γ_2 fractions versus immune γ_1 and γ_2 fractions or normal versus immune whole serum, there is always a striking difference, in spite of the fact that the normal guinea pig has probably just as much γ_1 and γ_2 in its serum. There is a striking quantitative difference between the immune serum and the normal serum, and I do not know what to make of that.

In addition, about 90% of the PMNs get γ_2 antibody on the surface, demonstrable by fluorescing antigen as well as antibody. But only 10 to 20% of cells get detectable γ_1. So there is another question of a possible subpopulation of PMNs. We do not really know what to conclude from that, especially whether immune γ_1 or γ_2 have a stronger cytophilic reactivity than just plain γ_1 or γ_2.

Dr. Wilkinson: Lymphocytes are much more difficult cells to work with than phagocytes. One of the things about lymphocytes is that they show much more pronounced chemokinetic reactions, and their locomotion is much more dependent on chemokinetic factors in the medium than that of phagocytes. And this is one of the reasons why I am rather concerned about the terminology, because I think we can get awfully mixed up.

The second thing is about the priming. All the work we have published has shown that lymphocytes must be stimulated or activated before they will show locomotor reactions to chemical stimuli. But I am not sure that is an absolute requirement. We are working on trying to sort out different cell populations. I think there are differences between different sorts of lymphocytes.

Dr. Jensen: The number of lymphocytes put in the chemotactic chambers is important. If you do not have enough cells, they will not get to the openings of the filters. There is much more space between the holes of the Nucleopore filter than there are holes. The holes have to be readily available for the lymphocytes to penetrate. Lymphoblasts, I suspect, will seek out a hole entrance, whereas unprimed cells will not.

Dr. Snyderman: I agree very fully with the chemokinetic behavior of lymphocytes. We have also looked at various mitogens, and they all cause lymphocytes to migrate across the filter. If you put them with the cells it is just as good if not better. If you look at individuals who have positive reactivity to PPD, PPD will also cause an increase in chemokinesis of the lymphocyte. All that we have seen that are actually chemotactic for lymphocytes have been the f-met peptides; however, it is confusing that although the f-met peptides are chemotactic for lymphocytes, we do not see anywhere nearly the degree of binding with lymphocytes that we do with polymorphonuclear lymphocytes.

Dr. Robert Clark: Dr. Jensen, about the PMN systems that are complement-dependent, it occurred to me that one potential explanation for the chemotaxis you observed was the local interaction of antigen-antibody and complement at the leading edge of the cell. This might result in continuous local generation of agents such as the C5 fragment. Is there anything in the data that is inconsistent with that?

Dr. Jensen: I do not think that could account for our observation. There are no free antigen-antibody complexes. While you may get a gradient of C5a, the C5a would be everywhere around the cell. So the cell would not have any incentive to migrate in a preferred direction.

Dr. Robert Clark: It seems to me that if the cell is in a gradient of complement, the largest amount of C5a would be generated on the side facing the higher concentration of complement, and migration in that direction would be expected.

Dr. Jensen: Yes, but if the leading edge of the cell were to generate C5a, any forward movement of the cell would be against the concentration gradient.

Leukocyte Chemotaxis, edited by John I. Gallin
and Paul G. Quie. Raven Press, New York
© 1978.

Chemotactic Lymphokines: A Review

Leonard C. Altman

*Division of Allergy and Infectious Diseases, Department of Medicine, University of
Washington, Seattle, Washington 98195*

Lymphocytes, as a consequence of appropriate stimulation, synthesize and release a number of biologically active substances known as lymphokines (32, 34,41).

Products of Activated Lymphocytes

Mediators Affecting Macrophages

1. Migration-inhibition factor (MIF)
2. Macrophage-activating factor (MAF)
3. Lymphocyte-derived chemotactic factor (LDCF)

Mediators Affecting Granulocytes

1. Chemotactic factors for polymorphonuclear leukocytes (PMNs), eosinophils, and basophils
2. Leukocyte inhibitory factor (LIF)

Mediators Affecting Lymphocytes

1. Chemotactic factor for lymphocytes
2. Mitogenic factor (MF)
3. Transfer factor (TF)

Other Factors

1. Lymphotoxin (LT)
2. Growth-inhibitory factors
   a. Clonal-inhibitory factor (CIF)
   b. Proliferation-inhibitory factor (PIF)
3. Osteoclast-activating factor (OAF)
4. Skin-reactive factor
5. Interferon

These soluble lymphocyte products are thought to be the mediators of delayed immune responses and may also play a role as effector substances in more immediate and accelerated types of immune reactions. Within this large group of lymphocyte mediators are a number of lymphokines with chemotactic activity for leukocytes. It is the purpose of this chapter to present a concise review of lymphokines that possess chemotactic activity. To this end, information will be presented regarding the methodology, physicochemical characterization, and *in vivo* activities of chemotactic lymphokines, as well as to review the role of these factors in human disease. Where appropriate, comparisons will be made between the chemotactic products of lymphocytes and other lymphokines as well as with nonlymphokine chemotactic agents. For convenience of presentation, this chapter will be divided into sections, each reviewing studies of lymphokines with chemotactic activity for a specific population of leukocytes, i.e., mononuclear leukocytes (MNLs), polymorphonuclear leukocytes (PMNs), eosinophils, basophils, and lymphocytes.

CHEMOTACTIC LYMPHOKINES AFFECTING MACROPHAGES

Experimental Studies

The first description of a chemotactic agent produced by lymphocytes was published in 1969 by Ward, Remold, and David (54). These investigators showed that antigen-stimulated lymph node lymphocytes produced a soluble factor that chemotactically attracted homologous (guinea pig) and heterologous (rabbit) peritoneal macrophages. The methods used by Ward and co-workers, although later modified, are worth reviewing, since the general principles are pertinent to most subsequent studies. Lymph node lymphocytes taken from guinea pigs previously immunized with antigen (o-chlorobenzoyl chloride—bovine gamma globulin, OCBC-BGG) were placed in culture in the absence of serum for 24 hr at 37°C either with the specific immunizing antigen or saline. Following incubation, the cells were removed by centrifugation and the cell-free culture supernatants tested for chemotactic activity in a Boyden-type chemotactic assay. One major technical change, soon made by Ward et al. and by other investigators, was, at the end of the incubation period, to add appropriate amounts of antigen or mitogen to the unstimulated (control) culture supernatants.

Using these techniques, Ward and co-workers showed that the production of a lymphokine chemotactic factor correlated with delayed skin reactivity and was dependent on the presence of both antigen and lymphocytes during the incubation period. Lymphocytes cultured without antigen or cultures to which antigen was added at the termination of the experiment were devoid of chemotactic activity. The chemotactic lymphokine was heat-stable (56°C for 30 min) and had an estimated molecular weight as determined by gel-filtration chromatography and sucrose gradient ultracentrifugation similar to bovine serum albumin (BSA, MW 67,000). In these earliest experiments, the investigators were unable to separate the chemotactic lymphokine from migration inhibitory factor (MIF). Subsequently Ward et al. (55) showed that the chemotactic lymphokine had a slower electrophoretic migration pattern and hence was more negatively charged than MIF. Further confirmation that MIF was distinct from the chemotactic agent was obtained from experiments that demonstrated that MIF-rich fractions did not interfere with lymphokine-promoted chemotaxis when mixed with either the cells or the lymphokine in the chemotactic chamber. In addition, both MIF and the chemotactic lymphokine were shown to have no significant effect on the chemotactic response of MNLs to bacterial chemotactic factor. It is important to note, for comparison with subsequent studies, that Ward et al. (55) separated their lymphocyte supernatants into five fractions by gel filtration but that fraction V, containing substances the size of lysozyme (MW 17,000), was not tested for chemotactic activity.

Extension of these studies to humans was initiated in 1971, when Rocklin and David showed that human blood, spleen, and tonsil lymphocytes could produce a factor chemotactic for heterologous (rabbit) macrophages (35). At this time, using Sephadex G-100 and G-75 gel filtration, these investigators failed to separate the human chemotactic lymphokine from human MIF (MW 25,000). In order to pursue studies of chemotactic lymphokines in man, Snyderman et al. (43) developed an assay to measure human MNL migration. By using polycarbonate filters (approximately 1/10 the thickness of nitrocellulose filters) and human peripheral MNLs, these investigators were able to use human peripheral blood for both the production of lymphokines and the measurement of MNL chemotaxis. Using this newly described assay, Snyderman and co-workers (43) demonstrated that human peripheral blood leukocytes, when stimulated with either phytohemagglutinin (PHA) or purified protein derivative of tuberculin (PPD), elaborated a soluble factor that would chemotactically attract homologous MNLs. Subsequently, Altman et al. (6), using the same methods, investigated various aspects of the production and characterization of this chemotactic lymphokine. In this report, the fact that antigen (PPD)- or mitogen (PHA)-stimulated human peripheral leukocytes could produce a soluble chemotactic factor was reconfirmed. Moreover, the production of this factor was shown: (a) to precede lymphocyte transformation, since chemotactic lymphokine activity was detectable as early as 6 hours after the initiation of culture; (b) to be a sensitive correlate of delayed hypersensitivity as measured by skin-testing; and (c) to be dependent on lymphocytes, since essentially pure populations of PHA-stimulated lymphocytes (> 99%) were capable of chemotactic lymphokine production.

Additional experiments showed that the chemotactic factor was heat-stable (56°C for 30 min), nondialyzable, and antigenically distinct from human C3 and C5, the precursors of two chemotactic peptides derived from complement. Further, these investigators demonstrated that the chemotactic lymphokine had an estimated molecular weight of 12,500 daltons, as determined by Sephadex gel filtration chromatography and sucrose density ultracentrifugation. Altman et al. named this substance lymphocyte-derived chemotactic factor of LDCF. This term has since been used to refer to the factor produced by lymphocytes which chemotactically attracts MNLs and will be used as such in the rest of this chapter; however, the restricted use of this definition does not indicate that the activity of LDCF is specific for MNLs.

Since these studies demonstrated that an ostensibly pure population of lymphocytes could produce LDCF, it was of interest to investigate more specifically what type of cell was responsible for the production of this mediator. For this purpose, Altman and Kirchner adapted the techniques of Snyderman et al. to study chemotaxis and lymphokine synthesis in the chicken. Using this experimental animal allowed these investigators to readily separate thymic-derived (T) from bursal-derived (B) lymphocytes. These investigators showed that concanavalin A (Con A) and pokeweed mitogen (PWM) stimulated lymphocytes from chemically bursectomized agammaglobulinemic chickens produced as much chemotactic lymphokine as did lymphocytes from normal chickens (2). From these studies, it was concluded that T lymphocytes in the absence of B cells could produce LDCF; however, these authors were careful to point out that their data did not exclude the possibility that B lymphocytes under appropriate circumstances might also produce this lymphokine. Subsequently Altman et al. (3) showed that PPD as well as Con A-stimulated chicken leukocytes could produce LDCF and that the production of this factor in the chicken, as previously demonstrated in man, was a correlate of delayed skin reactivity. Furthermore, leukocytes from the peripheral blood, spleen, and thymus of chickens were shown to produce LDCF; but bursal lymphocytes failed to make this factor. These findings were consistent with the previously noted observation that T lymphocytes produce LDCF. Physicochemical characterization of LDCF in the chicken showed that it was very similar to the human chemotactic lymphokine, in that chicken LDCF was a heat-stable nondialyzable factor of approximate MW 12,500. In addition, chicken (and human) LDCF was shown to be sensitive to treatment with pepsin and trypsin but resistant to neuraminidase, indicating that this chemotactic factor was a protein the activity of which was independent of a terminal sialic acid moiety. In spite of the remarkable physicochemical similarities between human and chicken LDCF, the activity of this factor was shown to exhibit species-specificity. Chicken LDCF was active in attracting homologous MNLs but failed to attract human, guinea pig, or rabbit cells, while human and guinea pig LDCF were inactive in chemotactically attracting chicken MNLs.

Since the original studies of Ward et al. were performed in the guinea pig, Wahl and co-workers (47) established a model to investigate further the production of LDCF production in that animal. The methods utilized were similar to those described by Snyderman et al., in that guinea pig leukocytes were used for both lymphokine production and as responder cells in the chemotactic assay. Using this approach, Wahl and co-workers extended the observations of Ward et al. by showing that not only lymph node lymphocytes but also splenic, peripheral blood, thymic, and peritoneal exudate lymphocytes could produce LDCF. Further, the production of this chemotactic lymphokine was shown to correlate with delayed skin reactivity and to be carrier-specific. Comparable to studies with human LDCF, chemotactic lymphokine synthesis in the guinea pig was evident in 6 to 8 hr and preceded lymphocyte proliferation. Furthermore, guinea pig LDCF was antigenically distinct from homologous C3 and C5, sensitive to digestion with proteolytic enzymes, resistant to neuraminidase, heat-stable (56°C for 30 min), and had an approximate MW of 12,500 daltons. These findings, while remarkably similar to those obtained in man and the chicken, differed slightly from the results of Ward and co-workers. Although the reasons for this discrepancy are not fully clear, it is possible (1) that more than one chemotactic lymphokine exists in the guinea pig; (2) that Ward et al. identified an aggregated form of the mediator; or (3) that Ward et al. did not detect this smaller factor because they did not test for chemotactic activity in those fractions containing molecules the size of lysozyme (MW 17,000) and smaller (see above). Postlethwaite and Snyderman, also using guinea pigs, examined the mechanisms of MNL accumulation and chemotactic lymphokine production *in vivo* (33). These investigators demonstrated that the intraperitoneal injection of antigen (horse radish peroxidase, HRPO) into previously immunized animals led to the local accumulation of large numbers of macrophages and that the peritoneal fluids from these animals contained a heat-stable, trypsin-sensitive chemotactic factor of approximate MW 12,500. This factor was shown to be antigenically unrelated to C5. Nonimmunized animals did not manifest these responses. Furthermore, splenic leukocytes from these animals cultured *in vitro* produced a chemotactic lymphokine with identical characteristics. These authors concluded that the factors produced *in vivo* and *in vitro* were LDCF.

Lymphocyte-derived chemotactic factors have been described in two other species. Boetcher and Meltzer showed that mouse spleen cells incubated with antigen (PPD) or mitogens (PHA, Con A, PWM) produced a chemotactic lymphokine which would attract homologous peritoneal macrophages (8,29). As previously observed in other species, lymphokine production was found to precede lymphocyte transformation; however, detectable LDCF production was first evident at 18 hr in contrast to 6 to 8 hr as seen in human subjects and guinea pigs. Furthermore, mouse splenocytes, in contrast to leukocytes from other species, failed to produce LDCF in serum-free media and required higher concentrations of mitogens to produce LDCF than for the induction of lymphocyte transformation. This is also at variance with studies in other species in which the optimal concentrations of lymphocyte stimulants have been the same for LDCF production and lymphocyte transformation. In a further contrast with data obtained in other species, preliminary studies by these workers suggest that mouse LDCF has an estimated MW of 40,000 daltons (30). Ward and Volkman have examined chemotactic lymphokine production in the rat (56). In this study, supernatants from mixed lymphocyte reactions (MLR), as well as soluble extracts from kidneys manifesting experimental graft versus host (GVH) reactions, were shown to contain MNL chemotactic activity. Characterization of this material by sucrose density ultracentrifugation showed a bimodal distribution with most of the activity sedimenting between a BSA marker and cytochrome C. A smaller peak was present between the BSA and human IgG markers. Although additional studies are necessary to define further the physico-chemical characteristics and the cell responsible for producing this factor, it seems reasonable to conclude that rat lymphocytes are able to produce an LDCF-type mediator.

The synthesis and measurement of LDCF *in vitro* has been used as a tool by various investigators to examine basic concepts, pharmacologic control, and maturation of the immune response. In previous studies, it had been established that T lymphocytes were capable of producing LDCF (2). Although this result fit the accepted doctrines of cellular immunity, it did not rule out the possibility that B lymphocytes under appropriate conditions might also produce LDCF. In order to investigate this question, Altman et al. (4) utilized a double-rosetting technique to separate human peripheral blood lymphocytes. B lymphocytes were identified and separated by their ability to form rosettes with sheep erythrocytes (E) and B lymphocytes by their ability to form rosettes with sheep erythrocytes coated with antibody and complement (EAC rosettes). Rosetted T or B cells were separated from nonrosetted leukocytes by centrifugation on Ficoll-Hypaque gradients. Using these methods, Altman et al. showed that T lymphocytes stimu-lated with either Con A or PHA produced a chemotactic lymphokine and that B lymphocytes cultured with their adherent EAC rosettes also produced a chem-otactic factor. The product of B lymphocytes was shown to be antigenically distinct from C3 and C5, and the separation of the EAC rosettes from B lympho-cytes with an anti-C3 globulin was shown to abrogate chemotactic lymphokine synthesis. Based on these studies, Altman et al. suggested that B lymphocytes could be activated to produce LDCF by binding at their C3 receptor. Subse-quently Mackler and co-workers (27) reported: (a) that binding of EA (sheep erythrocytes coated with 7S antibody) to the Fc membrane receptor of B lympho-cytes induced LDCF production; (b) that B lymphocytes dissociated from their EAC rosettes, if stimulated with Con A or PHA, were capable of LDCF synthe-sis; (c) that EAC-stimulated B lymphocytes produced LDCF in the absence of concomitant lymphocyte transformation; and (d) that T and B lymphocytes were both capable of elaborating another lymphokine, mitogenic factor (MF). These authors concluded that both T and B lymphocytes, if appropriately stimu-lated, could produce lymphokines, that stimulation of B lymphocytes at either their C3 or Fc receptors was a sufficient stimulus for lymphokine (LDCF and MF) synthesis but not DNA synthesis, and that B lymphocytes activated by binding at their C3 receptors could produce LDCF (and MF) following exposure to mitogens conventionally thought to stimulate only T lymphocytes. This last and rather unorthodox result was explained by suggesting that transient binding at the C3 receptor of B lymphocytes lowered the stimulation threshold of these cells so that they were able to respond to stimuli normally incapable B cell activation. To confirm that B lymphocytes were in fact producing LDCF, Altman et al. (1) characterized and compared the chemotactic factors produced by B and T lymphocytes. By use of Sephadex G-100 chromatography and isoelectric focusing, these investigators showed that B and T cells produced the same chemotactic product and that this product was identical to LDCF produced by unfractionated leukocyte populations. Furthermore, these authors showed that LDCF produced by B and T cells was distinct from C5a as determined by net molecular charge and antigenic differences. Wahl et al. (49), working with guinea pigs, confirmed the observation that binding at either the C3 receptor or the Fc receptor of B lymphocytes stimulated LDCF production. These investigators also demonstrated that B cells produced a chemotactic lymphokine following nylon column purification, incubation with polymerized flagellin (POL, a T independent B cell mitogen), lipopolysaccharide (LPS), lipid A, and anti-guinea pig immunoglobulin. Exposure of B lymphocytes to the monovalent Fab fragments of anti-immunoglobulin, however, failed to induce LDCF synthesis. These authors hypothesized that the basic mechanism responsible for initiating LDCF synthesis by B cells was cross-linking of lymphocyte surface receptors. In order to understand the mechanism(s) of B cell activation better, Sandberg et al. (39) and Koopman and co-workers (23) examined in greater detail the C3 stimulation of lymphocytes to produce LDCF. These studies showed that purified C3b could stimulate splenic lymphocytes and purified B cells to synthesize LDCF and that the C3a, C3c, and C3d fragments of the molecule were incapable of inducing lymphokine synthesis. Native C3 was shown to stimulate low levels of LDCF production. The authors suggested that stimulation by native C3 may have resulted from the cleavage of C3b from C3 by proteolytic enzymes released from leukocytes during incubation. These investigators confirmed the observation of Altman et al. that generation of LDCF by B lymphocytes occurs in the absence of concomitant lymphocyte proliferation.

Previous studies have shown that ostensibly pure populations of mitogen-stimulated human lymphocytes can produce LDCF (6). Wahl et al. re-examined and extended this observation by showing that antigen-stimulated guinea pig spleen or lymph node cells required viable macrophages to produce LDCF but that Con A- or LPS-stimulated lymphocytes were capable of LDCF production in the absence of macrophages (50). Carrying these studies one step further, these investigators showed that T lymphocytes required macrophages to produce LDCF following antigenic stimulation but that macrophage-deprived T cells produced LDCF when stimulated with nonspecific mitogens (Con A, PHA). B lymphocytes were shown to produce LDCF in response to the mitogen LPS with or without macrophage cooperation.

In a number of studies, the *in vitro* effects of pharmacologic agents on LDCF production have been examined. Ruhl and co-workers (37) showed that L-asparaginase (a drug capable of noncytotoxic depression of lymphocyte transformation) failed to depress LDCF synthesis by PHA-stimulated human lymphocytes, but that hydrocortisone was able to decrease both LDCF synthesis and concomitant lymphocyte transformation in a nontoxic dose-dependent fashion. Wahl, Altman, and Rosenstreich (48), working with guinea pigs, similarly showed that pharmacologic doses of glucocorticosteroids would inhibit LDCF synthesis and lymphocyte transformation but that these drugs did not interfere with the action of LDCF on macrophage responder cells. In addition, these investigators showed that corticosteroids were able to block the production of MIF by antigen-stimu-

TABLE 1. *Comparison of LDCF in various species*

Characteristic	Human	Guinea pig	Chicken	Mouse	Rat
Temperature stability	Stable (56°C, 30 min)	Stable (56°C, 20 hr)	Stable (56°C, 30 min)	nd[a]	nd
Approximate MW	12,500 (6)	(47)	12,500	40,000	30 to 60,000
	25,000 (35)	12,500 (33)			
		60–70,000 (54,55)			
Antigenic similarity to C3 or C5	None	None	nd	nd	nd
Proteolytic enzymes[b]	Sensitive	Sensitive	Sensitive	nd	nd
Neuraminidase	Resistant	Resistant	Resistant	nd	nd
Produced by T cells	Yes	Yes	Yes	Yes	nd
B cells	Yes	Yes	nd	no	nd

[a] Not determined
[b] Pepsin, trypsin, or chymotrypsin.

lated lymphocytes and the action of MIF on target macrophages. Foon and co-workers (13) recently demonstrated that lymphocytes stimulated with serotonin produce a chemotactic factor. In detail, this study showed that lymphocytes stimulated with serotonin produced this factor within 12 hours, that synthesis reached a maximum at 48 hours, and could be inhibited by methysergide, a specific serotonin antagonist. The chemotactic lymphokine produced by serotonin-stimulated cells was found to be identical in physical and chemical characteristics (heat-stable at 56°C for 30 min, nondialyzable, approximate MW 12,500) to that previously described (6). In order to study the maturational development of the immune response, Kretschmer and co-workers (24) examined the chemotactic responsiveness of MNLs and production of LDCF in human cord blood. These investigators found that newborn MNLs had a normal response to LDCF and that lymphocytes from cord blood were capable of generating normal amounts of this lymphokine. These data suggest that the mechanisms that mediate delayed immune function mature early in human development. Table 1 lists the comparative features of LDCF in all species in which its production has been studied.

Clinical Studies

The production of LDCF and the response of MNLs to this factor have been used by several investigators to study immunologic disorders in man. Snyderman et al. (42) found that MNLs from a patient with chronic mucocutaneous candidiasis (CMC) failed to respond normally to LDCF (or C5a) and that treatment with transfer factor (TF) restored the chemotactic responsiveness of the patient's MNLs to both chemotactic agents. Transfer factor therapy also restored delayed cutaneous reactivity and produced marked clinical improvement. Lymphocytes from the patient produced LDCF in response to PHA and streptolysin (SLO) but failed to synthesize this lymphokine in response to an antigenic extract from *Candida albicans.* These authors suggested that defective MNL chemotaxis may be a primary defect in certain patients with CMC and that enhancement of MNL chemotactic responsiveness might be one of the *in vivo* consequences of treatment with TF. Rosenberg and co-workers (36) examined LDCF production as well as the synthesis of lymphotoxin (LT, see list, above) and lymphocyte transformation in patients with recurrent herpes labialis in an effort to determine what host defense factors were of importance in preventing development and recurrence of this disease. These investigators showed that peripheral leukocytes from patients with antibodies to herpes simplex virus (HSV) produced LDCF, LT, and transformed in response to HSV antigens, while cells from antibody-negative patients failed to respond as measured by these parameters; however, these authors were unable to detect any significant differences in the production of LDCF and LT and only a small difference in the transformation response between lymphocytes from antibody-positive patients, with and without clinical disease. Ruhl et al. (38) examined the production of LDCF and DNA by PHA-stimulated lymphocytes from patients with Hodgkin's disease. They showed that lymphocyte transformation was depressed but that LDCF production was normal. Similar findings have been noted by Altman et al. *(unpublished observations)*. Ruhl et al. suggested two possible explanations for the observed dissociation between LDCF production and lymphocyte transformation: (a) two distinct populations of lymphocytes mediate these functions and one population is selectively depleted in Hodgkin's disease, or (b) a single population of lymphocytes synthesizes LDCF and DNA, and the abnormality in Hodgkin's disease is restricted to the latter function.

Altman et al. (5) studied LDCF production and MNL chemotaxis in children with Wiskott-Aldrich syndrome (WAS). This is an X-linked disease of children characterized by a perplexing spectrum of immune disorders, one of which is cutaneous anergy. These investigators found that mitogen (Con A, PHA, PWM) and antigen (SLO, Candida) stimulated lymphocytes from patients with WAS produced normal amounts of LDCF; however, spontaneous LDCF synthesis by unstimulated lymphocytes from these patients was significantly greater than normal. In addition, the authors found: (a) that MNL chemotactic responses were depressed in children with WAS; (b) that preincubation of normal MNLs in LDCF depressed the chemotactic responsiveness of these cells; and (c) that sera from patients with WAS had a similar inhibitory effect. Based on these data, Altman and co-workers hypothesized that regulation of LDCF synthesis was abnormal in WAS and that excessive elaboration of this mediator *in vivo* might be responsible for the depressed MNL chemotaxis and anergy evident in the disease. These observations, as well as data indicating (a) that the spontaneous synthesis of immunoglobulins is as much as 10 times normal in WAS, and (b) that B lymphocytes can produce LDCF, led these investigators to develop the unique hypothesis that B lymphocytes might be responsible for the hypersynthesis of both immunoglobulins and LDCF in WAS. Muchmore and co-workers (31) recently examined the ability of peripheral lymphocytes from patients with chronic lymphocytic leukemia (CLL) and Sézary syndrome to produce LDCF. Lymphocytes from CLL patients generally have the surface markers of B cells, while lymphoctyes from patients with the Sézary syndrome have T cell characteristics. Muchmore et al. showed that lymphocytes from patients with both diseases failed to produce LDCF when stimulated with nonspecific mitogens (PHA, Con A) or specific antigen (SLO). These reports demonstrate the usefulness of studying leukocyte chemotaxis and chemotactic lymphokine synthesis in the evaluation of human disease.

CHEMOTACTIC LYMPHOKINES AFFECTING POLYMORPHONUCLEAR LEUKOCYTES

Before reviewing the literature on this field, a few introductory comments are required. First, there have been significantly fewer studies of PMN chemotactic lymphokines than MNL chemotactic lymphokines, and second, although most investigators have studied the chemoattractant activity of lymphocyte products for a specific responder cell, i.e., MNLs, for the most part specificity of chemotactic activity has not been documented. In fact, although virtually all studies with LDCF have used MNLs as target cells in the hands of most investigators, activated lymphocyte supernatants will attract PMNs.

Ward and co-workers (55) were the first to describe a lymphocyte product with chemotactic activity for PMNs. These investigators reported that antigen (OCBC-BGG)-stimulated lymphocytes produced a PMN chemotactic factor that was different from both MIF and LDCF in its electrophoretic behavior on polyacrylamide gels. Based on this result, Ward et al. concluded that the PMN chemotactic factor was a distinct lymphokine; however, no other physicochemical studies were performed. More recently, Ward and Volkman (56), in their study of chemotactic lymphokine production during MLR and GVH reactions, reported that, although LDCF was generated during these reactions, negligible amounts of PMN chemotactic activity were produced. The authors point out that the specificity of the chemotactic factors detected was consistent with the observed histology (< 1% PMNs) seen in kidneys undergoing experimental GVH reactions. Transfer factor, although not truly a lymphokine in that it is a preformed mediator extractable from unstimulated lymphocytes, has been reported to be strongly chemotactic for PMNs and weakly chemotactic for MNLs (14). The chemotactic activity of TF is antigenically distinct from C3 and C5 and would appear unrelated to LDCF, since it is dialyzable and has an estimated MW of 5,000 daltons. Recently Yoshida et al. (58) reported that supernatants from continuous cell lines contained, among other lymphokines, a PMN chemotactic factor. Cell lines of T and B lymphocyte origin were both capable of producing this factor. Using Sephadex G-100 chromatography, these investigators reportedly separated the chemotactic factor from an MIF-like material present in the same supernatants and were able, with an antilymphokine serum, to remove the chemotactic but not the MIF-like activity. In contrast, a subsequent report from the same laboratory showed that MIF but not a PMN chemotactic factor produced by antigen-stimulated normal lymphocytes could be removed by antilymphokine serum (25). These data suggest that the lymphokine-like factors produced by continuous cell lines, although biologically active, may differ from the conventional lymphokines produced by normal lymphocytes. Foon and co-workers (13), in their recent report describing the production of LDCF by serotonin-stimulated lymphocytes, state that chemotactically active supernatants were capable of attracting PMNs as well as MNLs. Finally, I can support this observation of Foon et al., since my experience suggests that antigen- and mitogen-stimulated human lymphocyte culture supernatants that demonstrate LDCF activity are also active in attracting PMNs (Altman, L. C., *unpublished observations*).

CHEMOTACTIC LYMPHOKINES AFFECTING EOSINOPHILS

At least five factors are known that chemotactically attract eosinophils: (a) ECF-A (eosinophil chemotactic factor of anaphylaxis) (22); (b) ECF-C (C5a)

(19); (c) histamine (9); (d) bacterial chemotactic factor (52); and (e) a lymphokine chemotactic factor. Only studies of this last factor will be discussed. Cohen and Ward (10) were the first investigators to demonstrate that lymphocytes produced a factor with eosinophil chemotactic activity. For measurement of chemotaxis, these investigators utilized a modified Boyden assay and guinea pig peritoneal exudate cells rich in eosinophils. Lymphocyte supernatants from antigen-stimulated (OCBC-BGG) guinea pig lymph node cells were used as a source of chemotactic lymphokine. Using these methods, Ward et al. observed that antigen-stimulated lymphocytes from immune guinea pigs produced a soluble factor that could be activated by immune complexes to enhance eosinophil chemotaxis. This factor was not chemotactically active without the addition of immune complexes. Ward et al. also showed that immune complexes alone had no eosinophil chemotactic activity and that unstimulated lymphocyte culture fluids failed to show chemotactic activity with or without the addition of immune complexes. Generation of the lymphokine eosinophil chemotactic factor was antigen-specific in that the immune complexes used to activate the lymphocyte-derived factor had to contain the same antigen that was used to stimulate the lymphocyte cultures. Cohen and Ward also demonstrated that intradermal injection of the factor enhanced local eosinophil accumulation. It is important to note that this factor, although reportedly active in promoting eosinophil chemotaxis, also had significant PMN chemotactic activity (10). In a subsequent report, Torisu et al. (46) demonstrated that the production of this lymphocyte-derived chemotactic factor was carrier-specific, and that only immune complexes prepared with IgG_2 and not IgG_1 antibodies were able to produce eosinophil chemotactic activity. This mediator was heat-stable (56°C for 30 min) and had a bimodal distribution of activity when separated by sucrose density gradient ultracentrifugation and Sephadex G-100 chromatography. Neither method separated MIF from the eosinophil chemotactic factor. To characterize this lymphokine further, Torisu et al. (46) prepared columns of Sepharose beads coupled to either antigen (in this case, BGG—the antigen used for lymphocyte stimulation) or antibody (anti-BGG). Lymphocyte supernatants were passed through the columns before and after incubation with immune complexes. Prior to immune complex activation, the antibody-conjugated column, but not the antigen-conjugated column, was able to remove the chemotactic lymphokine. After incubation with immune complexes, neither column removed the eosinophil chemotactic factor. Neither column removed MIF activity. The authors concluded from these studies (a) that guinea pig MIF and eosinophil chemotactic factor are separable, (b) that the eosinophil chemotactic factor contains a fragment of the antigen responsible for its production, and (c) that perhaps the activation of this lymphokine by immune complexes results from cleavage of this antigenic fragment from the lymphokine molecule. Colley and co-workers (12,15,16), in a series of articles, have described a lymphokine with eosinophil chemotactic activity apparently distinct from that described by Ward et al. and Torisu and co-workers. This factor, called eosinophil stimulation promoter

(ESP), stimulates the migration of eosinophils as measured in an agarose droplet migration assay. In brief, the methods employed by these investigators involve the production of ESP by mouse spleen or lymph node lymphocytes and the use of eosinophil-rich mouse peritoneal exudate cells as responder cells. Using these techniques, Colley reported that ESP was produced by immune lymphocytes when stimulated with either specific antigens (PPD, schistosomal egg antigen) or PHA, and that this factor was heat-stable (56°C for 30 min) and nondialyzable (12). In a subsequent report, Greene and Colley showed that killing lymphocytes by repeated freeze-thawing or treatment with antithymocyte serum abrogated the ability of these cells to produce ESP as did treatment with puromycin, an inhibitor of protein synthesis (15). These investigators also reported that ESP was sensitive to chymotrypsin but resistant to neuraminidase and RNase. Peak ESP activity eluted from G-75 Sephadex gels with molecules of approximate molecular weight of 31,000 (range 24,000 to 56,000 daltons). Recently Greene and Colley utilized several experimental approaches to examine which cell population is responsible for ESP production (16). These studies showed: (a) Con A, a potent T cell mitogen, but not LPS, a B cell mitogen, induced ESP production; (b) treatment of lymphoid cells with anti-theta serum and complement eliminated ESP production; (c) thymocytes do not produce ESP; (d) lymphoid cells from nude mice fail to produce ESP; and (e) depletion of B lymphocytes and macrophages by nylon fiber adherence eliminated antigen-induced but not Con A-stimulated ESP production. These authors concluded that ESP production is a function of peripheral T lymphocytes and that macrophages are required for the antigen-induced production of this lymphokine. Further, although Greene and Colley did not show that B lymphocytes produce ESP, their studies do not rule out this possibility. It should be noted how remarkably similar these findings are to the observations of Altman and co-workers and other investigators in regard to LDCF. Why the findings of Ward et al. and Greene and Colley are different is not clear. It is true that different species were used by these two groups of investigators; however, it seems unlikely that immune complex activation would be needed to generate eosinophil chemotactic activity in one species and not another. It is also true that different methods for measuring eosinophil migration were utilized by these investigators. Lastly, it is possible that the lymphocyte supernatants studied by Greene and Colley contained immune complexes; however, they did not add exogenous antigen-antibody complexes to their cultures, and it seems unlikely that sufficient de novo antibody synthesis would have occurred *in vitro* to produce immune complexes. This explanation would also not account for those experiments in which PHA was used to stimulate ESP synthesis.

Kay et al. (21) examined the production of a lymphocyte-derived eosinophil chemotactic factor in six patients with Hodgkin's disease. Lymphocytes from five of the six produced supernatants that were more chemotactic for eosinophils than PMNs. In contrast, supernatants of lymph node cultures from two patients with lymphocytic lymphoma and four patients with reactive lymphatic hyper-

TABLE 2. *Comparison of eosinophil chemotactic factors*

Factor	Source	Characteristics	
ECF-A	Basophils, mast cells, PMNs	MW 500 heat-labile (100°C, 20 min) trypsin-resistant subtilisin-sensitive	
ECF-C	Complement (C5)	MW 15,000 heat-stable (56°C, 30 min) pI = 8.7	
Histamine	Basophils, mast cells	MW 111 $C_5H_9N_3$	
Bacterial chemotactic factor	Bacteria	MW 1,000–2,500 heat-stable (100°C, 30 min) trypsin, chymotrypsin-resistant pronase, subtilisin-sensitive	
Lymphokine chemotactic factor	T lymphocytes	MW 67,000, ? 12,500 heat-stable (56°C, 30 min)	Torisu et al. (46)
		MW 24,000–56,000 heat-stable (56°C, 30 min) chymotrypsin-sensitive RNase, neuraminidase-resistant	Greene et al. (15,16)

plasia had little eosinophil chemotactic activity. Supernatants with eosinophil chemotactic activity fractionated by gel filtration had four active peaks with approximate molecular weights of 30,000, 6,000, 2,000, and 500 daltons, respectively. Table 2 summarizes the data reviewed in this section regarding eosinophil chemotactic factors.

CHEMOTACTIC LYMPHOKINES AFFECTING BASOPHILS

The chemotaxis of basophils and the factors responsible for their migration have received little attention. Kay et al. (20) were the first to demonstrate that stimulated lymphocyte culture supernatants were chemotactic for basophils. These authors showed that antigen (streptokinase-streptodornase, SKSD)-stimulated human leukocytes produced a factor that chemotactically attracted homologous basophils. Indicator cells in these experiments were obtained from patients with chronic myelogenous leukemia and markedly elevated basophil counts; however, Kay et al. point out that other granulocytes present in the leukocyte preparations responded to the chemotactic lymphokine, indicating that the factor was not selective in its activity. Boetcher and Leonard (7) confirmed the work of Kay et al. and showed further that mitogen (PHA)-stimulated human lymphocytes also produced a factor with basophil chemotactic activity. In addition, their data shows that preincubation of basophils with chemotactically active lymphocyte supernatants augmented by 5- to 10-fold the subsequent response of these basophils to C5a. Preincubation of MNLs in active supernatants failed to augment their chemotactic responsiveness. The authors concluded from their data that the accumulation of basophils at sites of immune reactions may result from a two-step mechanism: priming of basophils by a product of stimulated lymphocytes followed by an augmented response to C5a. It is important to appreciate that the lymphocyte product used in these studies, although not characterized, was LDCF in that it had vigorous activity for MNLs as well as activity for basophils. Recent investigation from the same laboratory showed that the lymphocyte-derived basophil chemotactic factor was present in stimulated culture supernatants within 24 hr and was a heat-stable (56°C for 30 min), nondialyzable molecule of approximate MW of 12,500 daltons (26). Cultures stimulated with T cell mitogens (PHA, Con A, PWM), B cell mitogens (LPS, PWM), and antigens (SKSD, PPD) all produced the basophil chemotactic factor. Again, it is important to appreciate that this basophil chemotactic factor was quite active in attracting MNLs. Indeed, the physicochemical characteristics described by Boetcher and Leonard are identical to those previously reported by Altman et al. for LDCF. This strongly suggests that the same lymphokine is chemotactic for both types of leukocytes. Ward and co-workers (51) have examined the mechanisms of lymphocyte-dependent basophil chemotaxis in the guinea pig. This animal is particularly appropriate for the study of basophil chemotaxis, since the classic Jones-Mote reaction or cutaneous basophil hypersensitivity (CBH) is most evident in this species. These investigators showed that culture fluids from antigen (dinitrophenyl-bovine serum albumin, DNP-BSA)-stimulated lymphocyte cultures had chemotactic activity for blood and bone marrow basophils. Unstimulated supernatants were devoid of activity. The basophil chemotactic factor detected in this study was partially inactivated by heating (56°C for 1 hr), nondialyzable, and displayed a bimodal distribution on sucrose density gradients with most of the activity sedimenting coincident with a BSA marker. A lesser peak of activity was detected slightly ahead of (sedimented faster than) an IgG marker. Two other interesting aspects regarding basophil chemotaxis were reported: (a) that incubation of MNLs with chemotactically active lymphocyte supernatants significantly reduced the basophil but not the MNL chemotactic potential of the supernatants, and (b) that incubation of basophils with antigens used for the induction of basophilia markedly suppressed the subsequent response of these cells to either lymphokine or C5-related chemotactic factors. This suppression was specific, since exposure of basophils to only the same antigens used to induce basophilia and not unrelated antigens produced chemotactic suppression. These authors conclude (a) that in guinea pigs the lymphokines which attract MNLs and basophils are probably distinct, and (b) that their data may explain the mechanisms that regulate the accumulation of basophils *in vivo.* Two studies by Stadecker and Leskowitz also deserve mention (44,45). These investigators showed that the intradermal injection of antigens (egg albumin, EA, and BSA) or T cell mitogens (PHA, Con A, PWM) into normal guinea pigs produced basophil-rich skin reactions. Injection of *Escherichia coli* LPS, a B cell mitogen, although causing local induration and erythema, failed to stimulate *in vivo* basophil accumulation. Systemic treatment of guinea pigs with an anti-T cell serum markedly suppressed antigen and T cell mitogen-induced cutaneous basophil accumulation and produced a marked drop in circulating T cells. These data suggest that T lymphocytes are primarily responsible for mediating CBH responses. The authors hypothesize that T cells may effect this response by producing a basophil chemotactic factor.

CHEMOTACTIC LYMPHOKINES AFFECTING LYMPHOCYTES

Although *in vivo* studies and clinical observation suggest that lymphocytes do migrate, very little is known about chemotactic factors that attract lymphocytes. Early investigators reported that lymphocytes did not show chemotactic behavior (17,28). More recently, it has been reported that lymphocytes will respond to altered immunoglobulin (18) or to anti-immunoglobulin (40). It is unclear however if the migration observed in these studies was enhanced chemokinesis or chemotaxis. Wilkinson et al. (57) recently reported that human and mouse lymphoblasts could be chemotactically attracted by a diverse group of substances including casein, LPS-activated human serum, alkali-denatured albumin, oxazalone, and *Corynebacterium parvum.* Two reports describing a lymphokine with chemotactic activity for lymphocytes exist (11,53): Ward et al. (53) showed that antigen (OCBC-BGG)-stimulated guinea pig lymphocytes produced a soluble factor that chemotactically attracted rat lymphocytes. An 18-hour *in vitro* incubation period was necessary to demonstrate the chemotactic effect. Bacterial chemotactic factor and C5a failed to attract lymphocytes under these conditions. Furthermore, these investigators showed that abolishing the gradient in the chemotactic chamber markedly diminished lymphocyte migration. This experiment tends to confirm that these investigators measured true chemotaxis and not enhanced chemokinesis. Subsequently Cohen et al. (11) examined extracts of delayed hypersensitivity skin sites for evidence of *in vivo* production of a lymphocyte chemotactic factor. In this study, guinea pigs were immunized with antigens (EA, BGG), skin-tested, and pieces of skin from the test sites removed, homogenized, and supernatants prepared. The soluble skin extracts were then tested for chemotactic activity. Using these methods, Cohen et al. showed that supernatants from delayed hypersensitivity skin sites had chemotactic activity for lymphocytes and MNLs. Extracts from nonimmunized animals were devoid of activity. These investigators then characterized the lymphocyte chemotactic factor by sucrose density gradient ultracentrifugation. Two peaks of activity were detected: one near a BSA marker and the other near an IgG marker. Finally, these investigators showed that injecting these chemotactically active extracts into guinea pig skin produced erythema, induration, and a characteristic mononuclear leukocyte infiltrate. Control extracts failed to produce this response. This report supports the contention that there is a lymphokine with chemotactic activity for lymphocytes and suggests that this factor plays a role in mediating delayed hypersensitivity reactions.

SUMMARY

Lymphocytes produce a variety of biologically active factors (lymphokines), of which a number have chemotactic activity. Chemotactic lymphokines have been described which attract MNLs, PMNs, eosinophils, basophils, and lymphocytes; and extensive physicochemical characterization of these factors has been carried out. The best defined factor is LDCF, which is active in the attraction of MNLs. This chemotactic agent is a small molecular weight (12,500) noncomplement-derived protein that can be produced by both T and B lymphocytes. Studies of other chemotactic lymphokines are less advanced: however, there are substantial data to indicate that lymphokine chemotactic factors which promote basophil and eosinophil chemotaxis are similar to LDCF. Abnormalities in the synthesis of chemotactic lymphokines have been implicated in the pathophysiology of various human diseases (e.g., Wiskott-Aldrich syndrome, chronic mucocutaneous candidiasis, Hodgkin's disease).

ACKNOWLEDGMENTS

The investigation of this laboratory is supported in part by NIH Grants GM 22550 and AI07763.

REFERENCES

1. Altman, L. C., Chassy, B., and Mackler, B. F. (1975): Physicochemical characterization of chemotactic lymphokines produced by human T and B lymphocytes. *J. Immunol.,* 18–21.
2. Altman, L. C., and Kirchner, H. (1972): The production of a monocyte chemotactic factor by agammaglobulinemic chicken spleen cells. *J. Immunol.,* 109:1149–1151.
3. Altman, L. C., and Kirchner, H. (1974): Mononuclear leucocyte chemotaxis in the chicken: Definition of a phylogenetically specific lymphokine. *Immunology,* 26:393–405.
4. Altman, L. C., and Mackler, B. F. (1974): Chemotactic lymphokine production by human thymus-derived (T) and bone marrow derived (B) lymphocytes. *Fed. Proc.,* 33:3033.
5. Altman, L. C., Snyderman, R., and Blaese, R. M. (1974): Abnormalities of chemotactic lymphokine synthesis and mononuclear leukocyte chemotaxis in Wiskott-Aldrich syndrome. *J. Clin. Invest.,* 54:486–493.
6. Altman, L. C., Snyderman, R., Oppenheim, J. J., and Mergenhagen, S. E. (1973): A human mononuclear leukocyte chemotactic factor: Characterization, specificity and kinetics of production by homologous leukocytes. *J. Immunol.,* 110:801–810.
7. Boetcher, B. A., and Leonard, E. J. (1973): Basophil chemotaxis: Augmentation by a factor from stimulated lymphocyte cultures. *Immunol. Commun.,* 2:421–429.
8. Boetcher, D. A., and Meltzer, M. S. (1975): Mouse mononuclear cell chemotaxis: Description of system. *J. Natl. Cancer Inst.,* 54:795–799.
9. Clark, R. A. F., Gallin, J. I., and Kaplan, A. P. (1975): The selective eosinophil chemotactic activity of histamine. *J. Exp. Med.,* 142:1462–1475.

10. Cohen, S., and Ward, P. A. (1971): In vitro and In vivo activity of a lymphocyte and immune complex-dependent chemotactic factor for eosinophils. *J. Exp. Med.,* 133:133–146.
11. Cohen, S., Ward, P. A., Yoshida, T., and Burek, C. L. (1973): Biologic activity of extracts of delayed hypersensitivity skin reaction sites. *Cell Immunol.,* 9:363–376.
12. Colley, D. G. (1973): Eosinophils and immune mechanisms: I. Eosinophil stimulation promoter (ESP): A lymphokine induced by specific antigen or phytohemagglutinin. *J. Immunol.,* 110:1419–1423.
13. Foon, K. A., Wahl, S. M., Oppenheim, J. J., and Rosenstreich, D. L. (1976): Serotonin-induced production of a monocyte chemotactic factor by human peripheral blood leukocytes. *J. Immunol.,* 117:1545–1552.
14. Gallin, J. I., and Kirkpatrick, C. H. (1974): Chemotactic activity in dialyzable transfer factor. *Proc. Natl. Acad. Sci. U.S.A.,* 71:498–502.
15. Greene, B. M., and Colley, D. G. (1973): Eosinophils and immune mechanisms: II. Partial characterization of the lymphokine eosinophil stimulation promoter. *J. Immunol.,* 113:910–917.
16. Greene, B. M., and Colley, D. G. (1976): Eosinophils and immune mechanisms: III. Production of the lymphokine eosinophil stimulation promoter by mouse T lymphocytes. *J. Immunol.,* 116:1078–1083.
17. Harris, H. (1953): The movement of lymphocytes. *Br. J. Exp. Pathol.,* 34:599–602.
18. Higuchi, Y., Honda, M., and Hayashi, H. (1975): Production of chemotactic factor for lymphocytes by neutral SH-dependent protease of PMN rabbit leucocytes from immunoglobulin especially IgM. *Cell Immunol.,* 114:809–814.
19. Kay, A. B., (1970): Studies on eosinophil leucocyte migration: II. Factors specifically chemotactic for eosinophils and neutrophils generated from guinea pig serum by antigen-antibody complexes. *Clin. Exp. Immunol.,* 7:723–737.
20. Kay, A. B., and Austen, K. F. (1972): Chemotaxis of human basophil leucocytes. *Clin. Exp. Immunol.,* 11:557–563.
21. Kay, A. B., McVie, J. G., Stuart, A. E., Krajewski, A., and Turnbull, L. W. (1975): Eosinophil chemotaxis of supernatants from cultured Hodgkin's lymph node cells. *J. Clin. Pathol.,* 28:502–505.
22. Kay, A. B., Stechschulte, D. J., and Austen, K. F. (1971): An eosinophil leukocyte chemotactic factor of anaphylaxis. *J. Exp. Med.* 133:602.
23. Koopman, W. J., Sandberg, A. L., Wahl, S. M., and Mergenhagen, S. E. (1976): Interaction of soluble C3 fragments with guinea pig lymphocytes: Comparison of effects of C3a, C3b, C3c, and C3d on lymphokine production and lymphocyte proliferation. *J. Immunol.* 117:331–336.
24. Kretschmer, R. R., Stewardson, P. B., Papierniak, C. K., and Gotoff, S. P. (1976): Chemotactic and bactericidal activities of human newborn monocytes. *J. Immunol.,* 117:1303–1307.
25. Kuratsuji, T., Yoshida, T., and Cohen, S. (1976): Anti-lymphokine antibody: II. Specificity of biological activity. *J. Immunol.* 117:1985–1991.
26. Lett-Brown, M. A., Boetcher, D. A., and Leonard, E. J. (1976): Chemotactic responses of normal human basophils to C5a and to lymphocyte-derived chemotactic factor. *J. Immunol.,* 117:246–252.
27. Mackler, B. F., Altman, L. C., Rosenstreich, D. L., and Oppenheim, J. J. (1974): Induction of lymphokine production by EAC and of blastogenesis by soluble mitogens during human B-cell activation. *Nature,* 249:834–837.
28. McCutcheon, M. (1924): Studies on the locomotion of leucocytes: III. The rate of locomotion of human lymphocytes *in vitro. Am. J. Physiol.,* 69:279–282.
29. Meltzer, M. S. (1976): Chemotactic response of mouse macrophages to culture fluids from mitogen stimulated spleen cells. *Clin. Immunol. Immunopathol.,* 6:238–247.
30. Meltzer, M. S., Stevenson, M. M., and Leonard, E. J. (1976): Tumor cell chemotactic factor for mouse macrophages. *Fed. Proc.,* 35:406.
31. Muchmore, A. V., Blaese, R. M., and Altman, L. C. (1978): Submitted for publication.
32. Pick, E., and Turk, J. L. (1972): The biologic activities of soluble lymphocyte products. *Clin. Exp. Immunol.,* 10:1–23.
33. Postlethwaite, A. E., and Snyderman, R. (1975): Characterization of chemotactic activity produced *in vivo* by a cell-mediated immune reaction in the guinea pig. *J. Immunol.,* 114:274–278.
34. Rocklin, R. E. (1976): Mediators of cellular immunity, their nature and assay. *J. Invest. Dermatol.,* 67:372–380.

35. Rocklin, R. E., and David, J. R. (1971): Studies on the characterization of mediators produced by antigen-stimulated human lymphocytes. *Fed. Proc.,* 30:1128.
36. Rosenberg, G. L., Snyderman, R., and Notkins, A. L. (1974): Production of chemotactic factor and lymphotoxin by human leukocytes stimulated with herpes simplex virus. *Infect. Immunity,* 10:111–115.
37. Ruhl, J., Vogt, W., Bochert, G., Schmidt, S., Moelle, R., and Schaoua, H. (1974): Effect of L-asparaginase and hydrocortisone on human lymphocyte transformation and production of a mononuclear leucocyte chemotactic factor *in vitro. Immunology,* 26:989–994.
38. Ruhl, H., Vogt, W., Bochert, G., Schmidt, S., Schaoua, H., and Moelle, R. (1974): Lymphocyte transformation and production of a human mononuclear leucocyte chemotactic factor in patients with Hodgkin's disease. *Clin. Exp. Immunol.,* 17:407–415.
39. Sandberg, A. L., Wahl, S. M., and Mergenhagen, S. E. (1975): Lymphokine production by C3b-stimulated B cells. *J. Immunol.,* 115:139–144.
40. Schreiner, G. F., and Unanue, E. R. (1975): Anti-Ig triggered movements of lymphocytes: Specificity and lack of evidence for directional migration. *J. Immunol.,* 114:809–814.
41. Snyderman, R., and Altman, L. C. (1974): Mediators of delayed hypersensitivity. In: *Annual Review of Allergy,* edited by Claude A. Frazier, pp. 377–387. Medical Examination Publishing Co., New York.
42. Snyderman, R., Altman, L. C., Frankel, A., and Blaese, R. M. (1973): Defective mononuclear leukocyte chemotaxis: A previously unrecognized immune dysfunction. *Ann. Intern. Med.,* 78:509–513.
43. Snyderman, R., Altman, L. C., Hausman, M. S., and Mergenhagen, S. E. (1972): Human mononuclear leukocyte chemotaxis: A quantitative assay for humoral and cellular chemotactic factors. *J. Immunol.,* 108:857–860.
44. Stadecker, M. J., and Leskowitz, S. (1974): The cutaneous basophil response to mitogens. *J. Immunol.,* 113:496–500.
45. Stadecker, M. J., and Leskowitz, S. (1976): The inhibition of cutaneous basophil hypersensitivity reactions by a heterologous anti-guinea pig T cell serum. *J. Immunol.,* 116:1646–1651.
46. Torisu, M., Yoshida, R., Ward, P. A., and Cohen, S. (1973): Lymphocyte-derived eosinophil chemotactic factor: II. Studies on the mechanism of activation of the precursor substance by immune complexes. *J. Immunol.,* 111:1450–1458.
47. Wahl, S. M., Altman, L. C., Oppenheim, J. J., and Mergenhagen, S. E. (1974): *In vitro* studies of a chemotactic lymphokine in the guinea pig. *Int. Arch. Allergy Appl. Immunol.,* 46:768–784.
48. Wahl, S. M., Altman, L. C., and Rosenstreich, D. L. (1975): Inhibition of *in vitro* lymphokine synthesis by glucocorticosteroids. *J. Immunol.,* 115:476:480.
49. Wahl, S. M., Iverson, G. M., and Oppenheim, J. J. (1974): Induction of guinea pig B-cell lymphokine synthesis by mitogenic and nonmitogenic signals to Fc, Ig, and C3 receptors. *J. Exp. Med.,* 140:1631–1645.
50. Wahl, S. M., Wilton, J. M., Rosenstreich, D. L., and Oppenheim, J. J. (1975): The role of macrophages in the production of lymphokines by T and B lymphocytes. *J. Immunol.,* 114:1296–1301.
51. Ward, P. A., Dvorak, J. F., Cohen, S., Yoshida, T., Data, R., and Selvaggio, S. S. (1975): Chemotaxis of basophils by lymphocyte-dependent and lymphocyte-independent mechanisms. *J. Immunol.,* 114:1523–1531.
52. Ward, P. A., Lepow, I. H., and Newman, L. J. (1968): Bacterial factors chemotactic for polymorphonuclear leukocytes. *Am. J. Pathol.,* 52:725–736.
53. Ward, P. A., Offen, C. D., and Montgomery, J. R. (1971): Chemoattractants of leukocytes, with special reference to lymphocytes. *Fed. Proc.,* 30:1721–1724.
54. Ward, P. A., Remold, H. G., and David, J. R. (1969): Leukotactic factor produced by sensitized lymphocytes. *Science,* 163:1079–1081.
55. Ward, P. A., Remold, H. G., and David, J. R. (1970): The production by antigen-stimulated lymphocytes of a leukotactic factor distinct from migration inhibitory factor. *Cell Immunol.,* 1:162–174.
56. Ward, P. A., and Volkman, A. (1975): The elaboration of leukotactic mediators during the interaction between parental-type lymphocytes and F_1 hybrid cells. *J. Immunol.,* 115:1394–1398.
57. Wilkinson, P. C., Russell, R. J., Pumphrey, R. S. H., Sless, F., and Parrott, D. M. V. (1976): Studies of chemotaxis of lymphocytes. *Agents Actions,* 6:243–247.
58. Yoshida, T., Kuratsuji, A., Takada, Y., Takada, J. M., and Cohen, S. (1976): Lymphokine-

like factors produced by human lymphoid cell lines with B or T cell surface markers. *J. Immunol.,* 117:548–554.

DISCUSSION

Dr. Snyderman: Drs. Postlethwaite, Kang, and I have recently shown that lymphocytes also release a factor that is chemotactic for fibroblasts. I think this has some interesting implications for wound-healing. We started using the term *LDCF* in 1972 and a lot of people are now using it. Perhaps we could use the term *LDCF* plus whatever cell type is attracted. We could start talking about LDCF-M, monocytes or macrophages as opposed to LDCF-F for fibroblasts.

Dr. Altman: I thought about that approach for distinguishing between the different chemotactic lymphokines. The problem is that one factor may be capable of attracting more than one type of responder cell; for example, the work of Dr. Boetcher and Dr. Leonard, indicates that the chemotactic lymphokine that attracts monocytes also attracts basophils. What should we call this factor— LDCF-M for monocytes or LDCF-B for basophils? Obviously, there is no ideal form of nomenclature.

Dr. Ward: The lymphocyte chemotactic factors are lymphokines. By and large, they specifically attract T cells; they will not attract B cells. They can be produced by stimulation of T cells with CON-A, PHA, or specific antigen. Functionally similar material, but not necessarily structurally identical material, can be produced by macrophages, that have been activated via phagocytosis. I think that is really as much as one can say. These studies are in a relatively early stage, but they do provide some explanation for the accumulation of T cells in some kinds of hypersensitivity states.

Dr. Lynn: I seem to get the impression that all cells are attracted by lymphokines. Are the lymphokines secreted? What fraction of this material is actually stored in granules? Is lymphokine release a reflection of cell death?

Dr. Altman: I think that most of the chemotactic activity present in lymphocyte culture supernatants is actively synthesized and released by viable cells and does not reflect cell death. If you repeatedly freeze and thaw lymphocytes and examine the soluble fraction obtained, it does not contain very much chemotactic activity. Also, supernatants from lymphocytes cultured in the absence of antigens or mitogens contain only small amounts of chemotactic activity. In these cultures, cell death is certainly occurring. Furthermore, kinetic studies have shown that chemotactic lymphokine production is maximal at approximately 48 hr and that culture supernatants from later time points contain less activity. This suggests, if anything, that *in vitro* cell death (which increases with time) may nonspecifically destroy or catabolize LDCF. I know from personal conversation that Dr. Snyderman has data that suggest a small amount of LDCF is stored in unstimulated lymphocytes. Dr. Snyderman, do you wish to comment?

Dr. Snyderman: I agree with you fully. In some work that we did, where we tried to dissect the initial secretion from synthesis, we had cells incubated with and without cycloheximide. If you look at cells that are stimulated with CON-A, without cycloheximide, within 3 hr, significant amounts of chemotactic activity are present in the supernatant. The chemotactic activity then increases with time and levels off at 48 hr. If you preincubate the cells with cycloheximide, there is an initial release on contact with the mitogen or antigen and then nothing more is released. We could show with ^{14}C leucine that under those conditions there is no protein synthesis whatsoever. I therefore think there is *some* preformed material initially released by stimulated cells but *most* is newly synthesized and then released.

Dr. Nelson: When you isolated a population of B lymphocytes did you not also get monocytes? How can you be sure the chemotactic materials are lymphocyte- and not monocyte-derived?

Dr. Altman: The monocyte contamination was small (about 2%) in our B cell populations. It seems unlikely that this would account for the observed results, but you are correct; it is a remote possibility.

Leukocyte Chemotaxis, edited by John I. Gallin
and Paul G. Quie. Raven Press, New York
© 1978.

Lipid Molecules as Chemotactic Factors

Stephen R. Turner and William S. Lynn

*Department of Medicine, Duke University Medical Center,
Durham, North Carolina 27710*

Recent progress in the isolation of well-defined chemotactic molecules has led to a clearer understanding of the chemical nature of leukocyte chemotaxis. It is now well established that low concentrations of well-defined peptides and lipids can attract leukocytes under controlled conditions *in vitro.* Many examples of chemotactic peptides can be drawn from the *N*-formylated peptides (21,25) and eosinophilic tetrapeptides (5,6). Although these studies have greatly strengthened the contention that peptides are major chemotactic mediators *in vivo,* several classes of nonpeptides (lipids) have been shown to exhibit chemotactic effects similar to those traditionally associated with peptides.

The concept of chemotactic lipids is in consonance with the suggestion by Wilkinson (33) that hydrophobic interactions may be a major determinant of chemotactic properties as a consequence of increased hydrophobicity accompanying denaturation or synthetic alkylation. The highly chemotactic peptides described by Schiffmann and co-workers (21,25) are quite hydrophobic, e.g., *N*-formyl-Met-Phe is more soluble in methanol than in water, and the eosinophilic tetrapeptides also seem to require nonpolar amino acid residues for maximum effectiveness (6).

If hydrophobicity is a hallmark of chemotactic factors, it would not be unexpected to identify lipids that possess chemotactic properties. This potential for chemotactic function seems to be realized in HETE, a hydroxy fatty acid (described in detail in following sections), prostaglandins (PGs), and lipid constituents of bacterial chemotactic factors.

The Chemotactic Lipids

Prostaglandin E_1 (PGE_1) was the first simple lipid to be implicated in leukocyte chemotaxis. Prostaglandins (PGs) have many inflammatory actions and would be a logical class of compounds to examine for chemotactic members. Two groups (12,13) have observed that PGE_1 is chemotactic for rabbit PMN cells at concentrations of 0.01 to 1.0 μg/ml. These results could not be duplicated by investigators who used human (28) or rat (2) PMN cells; however, PGE_1 solutions that were "aged" for 12 hours became chemotactic for rat PMN cells

(2). The presumed degradation of PGE_1 to a chemotactic product underscores the need for extreme care in the handling of lipids and may in part explain the conflicting data. Species-specificity of PGE_1 for rabbit cells must also be considered in any evaluation of chemotactic properties. The picture of PG effects on leukocyte migration is further clouded by reports that rather than being chemotactic, PGs stimulate random movement (23) or amplify the chemotactic effects of other agents (17).

Bacterial culture filtrates are another souce of chemotactic lipids. Lipid-like materials were shown to account for at least some of the chemotactic properties of *Escherichia coli* culture filtrates (22,27). The target cell specificity of *E. coli* lipids appears to be subject to modulation by association with protein moieties (27), though the nature of the lipid protein interaction has not been determined. The chemotactic lipid component exhibited chromatographic behavior similar to that of an oxidized fatty acid.

Coryneform bacteria synthesize a chemotactic lipid fraction that has been tentatively identified as phospholipid by its chromatographic behavior (20). This material was preferentially chemotactic for monocytes as opposed to neutrophils.

The most recent class of chemotactic lipids to be reported is represented by HETE, a hydroxy fatty acid generated from arachidonic acid by the action of an aggregation-activated blood platelet lipoxygenase (19). Platelets also contain an aggregation-activated cyclo-oxygenase which metabolizes arachidonic acid into prostaglandins (16) and thromboxanes (10). The cyclo-oxygenase is inhibited by nonsteroid anti-inflammatory drugs such as aspirin and indomethacin, while the lipoxygenase is unaffected or stimulated by such agents (19). In the following sections, we will review what is known of HETE's chemotactic properties and try to make a reasonable case for the participation of HETE in inflammatory reactions.

A Chemotactic Metabolite of Arachidonic Acid

Our attempts to identify the chemotactic constituents of crude casein led to the observation that chemotactic activity was easily extracted from casein by organic solvents. Gas liquid chromatography (GLC) of butanol-acetic acid extracts of casein revealed the presence of many free fatty acids. Purified samples of these and other fatty acids were tested for chemotactic activity in the Boyden assay system using human PMN indicator cells. We found that arachidonic acid uniquely attracted large numbers of cells into well-defined circular clusters that were nonuniformly distributed over the surface of the micropore filter of the Boyden chamber (28). These clusters were apparently sites where droplets of arachidonic acid had become embedded in the filter and had partially oxidized into a chemotactic product that diffused to form a localized gradient. In subsequent experiments, we found that addition of arachidonic acid to the incubation buffer as an ethanolic solution or as the sodium salt abolished both the formation of cell clusters and oil droplets (S. R. Turner and W. S. Lynn, *unpublished*

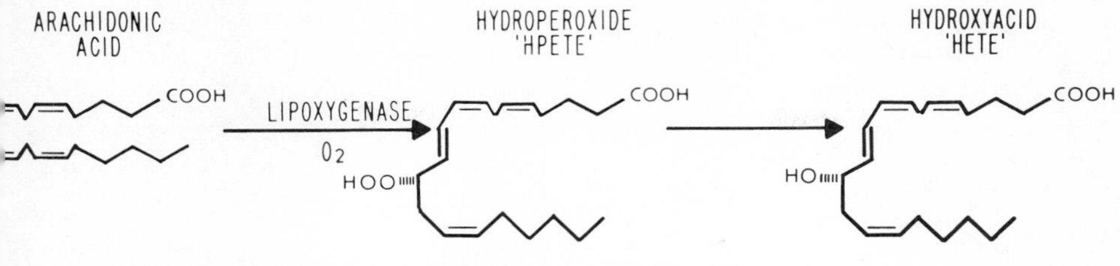

ARACHIDONIC ACID HYDROPEROXIDE 'HPETE' HYDROXYACID 'HETE'

FIG. 1. HETE synthesis by platelet lipoxygenase.

observations). Furthermore, controlled exposure of arachidonic acid to oxygen or ultraviolet (UV) radiation yielded a chemotactic product that attracted PMN cells without forming cell clusters. The active component of the oxidation products had the properties of a monohydroxy fatty acid, as evidenced by data from GLC, thin layer chromatography (TLC), and UV spectrophotometry.

Further progress in our study of arachidonic acid was greatly facilitated by the elegant studies by Samuelsson and co-workers (10,16) and Nugteren (19), which delineated the basic metabolism of unsaturated fatty acids by blood platelet enzymes. The central role of arachidonic acid in the biosynthesis of nonpeptide inflammatory mediators particularly intrigued us. The platelet cyclo-oxygenase responsible for the synthesis of prostaglandin endoperoxides and thromboxanes co-exists with a lipoxygenase that transforms arachidonic acid into the hydroxy fatty acid known variously as HETE, 12-ho-20:4, and 12L-OH-5,8,10,14-eicosatetraenoic acid. (We will use HETE for the sake of brevity, though a descriptive, euphonic name for this compound has not been introduced.) The synthesis of HETE in platelets is outlined in Fig. 1. The postulated hydroperoxide intermediate is probably immediately reduced to the hydroxy acid by glutathione and has not been isolated from platelet incubations.

In a study which predates the discovery of the role of arachidonic acid in platelet aggregation, Weksler and Coupal (32) described the generation of chemotactic activity by aggregated blood platelets. Evaluation of their work in light of the new information on platelet metabolism compelled us to hypothesize that HETE or a similar metabolite of arachidonic acid might be an example of a chemotactic lipid. To test this hypothesis, we isolated HETE from human blood platelets incubated with arachidonic acid. HETE was identified by its UV absorption spectrum, behavior on GLC and TLC, and by its mass spectrum (30). Solutions of HETE proved to be strongly chemotactic for human PMN cells at concentrations between 10^{-4} and 10^{-7} M, with activity persisting to 10^{-8} or 10^{-9} M. Additions of 10^{-5} M HETE to both sides of the Boyden chamber resulted in no net chemotaxis of PMN cells, suggesting that the cell response is at least partly chemotactic, as opposed to chemokinetic. Mass spectral analysis also confirmed the presence of HETE in the chemotactic autoxidation products of arachidonic acid (30), which proved to be a mixture of positional isomers of HETE having the general formula n-ho-20:4 where n is the position

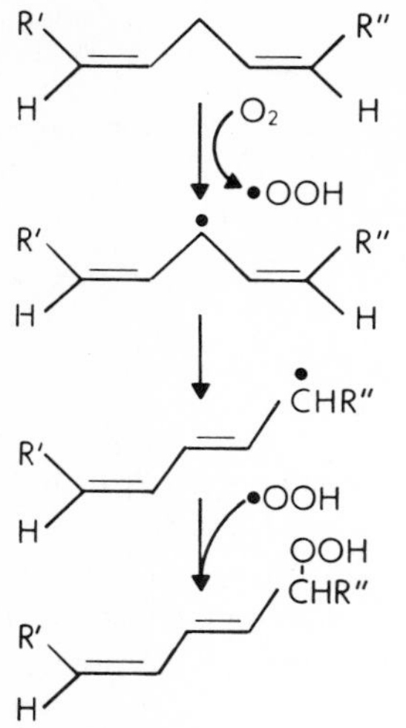

FIG. 2. Proposed mechanism for lipid peroxidation.

of the hydroxyl function counting from the carboxyl end. Only the isomers with n = 5,8,9,11,12, and 15 were present in significant amounts (29). These are the isomers anticipated if peroxidation follows the proposed mechanism (7) shown in Fig. 2, in which oxygen abstracts a methylene hydrogen atom to form a free radical that is stabilized by rearrangement to a conjugated diene. The stabilized radical combines with a hydroperoxy radical to yield the hydroperoxy acid. Subsequent reduction of the hydroperoxide would yield the corresponding hydroxy fatty acid. Dilution of HETE by its isomers may account for the observation that HETE from photoxidation has a lower specific chemotactic activity than purified HETE obtained from platelet incubations (S. R. Turner and W. S. Lynn, *unpublished observation*).

The target cell spectrum of HETE seems to be rather broad. We have noted that HETE attracts human neutrophils (30) and alveolar macrophages from both human (J. A. Tainer and W. S. Lynn, *unpublished observation*) and rabbit (27). Recently, Goetzl (4) has reported that HETE is also an effective cytotoxin for human peripheral monocytes and eosinophils.

We should note that HETE is a highly labile material for which adequate storage procedures have not been developed. This lability is not shared by the analog 15-ho-20:4, which in our hands is quite stable when stored under argon at $-70°C$.

OBSERVATIONS ON THE STRUCTURE OF HETE

A well-defined chemotactic agent such as *N*-formyl-Met-Leu-Phe (21) or Val-Gly-Ser-Glu (6) is invaluable for studying structure-function relationships. At present, our rudimentary data for HETE cannot provide the insights that have been gained from the study of the chemotactic peptides, but we can outline in broadest terms some of the features of HETE that seem to be involved in its chemotactic actions.

As simple as the structure of HETE appears, there are still many structural variations that may be manifested. We consider here the available data pertinent to a few structural parameters.

In unpublished studies, we have obtained several lines of evidence that suggest that the n-9 position of the hydroxyl group in HETE is essential for chemotactic activity. We prepared the n-6 isomer (15-ho-20:4) using soybean lipoxygenase (E.C. 1.13.1.13) and arachidonic acid (8). This isomer exhibited chemotactic properties only at concentrations greater than 10^{-4} M and maximal chemotactic response never exceeded 10% of that attainable with HETE. This behavior of 15-ho-20:4 is consistent with the idea stated above, that the chemotactic activity of autoxidized arachidonic acid is a result primarily of the presence of HETE in a mixture of inactive or weakly active isomers. It is possible, however, that the isomer mixture obtained by autoxidation consists of inhibitory and chemotactic components, whose effects largely offset each other. We are testing the validity of this possibility by isolating all members of the isomer series and assaying each of them for stimulation and inhibition of chemotaxis.

Preliminary studies of 12-ho-20:3 the n-9 hydroxy derivative of dihomo-γ-linolenic acid (8,11,14–20:3) obtained by platelet lipoxygenase indicate that this compound is the major product and is chemotactic for human neutrophils. On the other hand, the monohydroxy fatty acids derived from the autoxidation of 11,14,17-20:3 had no chemotactic activity at any concentration. This result is expected if the n-9 isomer is required for chemotactic activity. In the case of 11,14,17–20:3, the n-9 hydroxy isomer is not available through the proposed peroxidation mechanism (Fig. 2), which predicts only the isomers at n-3, n-6, n-7, and n-10.

The stereochemistry of the carbon atom bearing the hydroxyl group may be of importance in determining chemotactic function, although the racemic mixture produced by autoxidation of arachidonic acid does not appear to contain any strongly inhibitory enantiomers. HETE belongs to the L series (19) as does 15-ho-20:4 (8). The D enantiomer of 11-ho-20:4 (available through the action of potato lipoxygenase) is currently in preparation (3) for evaluation of its chemotactic properties.

Unsaturation is required for chemotactic activity in HETE, as evidenced by the complete loss of activity following catalytic reduction to 12-ho-20:0 with hydrogen-palladium in methanol-acetic acid (29). α-hydroxy arachidic acid (2-ho-20:0) was likewise void of chemotactic activity. Addition of one double bond at n-3 is also without apparent effect on chemotactic activity, as witnessed by the generation of chemotactic activity from 5,8,11,14,17–20:5 (28). We do not know which double bonds are absolutely essential for chemotaxis, but the preliminary results for 12-ho-20:3 described above would imply that the n-15 double bond is not critical.

Unequivocal evidence is not yet available to determine the role of the carboxyl group in HETE's chemotactic properties. In our hands, methylation of the carboxyl group by diazomethane has resulted in decreased chemotactic effectiveness of variable degrees, ranging from complete inhibition to 50% reduction. A similar loss of chemotactic activity was observed when *N*-formyl-Met-Phe was subjected to the same methylation procedure. It is conceivable that a phagocyte esterase (25) releases the free carboxyl group from the methyl esters.

Endogenous HETE in Chemotaxis

There is increasing support for the contention that HETE may be a biologically significant mediator of chemotaxis. Besides its demonstrated chemotactic activity *in vitro,* HETE is a potential metabolite in most mammalian tissues because of the presence of arachidonic acid esters in plasma membranes. Arachidonic acid comprises by weight approximately 20% of erythrocyte lipids and 27% of total plasma lipids in the rat (24). The phospholipids of human neutrophils, monocytes, and lymphocytes consist of 12 to 20 mole percent arachidonic acid (26). Esterified forms of arachidonic acid do not seem to be chemotactic, as we have observed for methylarachidonate (28). We have also found, in unpublished work, that diarachidonyl phosphatidyl choline and cholesterol arachidonate are not chemotactic for human PMN cells at concentrations of 10^{-4} to 10^{-9} M. Esterified arachidonic acid, though not a substrate for platelet lipoxygenase (19), can be oxidized by microsomal enzymes to yield malondialdehyde and other unidentified oxidation products (18). The chemotactic activity of these products has not been reported.

In tissues, the free arachidonic acid required for HETE synthesis could be obtained from membrane esters through the action of phospholipases. Such a course of action might follow tissue damage and activation of endogenous phospholipases. In support of this scheme is the observation by Hamberg (9) that guinea pig tissue homogenates produce HETE when they are incubated at 37°C. Lung and spleen, respectively, yielded approximately 15 and 30 μg of HETE per g of tissue, while kidney and whole blood were less than one-tenth as efficient in producing HETE. Lipoxygenase inhibitors blocked the appearance of HETE in all tissue homogenates, indicating that HETE was formed by enzymic action. Elevated levels of HETE have also been found in the lesional epidermis of psoriasis (11). The significance of HETE in this pathology is unknown.

We feel that the data presented here support the proposition of a new mechanism for the endogenous production of chemotactic mediators, namely, the transformation of arachidonic acid into HETE. As shown in Fig. 3, we propose that the disruption of plasma membrane integrity exposes arachidonate-rich phospholipids to the action of phospholipases which split off free arachidonic acid. Tissue lipoxygenase metabolizes the arachidonic acid to HETE, which in turn aids in the recruitment of phagocytes. Aggregated blood platelets represent another major source of endogenous HETE, though at least two other chemotactic mediators are released by platelets in the presence of serum: complement component C5a (31,32) and fibrinopeptide B (15).

MEMBRANE DISRUPTION

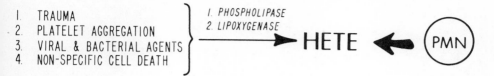

FIG. 3. Proposed scheme for the production of chemotactic lipids *in vivo*.

One application of the proposed scheme for the formation of chemotactic lipids is partial rationalization of the phenomenon called necrotaxis. Bessis (1) has described necrotaxis in a system in which laser-injured erythrocytes were recognized and phagocytized by neighboring leukocytes. Presumably, chemotactic signals released by the damaged erythrocytes guided the leukocytes to their targets. These experiments were performed in the absence of both serum and complement, which implies that chemotactic signals were generated from the structural material of the erythrocytes. These signals may well result from both oxidized arachidonic acid derived from the erythrocyte membrane, and from denatured proteins, which must certainly be released by the disrupted erythrocytes. Chemical analysis of necrotic erythrocytes is not available to ascertain the presence of chemotactic lipids or proteins, but the chances seem great for the presence of both classes of mediators.

The identification of chemotactic lipids raises many new questions about the interaction of leukocytes with their cytotaxins. Of particular importance is the nature of the putative chemotactic binding sites on leukocyte membranes. It is not known whether or not lipid and peptide chemotactic factors are recognized by the same binding sites. The demonstration of separate receptors for lipids and peptides may have important implications about the control of chemotaxis *in vivo*. HETE metabolism by phagocytes is another process that is virtually unexplored. It seems unlikely that a fatty acid such as HETE would be a substrate for the esterases that act upon the *N*-formyl peptides (25). More probably, HETE metabolism would be analogous to that of PGs, e.g., conversion of the hydroxyl group to a keto function by a dehydrogenase, double-bond isomerization and reduction, and β- and ω-oxidation (14). Improved understanding of the interactions of peptides and lipids in the control of chemotaxis should facilitate better management of pathologic conditions that involve dysfunction of the phagocytic defense system.

ACKNOWLEDGMENTS

The work of this laboratory was supported in part by National Institutes of Health Training Grant ES 0024, and grants from the Veterans Administration and the Walker P. Inman Fund (SRT).

We thank the Durham County Chapter of the American Red Cross for the donation of outdated blood platelets used in the lipoxygenase studies.

REFERENCES

1. Bessis, M. (1973): Necrotaxis: Chemotaxis towards an injured cell. *Nouv. Rev. Fr. Hematol.* 13:887.
2. Ford-Hutchinson, A. W., Smith, M. J. H., and Walker, J. R. (1976): Chemotactic activity of solutions of prostaglandin E_1. *Proc. Br. Pharmacol. Soc.,* 56:345.
3. Galliard, T., and Phillips, D. R. (1971): Lipoxygenase from potato tubers. *Biochem. J.,* 124:431.
4. Goetzl, E. J. (1976): Modulation of human eosinophil polymorphonuclear leukocyte migration and function. *Am. J. Pathol.,* 85:419.
5. Goetzl, E. J., and Austen, K. F. (1975): Purification and synthesis of eosinophilotactic tetrapeptide of human lung tissue: Identification as eosinophil chemotactic factor of anaphylaxis. *Proc. Natl. Acad. Sci. U.S.A.,* 72:4123–4127.
6. Goetzl, E. J., and Austen, K. F. (1976): Structural determinants of the eosinophil chemotactic activity of the acidic tetrapeptides of eosinophil chemotactic factor of anaphylaxis. *J. Exp. Med.,* 144:1424.
7. Gurr, M. I., and James, A. T. (1975): *Lipid Biochemistry.* Chapman and Hill, London.
8. Hamberg, M. (1971): Steric analysis of hydroperoxides formed by lipoxygenase oxygenation of linoleic acid. *Anal. Biochem.,* 43:515.
9. Hamberg, M. (1976): On the formation of thromboxane B_2 and 12L-hydroxy-5,8,10,14-eicosatetraenoic acid (12-ho-20:4) in tissues from the guinea pig. *Biochim. Biophys. Acta,* 431:651.
10. Hamberg, M., Svensson, J., and Samuelsson, B. (1975): Thromboxanes: A new group of biologically active compounds derived from prostaglandin endoperoxides. *Proc. Natl. Acad. Sci. U.S.A.* 72:2994.
11. Hammarström, S., et al. (1975): Increased concentrations of nonesterified arachidonic acid, 12L-hydroxy-5,8,10,14-eicosatetraenoic acid, prostaglandin E_2, and prostaglandin $F_{2\alpha}$ in epidermis of psoriasis. *Proc. Natl. Acad. Sci. U.S.A.* 72:5130.
12. Higgs, G. A., McCall, E., and Youlten, L. J. F. (1975): A chemotactic role for prostaglandins released from polymorphonuclear leukocytes during phagocytosis. *J. Pharmacol.,* 53:539–546.
13. Kaley, G., and Weiner, R. (1971): Prostaglandin E_1: A potential mediator of the inflammatory response. *Ann. N.Y. Acad. Sci.,* 180:338–350.
14. Karim, S. M. M. (1976): *Prostaglandins: Chemical and Biochemical Aspects.* University Park Press, Baltimore.
15. Kay, A. B., Pepper, D. S., and McKenzie, R. (1974): The identification of fibrinopeptide B as a chemotactic agent derived from human fibrinogen. *Br. J. Haematol.,* 27:669.
16. Malmsten, C., Hamberg, M., Svensson, J., and Samuelsson, B. (1975): Physiological role of an endoperoxide in human platelets: Hemostatic defect due to platelet cyclo-oxygenase deficiency. *Proc. Natl. Acad. Sci. U.S.A.,* 72:1446.
17. McClatchey, W., and Snyderman, R. (1976): Prostaglandins and inflammation: Enhancement of monocyte chemotactic responsiveness by prostaglandin E_2. *Prostaglandins* 12:415.
18. Niehaus, W. G., and Samuelsson, B. (1968): Formation of malonaldehyde from phospholipid arachidonate during microsomal lipid peroxidation. *Eur. J. Biochem.,* 6:126.
19. Nugteren, D. H. (1974): Arachidonate lipoxygenase in blood platelets. *Biochim. Biophys. Acta,* 280:299.
20. Russel, R. J., McInroy, R. J., Wilkinson, P. C., and White, R. G. (1975): Identification of a lipid chemo-attractant (chemotactic) factor for macrophages from anaerobic coryneform bacteria. *Behring Inst. Mitt.* 57:103.
21. Schiffmann, E., et al. (1975): N-formylmethionyl peptides as chemoattractants for leukocytes. *Proc. Natl. Acad. Sci. U.S.A.,* 72:1059–1062.
22. Schiffmann, E., et al. (1975): The isolation and partial characterization of neutrophil chemotactic factors from *Escherichia coli. J. Immunol.,* 114:1831.
23. Shibuya, E., Masuda, K., and Izawa, Y. (1976): Effects of prostaglandins on leukocyte migration. *Prostaglandins,* 12:165.
24. Shimasaki, H., and Privett, O. S. (1975): Studies on the role of vitamin E in the oxidation of blood components by fatty hydroperoxides. *Biochem. Biophys.,* 169:506.

25. Showell, H. J., Freer, R. J., Zigmond, S. H., Schiffmann, E., Aswanikumar, S., Corcoran, B., and Becker, E. L. (1976): The structure-activity relations of synthetic peptides as chemotactic factors and inducers of lysosomal enzyme secretion for neutrophils. *J. Exp. Med.,* 143:1154.
26. Stossel, T. P., Mason, R. J., and Smith, A. L. (1974): Lipid peroxidation by human blood phagocytes. *J. Clin. Invest.,* 54:638.
27. Tainer, J. A., Turner, S. R., and Lynn, W. S. (1975): New aspects of chemotaxis: Specific target cell attraction by lipid and lipoprotein fractions of *Escherichia coli* chemotactic factor. *Am. J. Pathol.,* 81:401–410.
28. Turner, S. R., Campbell, J. A., and Lynn, W. S. (1975): Polymorphonuclear leukocyte chemotaxis toward oxidized lipid components of cell membranes. *J. Exp. Med.,* 141:1437.
29. Turner, S. R., and Lynn, W. S. (1977): Structure-function correlations in chemotactic fatty acids. In preparation.
30. Turner, S. R., Tainer, J. A., and Lynn, W. S. (1975): Biogenesis of chemotactic molecules by the arachidonate lipoxygenase system of platelets. *Nature,* 257:680.
31. Ward, P. A. (1971): Complement derived chemotactic factors and their interaction with neutrophil granulocytes. In: *Proceedings of the International Symposium on the Biological Activity of Complement,* Vol. 180, edited by D. G. Ingraham, Karger, Basel.
32. Weksler, B. B., and Coupal, C. E. (1973): Platelet-dependent generation of chemotactic activity in serum. *J. Exp. Med.,* 137:1419.
33. Wilkinson, P. C. (1976): Recognition and response in mononuclear and granular phagocytes. *Clin. Exp. Immunol.,* 25:355.

DISCUSSION

Dr. Becker: Dr. Turner, how stable is the HETE? How easily is it radiolabeled? In other words, how feasible is it to do binding studies with HETE?

Dr. Turner: Stability is a problem with these compounds. Researchers at Upjohn have had trouble storing HETE longer than a week and have tried various methods to stabilize it. But if it is prepared and used promptly, I do not think there is any problem. Competitive binding studies of HETE and other chemotactic factors would be of great interest.

Dr. Ward: How do you deal with the solubility problems of these fatty acids and their derivatives? How reliable are your estimates of concentration?

Dr. Turner: I think the concentrations are quite reliable when we see a uniform distribution of cells responding in the Boyden chamber. When we see clusters of cells, we know that the formal concentration does not mean anything.

Dr. Wilkinson: We have done quite a lot of work with fatty acids and it is tremendously difficult. I certainly have the impression that a much wider range is active than you have mentioned. A lot of the fatty acids are weakly active when you use the leading-front technique. I do not know whether the cells will move all the way through the filter. There is an incredible problem with solubility. I do not think you mentioned this, but you get very "bumpy" dose-response curves. You have to check the thing over an enormously wide dose range.

Dr. Snyderman: Considering the problem dealing with these materials and chemotaxis, I wonder if it would not be worthwhile to look at some other function of the factors such as lysosomal enzyme release or as we have done, calcium fluxes. It might be a lot easier to measure things that occur instantaneously.

Dr. Quie: Dr. Elaine Mills and Dr. Jon Gerrard at Minnesota have shown that when arachidonic acid or other fatty acids are incubated with platelets, there is a tremendous burst of chemoluminescence. This reaction suggests that platelet metabolic by-products may be chemotactic or have other effects on leukocytes.

Dr. Schiffmann: Dr. Turner, did you test whether or not these factors can compete with fMet peptides or C5a?

Dr. Turner: A preliminary study in collaboration with Dr. Ralph Snyderman suggests that HETE does not block the binding of the fMet peptides.

Dr. Schiffmann: The other question concerns the instability of HETE. Is there any evidence that HETE, when interacting with the cells, goes to a more stable compound which is a true chemoattractant?

Dr. Turner: I can not say whether HETE is a cytotaxinogen or a cytotaxin. Understanding the metabolism of the compound will be essential to answering your question.

Dr. Jensen: Could you comment further on what lipid material you have extracted from casein that has chemotactic activity.

Dr. Turner: The soluble lipid obtained from casein consisted of a series of common fatty acids including predominantly palmitic and oleic acid. The chemotactic constituents of the extract have not been identified.

Dr. Robert Clark: Dr. Turner, neutrophils themselves are a source of oxidases and peroxidases. Have you any thoughts about whether these neutrophil enzymes might be capable of oxidizing the lipids to form chemotactic agents?

Dr. Turner: Generation of chemotactic lipids requires a relatively specific type of oxidation reaction catalyzed by a lipoxygenase enzyme. We are unable to obtain chemotactic products from arachidonic acid using nonspecific oxidizers such as hydrogen peroxide, iodine, and permanganate.

Dr. Goetzl: You had shown earlier, with Dr. Lynn, that addition of certain proteins to bacterial lipids would change their cellular preferential chemotactic activity. Do proteins alter HETE activity? Have you found that the addition of arachidonic acid to the polymorphonuclear leukocytes generates any chemotactic activity in the lipid?

Dr. Turner: We have not incubated polymorphonuclear leukocytes with arachidonic acid.

Leukocyte Chemotaxis, edited by John I. Gallin
and Paul G. Quie. Raven Press, New York
© 1978.

Characterization of Chemotactic Agents Produced in Experimental Pleural Inflammation

William S. Lynn, R. S. N. Somayajulu, Saura Sahu, and Jeff Selph

Department of Medicine, Duke University Medical Center, Durham, North Carolina 27710

For some time, it has been clear that activation of proteolysis in blood leads to the proteolytic production of several peptides, i.e., C_{5a}, C_{567}, and fibrinopeptides (1,5,12), which are chemotactically active for most types of inflammatory cells. Recently, we have demonstrated that blood platelets, when activated by collagen, arachidonic acid, or by lysis, rapidly synthesize a potent fatty acid chemotaxin from arachidonic acid, which was shown to be HETE (12-hydroxy, $\Delta 5,8,10,15$ eicosatetraenoic acid) (10). None of the other many fatty acid mediators produced by these activated platelets was chemotactically active. Another blood factor, which is produced by phagocytizing neutrophils, is an unusual small glycopeptide (apparent mol. wt. of 8,500) containing only one tyrosin residue/mole (9). Thus, it is clear that blood possesses three different systems for rapidly synthesizing chemotactically active molecules.

To ascertain which, if any, of the above three vascular systems play a role in *in vivo* neutrophil chemotaxis, the carrageenan model of pleurisy in rats (11) was chosen for study. Pleural fluid and cells were removed at different times after intrapleural injection of either carrageenan or kaolin (aluminum silicate), and all lipids were isolated from both cells and exudate fluid, separated as before (7,10), and assayed for chemotactic activity, using human neutrophilis (10). Similarly, peptides and proteins were isolated from both fractions (9) and all fractions assayed for chemotactic activity. Most (90%) of the activity that accumulates in these pleural exudates, as well as that present in the exudate cells, could be accounted for in the protein and peptide fractions. The active peptide fraction has properties similar to the peptide previously isolated from phagocytizing neutrophils (9).

Chemotactic peptides can also be produced by digestion of soluble proteins obtained from cell extracts of these pleural neutrophils with either pronase or chymotrypsin.

A small amount of the chemotactic activity was found in a lipid fraction containing an oxidized hydrocarbon which, upon reduction with H_2 under anhydrous conditions, could be converted to squalene. No HETE could be recovered from these inflammatory fluids at any time.

These data support the concept that the major chemotactic signals for neutrophil influx into rat pleura, after injecting either carrageenan, kaolin, or lysolecithin, are proteins and peptides. These peptides are synthesized and liberated by the neutrophils which are present at all times in the rat pleural cavity. The relationship of this neutrophil peptide to chemotactic peptides derived by proteolysis of serum complement (12) is not yet known.

METHODS

Experimental Pleurisy

Sprague Dawley Rats of 200 gm were injected with either 200 μg carrageenan, 200 μg 1-palmitoyl lysolecithin, or 800 μg kaolin in 0.3 ml of sterile isotonic saline as previously described (11). Pleural fluid was removed at 0 time, 1 hr, 3 hr, 7 hr, or 10 hr and the pleural cavity washed with 2 ml of isotonic saline. Cells were removed by centrifugation at 200 $\times$ g for 10 min and were washed $\times$ 2 with isotonic saline.

Cell extracts were made by freezing and thawing 5×10^8 rat cells obtained from pleura injected 7 hr previously with one of the above irritants. In all cases, the cells were approximately 90% neutrophils. The rest of the cells were large mononuclear cells.

Isolation of Lipid and Peptide Chemotaxins

After dialysis of the cellular extracts and the exudate fluid for 6 hr at 0° against distilled water, each fraction was freeze-dried and all lipids removed by extraction of the dry powders with chloroform-methanol as before (7). No chemotactic activity was lost during dialysis.

These extracts were separated into four fractions by silicic acid column chromatography, as before (7). Since all chemotactic activity was present in fraction I (neutral lipid) from the silicic acid column, activity was subsequently removed by extraction of the aqueous extracts with ethyl ether at pH 3.0. The ether extracts were further separated by silica gel TLC using chloroform-methanol-acetic acid-water (90:8:1:0.8 by volume) as solvent. (6,7). Lipids were detected by I_2 or by charring with H_2SO_4 and all areas (1 cm) on the TLC plate assayed for chemotactic activity, using both Boyden chamber system with human neutrophils (10) and *in vivo* rat pleural assay (11). The dried lipid fractions were all suspended by vigorous shaking of microgram quantities per milliliter in Hanks' buffer containing 0.1% serum albumin for assay.

Peptides in the soluble cell extracts and exudate were separated from proteins and smaller molecules by gel filtration by use of a column of Sephadex G50 (1 $\times$ 90 cm) and isotonic saline solution. The column was standardized using serum albumin, trypsin, cytochrome C, insulin, and adenylic acid as indicators of apparent molecular weight. All fractions were pooled and assayed for chemotactic activity in the two assay systems outlined above. All fractions were treated with pronase (3 μg/ml) for either 30 min at 37°C, pH 7.5 or for 6 hr, and chemotactic activity reexamined. As control, pronase was also assayed for chemotactic activity in each assay system.

In addition, lipid was removed from each of the active protein fractions before and after pronase treatment by extraction with chloroform-methanol (2:1 by volume) as before (7), and the extracted lipid assayed for chemotactic activity in the Boyden assay system.

Peptide fractions (apparent mol. wt. of 10,000 to 5,000) obtained from the neutrophil extracts (after 30-min exposure to pronase (3 μg/ml)) or from the acellular pleural exudate were further separated after reduction with mercaptoethanol and delipidation with chloroform-methanol (2:1) on polyacrylamide gel electrophoresis with and without sodium dodecyl sulfate, as before (2), and by high-voltage paper electrophoresis on a Camag Instrument, as before (7). Several peptides were shown to be present in each fraction, and after elution from the gels or the paper were found to be chemotactically active. Since so many active peptides were present in each fraction, they have not yet been fully resolved.

RESULTS AND DISCUSSION

Injection of kaolin (800 μg) or the sulfated polysaccharide, carrageenan (200 μg) into rat pleura results in accumulation of fluid and cells, both of which contain chemotactic agents for human neutrophils, when assayed both *in vivo* and *in vitro* (Fig. 1).

The relative activity in the exudates when expressed on a volume of fluid basis, fluctuates with time, apparently because of the disproportionate rates of ingress of fluid and cells into the pleural space (11). Since neither kaolin

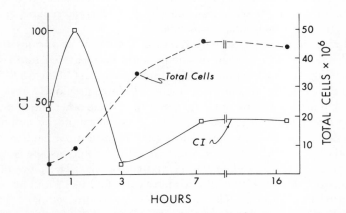

FIG. 1. Total cells were counted by hemocytometer in rat pleural exudate at various times following injection of 200 μg carrageenan ●------●. Chemotactic index (CI) was estimated in Boyden Chambers using 10% of the total cellular exudate (400 X g for 15 min) present in each rat □———□.

TABLE 1. *Isolation of chemotactic factors from rat pleural exudate*

| | % of Chemotactic activity | | | |
| | Isolated lipids | | Isolated peptides | |
Time after injection (hr)	HETE fraction	Oxidized squalene fraction	Control	Pronase treated
0	0	6 ± 2	94	0
1	0	11 ± 3	89	ND
3	0	8 ± 2	92	10
7	0	3 ± 2	97	ND
10	0	0 ± 1	100	0

ND = not done.
Note: Pleural fluid was obtained after injection of carrageenan, 200 µg/per rat, at at the times indicated. The lipid and peptide fractions (5,000 to 10,000 mol. wt.) were isolated and tested for chemotactic activity (see Methods). All activity was expressed as relative amounts per rat. The peptide fraction was treated with pronase, 3µg/ml for 6 hr at 25°C before assaying.

nor carrageenan possesses any chemotactic activity in the *in vitro* assay, an effort was made to characterize the chemotactic agent that was generated in the pleural space after injection and to identify its cellular source. Since both fluid and cells (which are 25% neutrophils) and a chemotactic agent are present in rat pleura at 0 time (Fig. 1 and Table 1), it is probable that carrageenan and kaolin act by stimulation of an already active process. As indicated in Table 1, both the lipid and the pronase-sensitive chemotactic factors are present in normal rat pleura. The peptide factor accounts for most of the chemotactic factor at all times. These two types of factors showed the same relative activities on neutrophil migration when assayed either in the rat pleural assay or in Boyden chambers, using human neutrophils.

The peptide chemotactic activity found at 0 time or at various times after pleural injection of carrageenan or kaolin could be separated into two classes of peptides (Fig. 2). One fraction contained small peptides (5,000 to 8,000 molecular weight similar to the glycopeptide fraction, isolated previously from phagocytosing human neutrophils by Spilberg et al. (9), and the other fraction contained larger peptides (20,000 to 25,000 mol. wt.). The chemotactic activity of the latter fraction could be increased slightly (2X) by brief treatment with pronase or chymotrysin but not by trypsin. Similar fractions could also be isolated from soluble extracts of these exudate cells (91% neutrophils, Fig. 2), but the activity of the larger cellular fraction could be increased 6-fold to 10-fold by brief treatment with pronase (Fig. 3). The small-molecular-weight cellular fraction, like the cellular soluble fraction, could not be activated by brief treatment with pronase. Both peptide fractions could be destroyed by prolonged digestion with pronase or chymotrysin (Table 1).

Initially, in the course of the experimental pleural inflammation, a small

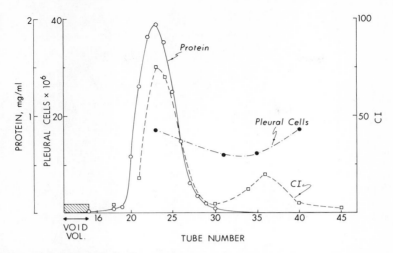

FIG. 2. Soluble exudate (after centrifugation at 400 X g for 15 min) obtained from rat pleura 7 hr after injection of 200 μg carrageenan was dialyzed, freeze-dried, and eluted from a Sephadex G-50 column (previously calibrated) with isotonic NaCl. Protein was estimated, using 260 and 280 mμ absorption o——o, relative chemotactic index was estimated for each fraction, using 0.3 ml of each eluate in Boyden chambers □····□, and total cells (Δ) counted in pleural exudates 3 hr after injection of 0.3 ml of each eluate. Total cells at 0 time was subtracted. Four rats were used for each experimental point with good agreement (10 to 15% variation) obtained in each group of rats.

amount of the chemotactic activity present was found to be associated with a nonacidic lipid fraction, which was shown to contain several unidentified periodic acid-Schiff positive (4) hydrocarbons, all of which, upon catalytic reduction with paladium and H_2, were shown by GC analysis to have been converted into a single hydrocarbon of 30 carbons containing no reactive carboxyl, acidic, aldehydic, or hydroxyl groups. (Potential carbonyl groups were reduced to hydroxyls using sodium borohydride before silylation.) These data, therefore, indicate that all of the above TLC bands represented several oxidized forms, possibly endoperoxides, of squalene. Considerable amounts of unoxidized squalene (11 to 16% of total ether-extractable lipid) was also present in all pleural washes. This squalene would not be separated from commercial squalence on three different TLC systems, including argentation TLC. Upon catalytic reduction with H_2 and palladium, the isolated squalene yielded one peak on GC (see Methods) which could not be separated, when different temperature programs were used, from authentic squalene. No wax or sterol was present in the squalene isolated from the TLC plates, as indicated by the fact that no fatty acid esters were seen by GC after transmethylation, nor were any sterol peaks seen after transmethylation and silylation (see Methods). No other chemotactic lipids were present and specifically no HETE could be detected either chemically or by chemotactic assay in any of the pleural exudates. This failure to observe chemo-

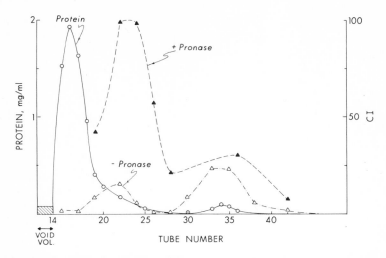

FIG. 3. Cell extracts (91% neutrophiles) isolated from rat pleural exudate 7 hr after injection of 200 µg carrageenan were prepared after dialysis and drying, and eluted from a Sephadex G-50 column as in Fig. 2. Protein o——o and the chemotactic index ▲---▲ were measured as in Fig. 2, using 0.3 ml of each fraction (each fraction contained 2.6 ml). In addition, 3 µg of pronase was present along with each fraction on the agent side during the 140-min assay.

tactic activity was unexpected, since we had previously shown that many unsaturated organic anions, such as arachidonic acid, prostaglandin A_2, prostaglandin E_2, etc., could be converted by nonenzymatic oxidation into many other unknown anions possessing considerable amounts of chemotactic activity (8). It is known that prostaglandin E_2 accumulates in these pleural exudates (11). Although many unidentified lipid anions were present in these exudates, none possessed any chemotactic activity when assayed either in rat pleura or in Boyden chambers.

SUMMARY AND CONCLUSIONS

These data therefore indicate that the major signal for migration of neutrophils into rat pleura following installation of foreign substances are peptides of varying molecular weights which are synthesized, at least in part, by rat neutrophils. These may be the same peptides previously observed which are produced by neutrophils during phagocytosis (9). Chemotactic peptides can also be produced by partial digestion of neutrophil extracts with pronase or chymotrysin, but not by trypsin. None of the active peptides found in the pleural exudate nor the ones produced from neutrophil extracts have been characterized. But it appears by analysis by gel filtration and gel electrophoresis (unpublished data) that many different peptides possessing chemotactic activity are produced. None of these peptides contained any extractable lipid with chemotactic activity, nor could the chemotactic fatty acid (HETE) which is synthesized by blood platelets (10) be detected at any time in these exudates. Moreover, no anionic lipids, which have been shown to possess chemotactic activity (8), were present.

Oxidized hydrocarbons with minimal chemotactic activity were found in the pleural extracts. These hydrocarbons appeared to be various oxidation products of squalene. Squalene was present as a major lipid in these exudates, both before and after stimulation of the inflammatory process.

These data strongly support the view that peptides are the major *in vivo* chemotactic mediators and that these active peptides can be produced in the absence of serum or complement by stimulated neutrophils (9). Active peptides can also be produced experimentally by incomplete digestion of soluble neutrophil extracts with pronase or chymotrypsin.

The role *in vivo* of lipid chemotaxins, especially HETE, remains obscure. HETE will promote the neutrophil inflammatory process in rat pleura (unpublished observation) and it may also be the cause of the sterile neutrophil abscesses seen in psoriasis (3). Since there is no evidence that cells, other than platelets, synthesize HETE and since platelets are not migratory, i.e., they remain within the vascular bed except with hemorrhage, it is unlikely that this platelet system is involved in extravascular inflammation, such as the experimental pleural system. It is more likely that the platelet system is primarily involved in the control of migration of inflammatory cells into the vascular bed, possibly from bone marrow or from other extravascular areas. Studies to assess the role of HETE and the other known lipid chemotaxins in leukocytosis are in progress.

REFERENCES

1. Becker, E. L., Showell, H. J., Henson, P. M., and Hsu, L. S. (1974): The ability of chemotactic factors to induce lysosomal enzyme release. *J. Immunol.,* 112:2047–2054.
2. Bhattacharyya, S. N., and Lynn, W. S. (1977): Structural studies on the oligosaccharides of a glycoprotein isolated from alveoli of patients with alveolar proteinosis. *J. Biol. Chem.,* 252:1172–1180.
3. Hammarström, S., et al. (1975): Increased concentrations of non-esterified arachidonic acid, 12-L-hydroxy-5,8,10,14-eicosatetraenoic acid, prostaglandin E_2 and prostaglandin $F_2\alpha$ in epidermis of psoriasis. *Proc. Nat'l. Acad. Sci. U.S.A.,* 72:5130–5134.
4. Kates, M. (1972): *Techniques of Lipidology in Lab. Techniques in Biochemistry and Molecular Biology,* edited by T. S. Work and E. Work, pp. 436–441. North-Holland Publishing Co., Amsterdam.
5. Kay, A. B., Pepper, D. S., and McKenzie, R. (1974): The identification of fibrinopeptide B as a chemotactic agent derived from human fibrinogen. *Br. J. Haematol.* 27:669–677.
6. Nugteren, D. H. (1975): Arachidonate lipoxygenase in blood platelets. *Biochim. Biophys. Acta,* 380:299–307.
7. Sahu, S., DiAugustine, R., and Lynn, W. S. (1976): Lipids found in pulmonary lavage of patients with alveolar proteinosis and in rabbit lung lamellar organelles. *Am. Rev. Resp. Dis.,* 114:177–185.
8. Sahu, S., and Lynn, W. S. (1977): Production of chemotactic lipid anions by non-enymatic oxidation and their occurrence in bacterial growth media. *Inflammation,* 2:47–54.
9. Spilberg, I., Gallacher, A., Mehta, J. M., and Manden, B. (1976): Urate crystal-induced chemotactic factor. *J. Clin. Invest.,* 58:815–819.

10. Turner, S., Tainer, J., and Lynn, W. S. (1975): Biogenesis of chemotactic molecules by the arachidonate lipoxygenase system of platelets. *Nature,* 257:680–681.
11. Vinegar, R., Traux, J. F., Selph, J. L., Welch, R. M., and White, H. L. (1976): The effect of caffeine on the pharmacology of aspirin and phenacetin. *Fed. Proc.,* 35:775.
12. Ward, P. A., and Newman, L. J. (1969): A neutrophil chemotactic factor from human C5. *J. Immunol.,* 102:93–99.

Leukocyte Chemotaxis, edited by John I. Gallin
and Paul G. Quie. Raven Press, New York
© 1978.

Clinical Manifestations of Disorders of Neutrophil Chemotaxis

Paul G. Quie and K. Lynn Cates

*Department of Pediatrics, University of Minnesota School of Medicine,
Minneapolis, Minnesota 55455*

The prompt accumulation of neutrophils in tissues invaded by bacteria is essential for suppression of bacterial growth and prevention of established infections. The experimental observations of Miles et al. (32) established that absence of neutrophils from tissue for as short a time as 2 to 4 hr enhances the infectivity of inoculated bacteria by as much as 100,000-fold. Therefore, rapid migration into tissues where surface defenses have been breached is a neutrophil function essential for host antibacterial defense. These experimental observations have been supported recently by several clinical observations which suggest an association between susceptibility to infection and depressed neutrophil chemotactic responsiveness in patients with recurrent severe infections (35). The clinical manifestations of patients with abnormal neutrophil chemotaxis will be described in this chapter and clinical situations with abnormal neutrophil chemotactic responsiveness will be reviewed.

Patients with granulocyte disorders have frequent infections, and the clinical manifestations are quite similar whether the disorder is insufficient numbers of cells or cell dysfunction. Infections tend to be prolonged, there is poor response to appropriate antibiotics, and recurrent infections are the rule. Patients with neutrophil chemotactic dysfunction or with other neutrophil dysfunction may be infected by any of a wide spectrum of microorganisms. *Staphylococcus aureus* is the most frequent bacterial species identified in infectious lesions in these patients, but gram-negative enteric bacteria and fungal species as well as *Staphylococcus epidermidis* are frequently responsible for recurrent and prolonged disease. Infections most typically involve soft tissues including skin, lungs, liver, and kidney. Patients with neutrophil dysfunction often have abscesses of the skin and subcutaneous tissue with regional adenopathy and adenitis. Pneumonia occurs frequently and deep tissue abscesses do occur but systemic bacterial disease is uncommon.

It is possible to contrast the etiologic agents and kinds of infections in patients with phagocytic disorders with those in patients with abnormal immunoglobulin response. Patients with hypogammaglobulinemia, for example, have frequent infections with *Streptococcus pneumoniae, Hemophilus influenzae,* and group A streptococci. Septicemia or meningitis may be recurrent in these patients before specific replacement therapy is applied, whereas septicemia and meningitis are rare in patients with granulocyte dysfunction.

Patients with defective leukocyte chemotaxis have purulent lesions and, indeed, there may be copious fluid in abscesses involving the lungs or subcutaneous tissue in these patients. Established infections occur because of delay in accumulation of leukocytes; however, subsequent systemic spread may be prevented by the eventual migration of neutrophils and monocytic cells.

An impressive list of clinical conditions with abnormal neutrophil chemotactic responsiveness has been described in the past decade. In most of these clinical situations, abnormal chemotaxis has been a result of an "intrinsic" neutrophil dysfunction, i.e., neutrophils function abnormally even when suspended in control serum, and serum from the patients does not compromise the chemotaxis of control neutrophils; however, defective generation of chemotactic factors (primarily complement components) has been described in a small group of patients and certain patients have demonstrated abnormal neutrophil chemotaxis because of circulating inhibitors. Clinical aspects of disorders of chemotaxis in these three categories will be discussed; however, major emphasis will be given to patients with "intrinsic" neutrophil dysfunction.

"INTRINSIC" NEUTROPHIL CHEMOTACTIC DEFECT

Ward and Schlegel described a patient in 1969 with defective leukotaxis and with recurrent infections (62). The neutrophils from this patient were deficient in bactericidal capacity for gram-negative bacteria as well as defective in chemotaxis, and the clinical syndrome described was similar to chronic granulomatous disease. Most patients with chronic granulomatous disease have normal neutrophil chemotaxis, but this patient demonstrated both abnormal chemotaxis and intracellular killing.

In 1971 Miller et al. reported two children with depressed neutrophil mobility and recurrent infection which was termed *Lazy Leukocyte syndrome* (38). These two children were severely neutropenic but had normal myeloid precursors and mature neutrophils in their bone marrow. Their illnesses were characterized by gingivitis and stomatitis and recurrent upper respiratory infections. The only immunologic or inflammatory abnormality identified in these children was defective chemotactic responsiveness and random mobility of their neutrophils. This neutrophil abnormality could not be corrected by fresh normal plasma and there was no lack of chemotactic factors and no inhibitor in the patient's plasma so there was an "intrinsic" neutrophil chemotactic defect. The patients' leukocytes demonstrated normal capacity for phagocytosis and bacterial killing, and abnormal membrane receptors for chemotactic factors was postulated.

Another patient with neutrophils defective in chemotaxis and intracellular killing was described by Singh et al. (51). A 58-year-old male with recurrent severe protracted subcutaneous infections and poor wound-healing was found to have defective neutrophil chemotaxis. Neutrophil abnormalities consistent with chronic granulomatous disease were also found, i.e., defective neutrophil bactericidal capacity and absent nitroblue tetrazolium reduction during phagocytosis. Chromosome analysis revealed deletion of a segment of chromosome 16, suggesting that chromosome 16 may be an important genetic locus for factors influencing leukocyte function.

Still another combination of intrinsic neutrophil functional defects was reported by Steerman et al. (56). These authors described a 4-year-old boy who suffered nine episodes of X-ray documented pneumonia before his second birthday. He also had delayed response to antibiotic therapy and frequent subcutaneous abscesses. The patient's neutrophils did not phagocytize staphylococci, and defective chemotaxis of his neutrophils was demonstrated *in vitro* and *in vivo* with little migration to skin windows. There was a paucity of neutrophils in the skin lesions and markedly delayed wound-healing complicated his clinical course. The patient also had X-linked hypogammaglobulinemia, and severe susceptibility to infections was probably a consequence of defective humoral as well as phagocytic function.

Patients with Chediak-Higashi syndrome have several functional abnormalities of their neutrophils including defective chemotaxis (10). The diagnosis of Chediak-Higashi syndrome is made by identification of leukocytes with giant cytoplasmic lysosomal granules, and the chemotactic defect has been postulated to result from the giant granules preventing the neutrophils from squeezing through small spaces. Recent evidence, however, suggests that there may be a metabolic defect in Chediak-Higashi leukocytes as well, which inhibits neutrophil migration. Boxer et al. found extremely elevated levels of intracellular cyclic adenosine monophosphate (AMP) in leukocytes of a patient with Chediak-Higashi syndrome (6). Ascorbic acid at 200 mg daily brought about a sharp reduction in the levels of leukocyte cyclic-AMP in this patient and there was convincing improvement in the patient's neutrophil chemotactic responsiveness. Ascorbic acid treatment also produced improved neutrophil bacterial killing in this patient.

Patients with defective neutrophil chemotaxis frequently have severe dermatologic abnormalities. Pincus et al. recently described a 4-year-old child with ichthyosis, severe subcutaneous abscesses, and depressed neutrophil chemotaxis (42). The organisms recovered from infected lesions included *S. aureus, Candida albicans,* and multiple gram-negative enteric bacteria. The frequent infections in this patient were probably related to the humoral epidermal barrier since "water-logged" skin was noted at birth, but the severity of the infectious process may have been related to defective neutrophil chemotaxis. The authors noted that only IgM was produced in response to antigenic challenge in this patient, and there was an extremely high level of serum IgE, which suggests that lymphocyte suppressor activity may have been present in this patient. The association of ichthyosis and depressed neutrophil chemotaxis was also noted by Miller et al. (37). The three children he described had persistent *Trichophyton rubrum* infections. One of the children suffered a pelvic abscess, and recurrent mild infections were noted in the other children. The fathers of these children also had chronic dermatitis, which was frequently infected, and depressed neutrophil chemotaxis.

Patients with extremely elevated levels of IgE and recurrent staphylococcal infections have been found to have defective neutrophil chemotaxis (11,23,24,59). In 1973, Clark et al. described an 11-year-old girl with depressed neutrophil chemotaxis and serum IgE levels ranging from 19,000 to 23,000 nanograms per milliliter. She had developed pustular dermatitis at 2 weeks of age and staphylococcal pneumonia at ages 3, 6, 7, and 9 years. Frequent subcutaneous abscesses and lymph node abscesses required surgical drainage. The patient also had monilial mouth lesions and immunologic abnormalities characteristic of the mucocutaneous candidiasis syndrome, i.e., a negative skin test and lack of *in vitro* lymphocyte responsiveness to Candida antigen (11).

In 1974, Harry Hill and I described three children, aged 18 months to 2 years, with depressed neutrophil chemotaxis, extremely elevated serum IgE, eczema, and recurrent staphylococcal abscesses (24). The age of onset and the skin disease were similar to those of the patient described by Clark et al. (11). Eczema developed within 2 months of age and abscesses requiring surgical drainage were present by 6 months of age. The children had extensive weeping dermatitis, with particularly extensive involvement of the face and scalp. Staphylococci and group A streptococci were frequently recovered from infected lesions. In addition to cellulitis and subcutaneous abscesses, staphylococcal pneumonia occurred in one child and a deep staphylococcal abscess of the gluteus muscle in another child. Candida lesions were not observed in these children, and all studies of humoral immune responses, lymphocyte response, and neutrophil phagocytic and bactericidal activities were normal.

Van Scoy et al. described a mother and daughter with extremely elevated serum IgE levels, eczema, and severe staphylococcal abscesses involving the lungs, retropharyngeal space and, in the mother, recurrent breast abscesses (59). A persistent Candida infection of the mouth and intertriginous areas of the body was also present. The daughter [patient No. 2 in report (59) of Van Scoy et al.] had recurrent staphylococcal lesions requiring incision and drainage during her first 18 months of life. A large staphylococcal lung abscess developed with only insidious respiratory symptoms. *S. aureus* was cultured from material obtained when the abscess was surgically drained and, after prolonged antimicrobial therapy, there was complete recovery (Fig. 1). This report and the report by Miller et al. (37) are evidence for the familial nature of some clinical conditions associated with defective chemotaxis.

Hill and our colleagues in Seattle studied neutrophil chemotactic function and measured serum IgE levels in four patients with Job's syndrome (23). This syndrome is characterized by recurrent severe staphylococcal abscesses and suppurative lymphadenitis without the usual concomitants of inflammation, redness, heat, and pain. A 16-year-old patient with Job's syndrome is shown in Fig. 2. This patient was 2 years old when treated by the author for a large "cold" abscess due to *S. aureus* involving the forehead. She has received nearly continu-

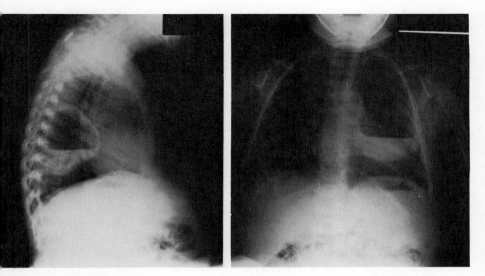

FIG. 1. Anterior and lateral chest X-ray of patient No. 2 described by Van Scoy et al. (59). The lesion shown developed after publication of the article describing findings in this patient.

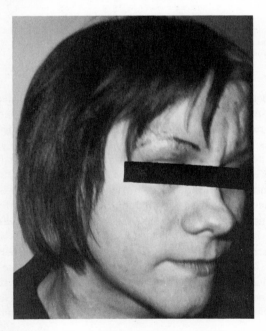

FIG. 2. A 16-year-old girl with Job's syndrome. There are numerous scars from staphylococcal lesions requiring surgical drainage. Although not appreciated from this semiprofile view, the patient has charactistic "broad" nasal bridge and features described in other patients with Job's syndrome. She has red hair.

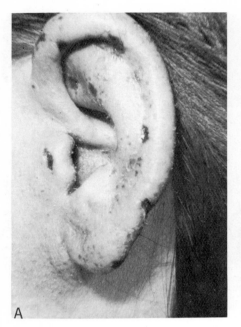 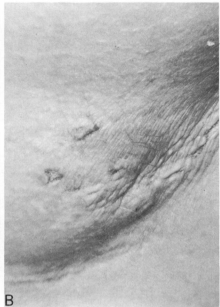

FIG. 3.A: Eczematoid lesions involving the skin of the external ear of the 16-year-old patient with Job's syndrome shown in Fig. 2. **B:** Lesions in the axillae of patient with Job's syndrome. Candida were grown from culture of these lesions.

ous antistaphylococcal therapy for the past 14 years and infections have been infrequent and superficial. Eczematoid lesions of her skin persist as shown in Fig. 3. She has recently developed Candida lesions of her mouth and changes in her fingernails typical of chronic Candida infection (Fig. 4).

The patients described with this syndrome have all been females with red hair and with severe atopic dermatitis. The serum IgE levels ranged from 6,000 to 19,500 IU, and a profound defect of neutrophil chemotaxis was present on repeated examination in patients with Job's syndrome. It is interesting to speculate that the clinical manifestation of "cold" abscesses and defective neutrophil chemotaxis may be related to the same circulating factor.

The initial distribution of lesions in patients with the hyperimmunoglobulin E syndrome is similar to that in many patients with atopic dermatitis with normal neutrophil chemotaxis, but the infections are more severe in patients with depressed neutrophil chemotaxis. As shown in Fig. 5, extensive abscess formation of soft tissue does occur, and there may be minimal local signs and symptoms.

There is little correlation between the levels of circulating IgE and leukocyte chemotactic responsiveness. Certain patients with elevated IgE levels may have normal neutrophil chemotaxis, and abnormal neutrophil chemotaxis may be

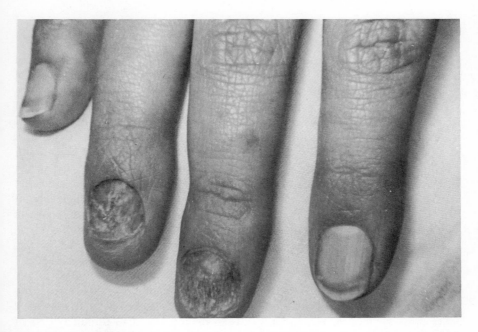

FIG. 4. Appearance of the fingernails of patient with Job's snydrome. These lesions are typically seen in patients with chronic mucocutaneous candidiasis.

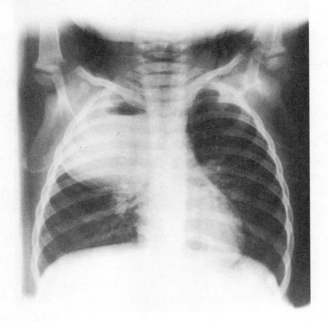

FIG. 5. Anterior view chest X-ray of a 14-month-old patient with extreme hyperimmunoglobulin E syndrome. *Staphylococcus aureus* was recovered from the abscess lesion in the right upper lobe and recovery was complete after prolonged antistaphylococcal therapy. This patient's father has had recurrent severe staphylococcal lesions his entire life.

present in patients with minimal or no elevation of immunoglobulin E levels. In the individual patient, there is a definite correlation between the severity of atopic dermatitis and depression of chemotaxis, however.

Patients with the hyperimmunoglobulin E syndrome are not rare. Dahl et al. (13) described 11 patients with depressed chemotaxis, eosinophilia, and recurrent staphylococcal abscesses, eczema, and hyperimmunoglobulin E. In the same issue of the *Archives of Dermatology,* Rogge and Hanifin described seven additional patients with severe atopic dermatitis and polymorphonuclear and mononuclear leukocyte chemotaxis deficiency (43). Rogge and Hanifin observed that patients with the most severe atopic dermatitis had the highest incidence of infection and the most severe abnormality of leukocyte function. Infections in their patients included *S. aureus,* dermatophytes, and *Herpes hominus* virus. The infections were persistent and frequently recurred, and in several patients depressed chemotaxis could be demonstrated only during severe flares of dermatitis.

We have made similar observations in our patients and it would appear that mechanisms involved in severe atopic dermatitis may also be related to depressed neutrophil chemotaxis. Histamine has been demonstrated to inhibit release of lysosomal enzymes from leukocytes, and these leukocyte enzymes are involved in the inflammatory response (27). Histamine has also been shown to be one of the compounds which can raise intracellular levels of cyclic-AMP and reduce the chemotactic response of human neutrophils. Unfortunately, it has not been possible to measure leukocyte histamine levels directly in these patients to date.

Björkstén and Lundmark reported defective neutrophil chemotaxis and recurrent infection in four siblings with increased levels of circulating IgA (5). All the patients had recurrent pneumonia in addition to recurrent skin infections, otitis media, and staphylococcal abscesses.

The association between depressed neutrophil chemotaxis, hyperimmuno-globulin A, and recurrent infections in the patients reported by Björkstén is especially interesting since it has recently been shown by Van Epps and Williams that polymeric molecules of IgA are cytophilic for human neutrophils and markedly suppress chemotaxis (58). The clinical observations of Björkstén coupled with the experimental observations of Van Epps suggest that the biology of the IgA immunoglobulin response should be studied in patients with neutrophil chemotaxis abnormalities.

In addition to the patients with extremely elevated levels of IgE and with elevated IgA mentioned above, Gallin et al. have described two patients with hypogammaglobulinemia with abnormal neutrophil chemotaxis (20). One of these patients had nodular hyperplasia of the small intestine, the other suffered repeated episodes of pneumonia and otitis media. These patients and the patients discussed earlier by Steerman et al. (56) suggest an association between abnormal granulocyte chemotaxis and abnormality of serum immunoglobulin. It is speculation, but it is extremely provocative, to suggest that exaggerated lymphocyte suppressor activity in certain patients may affect both immunoglobulin production and neutrophil function.

Patients with diabetes mellitus were shown by Mowat and Baum to have mildly depressed neutrophil chemotaxis (40). Chemotaxis in most of the diabetic patients studied was near normal, but many diabetic patients demonstrated depressed neutrophil chemotactic responsiveness that was 2 standard deviations below normal. We have observed a similar depression of chemotactic responsiveness in patients with juvenile-onset diabetes mellitus (25). There was much overlap between the chemotactic responsiveness of diabetic patients and normal controls but when 30 juvenile-onset diabetes mellitus patients were compared with 30 age-matched controls, the difference in chemotaxis was statistically significant. The decreased leukotactic response did not correlate with age of patients, degree of control, serum concentration of glucose, cholesterol, triglycerides or creatinine. We also confirmed the observation of Mowat and Baum (40) that incubation of diabetic leukocytes in 100 units of insulin in a glucose-containing medium improved the cells' responsiveness to a chemotactic stimulant.

The question concerning the role of exogenous insulin or metabolic abnormalities associated with diabetes on leukocyte function has been partially answered by a careful study recently reported by Molenaar et al. (39). These investigators examined 52 first-degree relatives of patients with diabetes. None of the first-degree relatives had diabetes or had ever received exogenous insulin. The chemotactic index was significantly lower in these first-degree relatives than in healthy persons who were not related to diabetics. This study suggests that a cellular membrane defect associated with diabetes also may be associated with abnormal neutrophil chemotactic responsiveness.

We have recently had an opportunity to study the immunologic function of a 3½-year-old white woman with mannosidosis (17). This storage disease results from deficiency of acidic alpha mannosidase activity, and mannose-rich material accumulates in cells including circulating leukocytes. The diagnosis of mannosidosis is made by demonstrating enzyme deficiency in plasma, leukocytes, and skin fibroblasts. Recurrent infections were a major problem in this patient. She had chronic otitis media with marked hearing loss and was hospitalized four times for severe upper respiratory infections before her second birthday. During her third year of life, she was nearly continuously hospitalized with otitis media and pneumonia, and her terminal illness was severe infiltrative lung disease with progressive respiratory failure. Viral cultures revealed adenovirus type 7 from urine, stool, and throat cultures, and from lung tissue obtained at autopsy.

There was a generally depressed immunologic response in this patient. Immunoglobulin levels were low and there was a decreased response of lymphocytes to phytohemagglutinin. The most striking defect was in neutrophil chemotactic responsiveness. There was also delayed phagocytosis of *S. aureus* and *E. coli.*

Normal nitroblue tetrazolium reduction by the patient's neutrophils was evidence that oxidative metabolic responsiveness was normal even though locomotion was abnormal. It is interesting to speculate that abnormal mannose material in this patient may have interfered with leukocyte membrane function or with the process of cell locomotion; however, it cannot be stated with certainty that the patient's systemic adenovirus did not contribute to the demonstrated neutrophil dysfunction.

"TRANSIENT" NEUTROPHIL CHEMOTACTIC DEFICIENCY

There have been several reports which give evidence that neutrophil chemotaxis may be transiently depressed. Anderson et al. found a marked depression of granulocyte chemotaxis and random migration in 35 children with measles (3). There was return of leukotactic function to normal approximately 10 days after onset of the measles rash. There was simultaneous improvement of leukocyte function with resolution of the measles rash and the patient's return to a normal clinical condition.

Hill et al. observed a depression of leukocyte chemotactic responsiveness in four patients with allergic rhinitis and severe staphylococcal furunculosis (26). These patients had normal concentrations of IgE and there was normal chemotaxis when the patients were clinically well. When allergic symptoms appeared, there was depressed neutrophil chemotaxis and a predictable onset of staphylococcal abscesses.

Certain patients who have undergone bone marrow transplantation for leukemia or aplastic anemia have severely depressed neutrophil chemotactic responsiveness (9). Depressed chemotaxis was found in 18 of 34 patients who had received transplants, and these 18 patients were the ones who were undergoing graft vs. host reactions or were receiving antithymocyte globulin. The patients with defective chemotaxis suffered significantly more severe bacterial infections than did patients with normal neutrophil chemotaxis.

McCall and his colleagues studied neutrophil chemotactic responsiveness and other neutrophil functions in a series of 22 patients with severe bacterial infections and a mortality rate of 30% (29). In all these patients, more than 90% of the peripheral leukocytes had toxic granulation (abnormally staining azurophil granules), Döhle bodies (aggregates of rough endoplasmic reticulum), or cytoplasmic vacuoles. All patients had a marked reduction in chemotactic responsiveness. In addition, there was reduction in random migration and in phagocytosis of staphylococci, reflecting a general depression of leukocyte locomotion.

We have studied an equal number of younger patients (mean age 11.5 yr) with less severe bacterial infections and have found that neutrophil chemotaxis is increased rather than depressed (22). In our patients, the bacterial infections responded to appropriate antibiotic therapy, there was no mortality, and, although not thoroughly documented, there was less morphologic abnormality in the peripheral neutrophils. The mean leukotactic index of the patients was more than twice that of age-matched, uninfected controls, and there was return to normal chemotactic response within 7 to 14 days after appropriate antibiotic therapy.

Patients with severe burns (greater than 30% second and third degree) have neutrophil chemotactic defects which persist for as long as several weeks (R. J. Faville and P. G. Quie, *unpublished observations*). As patients are grafted and return to a normal clinical state, there is improvement in neutrophil chemotactic responsiveness.

Depressed chemotactic responsiveness has also been observed in patients with chronic renal failure, especially after prolonged hemodialysis (21). This is not a constant phenomenon in all patients on chronic dialysis but there is a direct correlation between the number of dialysis treatments and the degree of depression of neutrophil chemotactic responsiveness. Patients receiving chronic hemodialysis are unusually susceptible to severe infections, and although there are several predisposing factors such as arteriovenous shunts which provide ready access for bacteria and fungi, defective neutrophil function may contribute to their susceptibility. It is of special interest that neutrophil chemotactic responsiveness returned to normal in three patients after they received kidney transplants.

Delayed chemotactic responsiveness has been reported in children with kwashiorkor (49). Clinically, these children have marked reduction in body weight, apathy, irritability, edema, hepatomegaly, and necrotizing skin lesions. Susceptibility to bacterial, fungal, and viral infections is increased (50), and there is frequently a paucity of leukocytes in lesions despite the presence of pyogenic microorganisms. Schopfer and Douglas have found diminished PMN chemotactic activity at early time intervals (30, 60, and 120 minutes), but a normal number of neutrophils had migrated completely through filters by 180 min incubation. The contribution of this chemotactic abnormality to susceptibility to infection is difficult to assess, since children with severe protein-calorie malnutrition may also have decreased antibody production, decreased cell-mediated immunity, low levels of complement components, and defective intraleukocyte killing of both gram-negative and gram-positive bacteria and of *C. albicans* (47,48,52).

Miller has reported decreased chemotactic responsiveness in newborn infants (33). Not only do neutrophils from newborns fail to migrate normally toward the usual attractants, but their serum fails to generate normal chemotactic activity. The cellular chemotactic defect may be related to decreased newborn PMN membrane deformability (34). Neonatal monocytes also have significantly decreased chemotactic responsiveness (28,41,64).

Other newborn phagocyte function studies, performed under varying experimental conditions, have resulted in conflicting results. Most workers, however, have found normal bacterial ingestion and killing by PMNs in full-term newborns, but both may be decreased in low-birth-weight or stressed infants (12, 18,19,30,65). There is decreased opsonic activity in newborn sera (especially from low-birth-weight infants) related to antibody and complement deficiency

(18,19,30). Abnormal leukocyte locomotion may contribute to the newborns' increased susceptibility to systemic infections; however, there is usually excellent resistance to bacterial invasion in most newborns, as they rapidly acquire a resident microbial flora uneventfully in spite of a generally immature inflammatory response.

DEFICIENCY OF CHEMOTACTIC FACTORS

Defects in the complement system have been described which result in diminished serum chemotactic factor production (46). Day et al. described recurrent infections and lupus erythematosus in two patients with congenital absence of Clr (15). When Gallin studied a Clr-deficient serum, he found that chemotactic activity was generated more slowly than in normal serum but eventually full chemotactic activity was generated (20). No relationship between delayed chemotactic factor generation and susceptibility to infection has been established in patients with dysfunction of the first two complement components; there is, however, an increased incidence of inflammatory disease such as systemic lupus erythematosus and dermatomyositis (46).

A patient with Klinefelter's syndrome, with a history of repeated pyogenic infections and a low serum C3 level, was found to lack serum chemotactic factor activity (1). Activity could be restored by addition of normal serum, but not by purified C3. Another patient with congenital absence of the third component of complement was described by Ballow et al. (4). This patient had serious infections with encapsulated gram-positive and gram-negative bacteria. Infections included otitis, diarrhea, and urinary tract infections. The patient's serum lacked chemotactic, opsonic, and bactericidal activity.

A 19-year-old female patient with C5 deficiency and with lupus erythematosus from age 11 has recently been described by Rosenfeld et al. (44,45). The patient's infections included oral and vaginal moniliasis, infected cutaneous and subcutaneous ulcers, chronically draining sinus tracts, sepsis, and meningitis. A markedly impaired ability to generate chemotactic activity was demonstrated in her serum. Family members heterozygous for C5 deficiency were able to generate normal chemotactic activity. Dysfunctional C5 has also been described in patients with recurrent infections whose sera were incapable of generating normal chemotactic activity (36).

Two patients with C7 deficiency have been reported (7,63). Serum from one of these patients did not generate chemotactic activity normally, but addition of C7 *in vitro* corrected the defect. Serum from the other patient was capable of normal chemotactic activity. Raynaud's phenomenon was noted in the patient with chemotactic deficiency but there was no history of increased susceptibility to infections.

From these clinical observations, it is possible to generalize that the most critical complement components in terms of chemotactic factor function are C3 and C5. A definite relationship between susceptibility to infection and deficiency of other complement components is difficult to establish; however, absence of other complement components may be associated with other diseases.

INHIBITORS OF CHEMOTAXIS

The clinical presentation of patients with circulating inhibitors of leukotaxis is similar to that of patients with intrinsically defective leukocyte mobility. Smith et al. describe a 7-year-old boy with recurrent pyoderma, otitis media, pneumonia, and purulent rhinitis from the age of one year (53). His neutrophils did not respond normally in chemotaxis assays when incubated with autologous serum, but migrated normally when washed and suspended in normal serum. In addition, there was depressed migration of neutrophils to skin windows. The inhibitor of leukotaxis was not identified in this patient, but it is of interest that he had extremely elevated levels of circulating IgA and IgG and a high titer of rheumatoid factor.

Soriano et al. described an 8-month-old child with cytomegalovirus infection, recurrent pneumonia, persisting pulmonary infiltrates, and staphylococcal skin lesions (55). The patient's neutrophils had markedly depressed chemotactic responsiveness when suspended in autologous plasma but responded normally when suspended in control plasma, thus demonstrating an inhibitor of leukotaxis. Both Smith et al. and Soriano et al. demonstrated that the inhibitory activity in their patients' plasma could be neutralized by normal plasma. When plasma was given to the patients, there was striking clinical improvement. Furthermore, neutrophils appeared in skin window chambers or vesicles after plasma therapy. The authors concluded that the patients lacked a normal antagonist of their respective serum inhibitors of chemotaxis.

Van Epps et al. noted an association between the presence of acute illnesses with leukocytosis, negative skin test response to recall antigens, and a serum chemotaxis inhibitor (57). Sixteen patients demonstrated this combination of clinical and laboratory findings during illness, with return of normal chemotactic activity and skin test responsiveness when clinical improvement occurred. The investigators used several techniques for separating serum fractions and identified serum inhibitor activity in fractions which had characteristics associated with immunoglobulin, especially with IgA.

Davis et al. have also described the association of elevated IgA, depressed neutrophil chemotaxis and recurrent infection (14). The patient was a 10-year-old black female with onset of eczema in the early months of life. Recurrent staphylococcal abscesses, gonococcal conjunctivitis, and repeated episodes of bronchopneumonia led to several surgical procedures including removal of a bronchiectatic lung segment at 2 years of age. The patient's IgG was 1.7 g/ml, IgM and IgE levels were normal, and IgA was markedly elevated at 1.2 g/ml. An IgA- and IgM-containing cryoglobulin was found in the patient's serum, and when separated this serum fraction inhibited chemotaxis of the patient's neutrophils as well as chemotaxis of neutrophils from 8 of 9 controls.

There was no inhibition of chemotactic factors by the patient's serum and the patient's neutrophil chemotaxis was restored by incubation in control plasma suggesting a cell-directed inhibitor of chemotaxis.

Cates et al. have studied a plasma inhibitor of chemotaxis in a patient with chronic mucocutaneous candidiasis (8). The patient's neutrophils had markedly depressed chemotactic responsiveness when suspended in her own plasma but were normal in control plasma. Normal neutrophils were also inhibited by the patient's plasma. Partial characterization of this inhibitor revealed that it had several properties in common with IgG, including the formation of identical precipitin arcs when immunoelectrophoresis of the plasma fraction containing the inhibitor was performed against anti-total-human-serum and anti-human IgG. Sucrose density ultracentrifugation was not done.

Altman et al. studied seven children with Wiskott-Aldrich syndrome and found that plasma from these patients inhibited chemotaxis of normal monocytes (2). Lymphocytes from patients with Wiskott-Aldrich syndrome produce much more lymphocyte-derived chemotactic factor than normal lymphocytes, and normal monocytes incubated in lymphocyte-derived chemotactic factor did not demonstrate normal locomotion. It is postulated that leukocytes in patients with Wiskott-Aldrich syndrome are constantly exposed to high levels of the lymphocyte-derived chemotactic factor and are "deactivated" and for that reason less able to respond to a chemotactic stimulus. There is also defective regulation of immune responsiveness in Wiskott-Aldrich syndrome which may contribute to severe eczema and recurrent severe infections.

The inhibitors of chemotaxis described above acted by directly affecting the neutrophils. Other inhibitors depress chemotaxis by inactivating circulating chemotactic factors. These inhibitors may be naturally occurring plasma proteins or products of an inflammatory response. It may be that chemotaxis is decreased only when these substances are present in high concentrations. For example, patients with Hodgkin's disease have 3 to 5 times higher levels of circulating chemotactic factor inhibitor with properties similar to inhibitors found in control serum (60). Patients with lepromatous leprosy and sarcoidosis also have increased levels of circulating chemotactic factor inactivator with similar properties to that in patients with Hodgkin's disease (31,61). Patients with Hodgkin's disease, leprosy, and sarcoidosis usually are incapable of developing delayed skin hypersensitivity responses that may be related to circulating inhibitors which prevent migration of leukocytes to inflammatory sites. Clinically, these patients are highly susceptible to bacterial, viral, and fungal infections, and it is probable that the combination of multiple intrinsic leukocyte defects as well as excessive circulating inflammatory inhibitors contribute to this increased susceptibility.

Patients with alcoholism and cirrhosis have a greatly increased susceptibility to serious bacterial infections, and DeMeo and Anderson identified serum inhibition of chemotaxis in patients with cirrhosis (16). Evidence for chemotactic factor inactivator activity in sera from patients with cirrhosis was the finding that their serum inhibited chemotactic activity in activated serum and also inhibited the chemotactic attractive properties of casein. The patients were not infected when their neutrophils and serum were studied, but there were serious infections in 7 of the 22 patients shortly after the studies were performed. Three of the patients had gram-negative bacterial sepsis, and others had peritonitis, meningitis, and *S. pneumoniae* pneumonia.

CONCLUSION

A comparison of capacity for neutrophil chemotactic responsiveness in patients with increased infections has been the subject of this chapter. One is impressed with the frequent association between abnormality of chemotaxis and unusual susceptibility to infection. This association is extremely interesting and it is tempting to speculate that there is a relationship between cellular dysfunction and disease. This relationship is far from proven by the largely *in vitro* observations that have been reviewed, and a great deal of research must be done before the role of leukocyte chemotaxis in host defense against microbial disease can be placed in proper perspective.

It is exciting to anticipate that practical measures for treatment or regulation of chemotaxis may be at hand once physiologic regulation mechanisms are known and the contribution of chemotaxis to host defense is better understood.

ACKNOWLEDGMENTS

This work was supported in part by United States Public Health Service Grants AI 08821, AI 06931 and AI 12402. Dr. Paul G. Quie is the American Legion Memorial Heart Research Professor. Dr. K. Lynn Cates is an N.I.H. National Research Service Awardee (AI 05478).

REFERENCES

1. Alper, C. A., Abramson, N., Johnston, R. B., Jr., Jandl, J. H., and Rosen, F. S. (1970): Increased susceptibility to infection associated with abnormalities of complement-mediated functions and of the third component of complement (C3). *N. Engl. J. Med.,* 282:349–358.
2. Altman, L. C., Snyderman, R., and Blaese, R. M. (1974): Abnormalities of chemotactic lymphokine synthesis and mononuclear leukocyte chemotaxis in Wiskott-Aldrich syndrome. *J. Clin. Invest.,* 54:486–493.
3. Anderson, R., Sher, R., Rabson, A. R., and Koornhof, H. J. (1974): Defective chemotaxis in measles patients. *S. Afr. Med. J.,* 48:1819–1820.
4. Ballow, M., Shira, J. E., Harden, L., Yank, S. Y., and Day, N. K. (1975): Complete absence of the third component of complement in man. *J. Clin. Invest.,* 56:703–710.
5. Björkstén, B., and Lundmark, K. M. (1976): Recurrent bacterial infections in four siblings with neutropenia, eosinophilia, hyperimmunoglobulinemia A, and defective neutrophil chemotaxis. *J. Infect. Dis.,* 133:63–71.
6. Boxer, L. A., Watanabe, A. M., Rister, M., Besch, H. R., Jr., Allen, J., and Baehner, R. L. (1976): Correction of leukocyte function in Chediak-Higashi syndrome by ascorbate. *N. Engl. J. Med.,* 295:1041–1045.
7. Boyer, J. T., Gall, E. P., Norman, M. E., Nilsson, U. R., and Zimmerman, T. S. (1975): Hereditary deficiency of the seventh component of complement. *J. Clin. Invest.,* 56:905–913.

8. Cates, K. L., Grady, P. G., Shapira, E., and Davis, A. T. (1977): Inhibition of polymorphonuclear leukocyte chemotaxis by serum from a patient with chronic mucocutaneous candidiasis. Submitted for publication.
9. Clark, R. A., Johnson, F. L., Klebanoff, S. J., and Thomas, E. D. (1976): Defective neutrophil chemotaxis in bone marrow transplant patients. *J. Clin. Invest.,* 58:22–31.
10. Clark, R. A., and Kimball, H. R. (1971): Defective granulocyte chemotaxis in the Chediak-Higashi syndrome. *J. Clin. Invest.,* 50:2645–2652.
11. Clark, R. A., Root, R. K., Kimball, H. R., and Kirkpatrick, C. H. (1973): Defective neutrophil chemotaxis and cellular immunity in a child with recurrent infections. *Ann. Intern. Med.,* 78:515–519.
12. Coen, R., Grush, O., and Kauder, E. (1969): Studies of bactericidal activity and metabolism of the leukocyte in full-term neonates. *J. Pediatr.,* 75:400–406.
13. Dahl, M. V., Greene, W. H., Jr., and Quie, P. G. (1976): Infection, dermatitis, increased IgE, and impaired neutrophil chemotaxis. *Arch. Dermatol.,* 112:1387–1390.
14. Davis, A. T., Grady, P. G., Shapira, E., and Pachman, L. M. (1977): Polymorphonuclear leukocyte chemotactic inhibition associated with a cryoglobulin. *J. Pediatr.* 90:225–229.
15. Day, N. K., Geiger, H., Stroud, R., DeBracco, M., Mancado, B., Windhorst, D., and Good, R. A. (1972): Clr deficiency: An inborn error associated with cutaneous and renal disease. *J. Clin. Invest.,* 51:1102–1108.
16. DeMeo, A. N., and Anderson, B. R. (1972): Defective chemotaxis associated with a serum inhibitor in cirrhotic patients. *N. Engl. J. Med.,* 286:735–740.
17. Desnick, R. J., Sharp, H. L., Grabowski, G. A., Brunning, R. D., Quie, P. G., Sung, J. H., Gorlin, R. J., and Ikonne, J. U. (1976): Mannosidosis: clinical, morphologic, immunologic, and biochemical studies. *Pediatr. Res.,* 10:985–996.
18. Dossett, J. H., Williams, R. C., Jr., and Quie, P. G. (1969): Studies on interaction of bacteria, serum factors and polymorphonuclear leukocytes in mothers and newborns. *Pediatrics,* 44:49–57.
19. Forman, M. L., and Stiehm, E. R. (1969): Impaired opsonic activity but normal phagocytosis in low birth weight infants. *N. Engl. J. Med.,* 281:926–931.
20. Gallin, J. I. (1975): Abnormal chemotaxis: Cellular and humoral components. In: *The Phagocytic Cell in Host Resistance,* edited by J. A. Bellanti and D. H. Dayton, pp. 227–248. Raven Press, New York.
21. Greene, W. H., Ray, C., Mauer, S. M., and Quie, P. G. (1976): The effect of hemodialysis on neutrophil chemotactic responsiveness. *J. Lab. Clin. Med.* 88:971–974.
22. Hill, H. R., Gerrard, J. M., Hogan, N. A., and Quie, P. G. (1974): Hyperactivity of neutrophil leukotactic responses during active bacterial infection. *J. Clin. Invest.,* 53:996–1002.
23. Hill, H. R., Ochs, H. D., Quie, P. G., Pabst, H. F., Klebanoff, S. J., and Wedgwood, R. J. (1974): Defect in neutrophil granulocyte chemotaxis in Job's syndrome of recurrent "cold" staphylococcal abscesses. *Lancet,* 2:617–619.
24. Hill, H. R., and Quie, P. G. (1974): Raised serum IgE levels and defective neutrophil chemotaxis in three children with eczema and recurrent bacterial infections. *Lancet* 1:183–187.
25. Hill, H. R., Sauls, H. S., Dettloff, J. L., and Quie, P. G. (1974): Impaired leukotactic responsiveness in patients with juvenile diabetes mellitus. *Clin. Immunol. Immunopathol.,* 2:395–403.
26. Hill, H. R., Williams, P. G., Krueger, G. G., and Janis, B. (1976): Recurrent staphylococcal abscesses associated with defective neutrophil chemotaxis and allergic rhinitis. *Ann. Intern. Med.,* 85:39–43.
27. Kelly, M. T., and White, A. (1973): Histamine release induced by human leukocyte lysates. *J. Clin. Invest.,* 52:1834–1840.
28. Klein, R. B., Rich, K. C., Biberstein, M., and Stiehm, E. R. (1976): Defective mononuclear and neutrophilic phagocyte chemotaxis in the newborn. *Clin. Res.,* 24:180A.
29. McCall, C. E., Caves, J., Cooper, R., and DeChatelet, L. (1971): Functional characteristics of human toxic neutrophils. *J. Infect. Dis.,* 124:68–75.
30. McCracken, G. H., Jr., and Eichenwald, H. F. (1971): Leukocyte function and the development of opsonic and complement activity in the neonate. *Am. J. Dis. Child.,* 121:120–126.
31. Maderazo, E. G., Ward, P. A., Woronick, C. L., Kubik, J., and DeGraff, A. C., Jr. (1976): Leukotactic dysfunction in sarcoidosis. *Ann. Intern. Med.,* 84:414–419.
32. Miles, A. A., Miles, E. M., and Burke, J. (1957): The value and duration of defense reactions of the skin to the primary lodgement of bacteria. *Br. J. Exp. Pathol.,* 38:79–96.

33. Miller, M. E. (1971): Chemotactic function in the human neonate: Humoral and cellular aspects. *Pediatr. Res.,* 5:487–492.
34. Miller,.M. E. (1975): Developmental maturation of human neutrophil motility and its relationship to membrane deformability. In: *The Phagocytic Cell in Host Resistance,* edited by J. A. Bellanti and D. H. Dayton, pp. 295–307. Raven Press, New York.
35. Miller, M. E. (1975): Pathology of chemotaxis and random mobility. *Semin. Hematol.,* 12:59–82.
36. Miller, M. E., and Nilsson, U. F. (1970): A familial deficiency of the phagocytosis-enhancing activity of serum related to dysfunction of the fifth component of complement (C5). *N. Engl. J. Med.,* 282:354–358.
37. Miller, M. E., Norman, M. E., Koblenzer, P. J., and Schonauer, T. (1973): A new familial defect of neutrophil movement. *J. Lab. Clin. Med.,* 82:1–8.
38. Miller, M. E., Oski, F. A., and Harris, M. B. (1971): Lazy-leucocyte syndrome: A new disorder of neutrophil function. *Lancet* 1:665–669.
39. Molenaar, D. M., Palumbo, P. J., Wilson, W. R., and Ritts, R. E., Jr. (1976): Leukocyte chemotaxis in diabetic patients with their nondiabetic first-degree relatives. *Diabetes* 25(Suppl. 2):880–883.
40. Mowat, A. G., and Baum, J. (1971): Chemotaxis of polymorphonuclear leukocytes from patients with diabetes mellitus. *N. Engl. J. Med.,* 284:621–627.
41. Orlowski, J. P., Siegar, L., and Anthony, B. F. (1976): Bactericidal capacity of monocytes of newborn infants. *J. Pediatr.,* 89:797–801.
42. Pincus, S. H., Thomas, I. T., Clark, R. A., and Ochs, H. D. (1975): Defective neutrophil chemotaxis with variant ichthyosis, hyperimmunoglobulinemia E and recurrent infections. *J. Pediatr.,* 87:908–911.
43. Rogge, J. L., and Hanifin, J. M. (1976): Immunodeficiencies in severe atopic dermatitis: Depressed chemotaxis and lymphocyte transformation. *Arch. Dermatol.,* 112:1391–1396.
44. Rosenfeld, S. I., Baum, J., Steigbigel, R. T., and Leddy, J. P. (1976): Hereditary deficiency of the fifth component of complement in man: II. Biologic properties of C5-deficient human serum. *J. Clin. Invest.,* 57:1635–1643.
45. Rosenfeld, S. I., Kelly, M. E., and Leddy, J. P. (1976): Hereditary deficiency of the fifth component of complement in man: I. Clinical, immunochemical and family studies. *J. Clin. Invest.,* 57:1626–1634.
46. Ruddy, S., Gigli, I., and Austen, K. F. (1972): The complement system of man. *N. Engl. J. Med.,* 287:592–596.
47. Schopfer, K., and Douglas, S. D. (1974): Immunological aspects of infantile protein-calorie malnutrition. *Bull. Schweiz. Akad. Med. Wiss.,* 31:327–334.
48. Schopfer, K., and Douglas, S. D. (1976): *In vitro* studies of lymphocytes from children with kwashiorkor. *Clin. Immunol. Immunopathol.,* 5:21–30.
49. Schopfer, K., and Douglas, S. D. (1976): Neutrophil function in children with kwashiorkor. *J. Lab. Clin. Med.,* 88:450–461.
50. Scrimshaw, N. S., Taylor, C. E., and Gordon, J. E. (1968): Interactions of nutrition and infection. WHO Monogr. Series 57:60–142.
51. Singh, H., Boyd, E., Hutton, M. M., Wilkinson, P. C., Peebles Brown, D. A., and Ferguson-Smith, M. A. (1972): Chromosomal mutation in bone marrow as a cause of acquired granulomatous disease and refractory macrocytic anemia. *Lancet* 1:873–879.
52. Sirisinha, S., Edelman, R., Suskind, R., Charupatana, C., and Olson, R. E. (1973): Complement and C3-proactivator levels in children with protein-calorie malnutrition and effect of dietary treatment. *Lancet* 1:1016–1020.
53. Smith, C. W., Hollers, J. C., Dupree, E., Goldman, A. S., and Lord, R. A. (1972): A serum inhibitor of leukotaxis in a child with recurrent infections. *J. Lab. Clin. Med.,* 79:878–885.
54. Snyderman, R., Pike, M. C., and Altman, L. C. (1975): Abnormalities of leukocyte chemotaxis in human disease. *Ann. N.Y. Acad. Sci.,* 256:386–401.
55. Soriano, R. B., South, M. A., and Goldman, A. S. (1973): Defect of neutrophil motility in a child with recurrent bacterial infections and disseminated cytomegalovirus infection. *J. Pediatr.,* 83:951–958.
56. Steerman, R. L., Snyderman, R., Leikin, S. L., and Colten, H. R. (1971): Intrinsic defect of the polymorphonuclear leukocyte resulting in impaired chemotaxis and phagocytosis. *Clin. Exp. Immunol.,* 9:939–946.

57. Van Epps, D. E., Palmer, D. L., and Williams, R. C., Jr. (1974): Characterization of serum inhibitors of neutrophil chemotaxis associated with anergy. *J. Immunol.*, 113:189–200.
58. Van Epps, D. E., and Williams, R. C., Jr. (1976): Suppression of leukocyte chemotaxis by human IgA myeloma components. *J. Exp. Med.*, 144:1227–1242.
59. Van Scoy, R. E., Hill, H. R., Ritts, R. E., Jr., and Quie, P. G. (1975): Familial neutrophil chemotaxis defect, recurrent bacterial infections, mucocutaneous candidiasis, and hyperimmuno-globulinemia E. *Ann. Intern. Med.*, 82:766–771.
60. Ward, P. A., and Berenberg, J. L. (1974): Defective regulation of inflammatory mediators in Hodgkin's disease. *N. Engl. J. Med.*, 290:76–80.
61. Ward, P. A., Goralnick, S., and Bullock, W. E. (1976): Defective leukotaxis in patients with lepromatous leprosy. *J. Lab. Clin. Med.*, 87:1025–1032.
62. Ward, P. A., and Schlegel, R. J. (1969): Impaired leukotactic responsiveness in a child with recurrent infections. *Lancet* 2:344–347.
63. Wellek, B., and Opferkuch, W. (1975): A case of deficiency of the seventh component of complement in man. *Clin. Exp. Immunol.*, 19:223–235.
64. Weston, W. L., Carson, B. S., Barkin, R. M., and Slater, G. E. (1976): Monocyte-macrophage function in the newborn. *Clin. Res.*, 24:182A.
65. Wright, W. C., Jr., Ank, B. J., Herbert, J., and Stiehm, E. R. (1975): Decreased bactericidal activity of leukocytes of stressed newborn infants. *Pediatrics* 56:579–584.

DISCUSSION

Dr. Gallin: Dr. Quie, your description of the facies of patients with hyperimmunoglobulin E syndrome is a helpful addition to our knowledge of this syndrome. I would like to add that we have identified two black girls with hyper IgE syndrome, with recurrent staphylococcal infections and facial characteristics similar to those described. Therefore, I think we should not limit this syndrome to a single racial group.

I would also like to mention that, in addition to chemotactic defects associated with deficient leukocyte locomotion and deficient chemotactic factor production, we have recently seen a somewhat different clinical syndrome with excessive chemotaxis. These are patients with a disease called erythema elevatum diutinum. A paper is in press in *Medicine* describing these patients. They have a massive accumulation of neutrophils in their skin and as a consequence have local skin destruction. The skin often gets infected. Many of the patients develop local infections which sometimes spread, causing local osteomyelitis. We have been able to show that in three of five of these patients their blister fluid contains very high amounts of chemotactic activity compared to normal blister fluid. Thus, these patients may have a new disorder of "chemotaxis" related to excessive chemotactic factor production.

Dr. Quie: Dr. Gallin, does the blister fluid have high activity before the neutrophils get there?

Dr. Gallin: Yes, blister fluid obtained from uninvolved areas has high chemotactic activity. We can treat this disease with dapsone. We do not understand how the drug works, but it does. When the patients are in remission (by dapsone), the chemotactic activity of their blister fluid returns to normal.

Dr. Hill: About the patients who appear to have hyperimmunoglobulin E syndrome but have normal chemotaxis when they are seen with active infections, a senior medical student working in our lab has shown that neutrophils from these patients, when they are asymptomatic, can be inhibited with ragweed antigen. When concentrations of 1 to 10,000 were used, which would be what is used in a skin test, neutrophil chemotaxis was depressed about 50%. We have not done cross-over studies with the patients' sera and normal cells as yet. It does appear, however, that there is direct or indirect interaction of antigen and neutrophils, or perhaps mediator release, which results in depressed chemotactic function. The findings are very consistent.

Dr. Williams: Which cells do you study?

Dr. Hill: Actually leukocyte-rich plasma is used in these studies.

Dr. Ward: Have you or has anyone measured plasma or urinary histamine to see if there is evidence of increased histamine release in the patients?

Dr. Quie: We postulate that abnormal histamine metabolism is related to this syndrome but unfortunately we still have not found a successful assay to answer that question. Dr. Hill, you may have had better luck.

Dr. Hill: We do not have an assay set for histamine determination either but another laboratory has done assays for us and the histamine levels in three of four patients with the syndrome have been significantly elevated.

Dr. Becker: Dr. Hill, all that you might be demonstrating is that these patients, in addition to eosinophilia, also have basophilia. And I think what you really want to do is to measure the excretion of histamine metabolites.

Dr. Miller: Dr. Quie, there are certainly patients with hyper-IgE, eczema, eosinophilia, in whom we do not find chemotactic defects. What do you suppose might be the possible difference between patients with chemotactic defects and patients without chemotactic defects?

Dr. Quie: Yes, we have seen several patients with the typical syndrome but with normal neutrophil chemotaxis. Dr. Hill may have given us a clue to this with his observation that neutrophils from these patients are inhibited in the presence of reagenic antigens. We have only measured responsiveness of washed cells from these patients and it is highly probable that they are more sensitive to histamine, etc., than normal. In short, these patients may all be part of the same syndrome. In some, the neutrophils are abnormal as is and in others the abnormality can only be identified with a challenge such as ragweed antigen or perhaps staphylococcal antigen.

Dr. Snyderman: We have been very interested in these patients and also in children with severe chronic eczema. Dr. Buckley and I have looked at 14 children with severe chronic eczema and about 7 or 8 children with severe hyper-IgE and undue susceptibility to infection. The only thing I would like to add is that if both monocyte function and neutrophil function are examined, abnormalities are not found in 100% of these individuals. Several children have abnormalities of both polymorphonuclear leukocyte and monocyte responses, and several, especially with the hyper-IgE syndrome and staphlococcal infections, have monocyte abnormalities but they have normal polychemotaxis.

Dr. Altman: I was wondering how frequently patients with the syndrome of hyper-IgE and recurrent infections have other manifestations of atopic disease that is, allergic rhinitis and asthma. Also, do those individuals who have the syndrome, with apparently normal chemotaxis, have defects of either neutrophil chemoluminescence or bactericidal activity?

Dr. Quie: The patients with hyperimmunoglobulin E syndrome have had early-onset eczema, and family members have allergic manifestations. Some of the patients, especially those with Candida infections, have problems with other immune responses, such as depressed lymphocyte functions.

We have searched for defects of other neutrophil functions in these patients and have found normal phagocytosis of bacteria, normal intracellular killing, and normal chemoluminescence. We are excited about some recent preliminary studies which show depressed uptake of radiolabled *C. albicans.* This function may be more related to chemotaxis than bacterial phagocytosis. We are puzzled that neutrophils from a few patients with the hyperimmunoglobulin E syndrome seem to have less neutrophil alkaline phosphatase than neutrophils from patients with "ordinary" infections.

Dr. Stossel: What about the total leukocyte count in patients with the hyperimmunoglobulin E syndrome?

Dr. Quie: These patients usually have leukocytosis and eosinophilia.

Dr. Stossel: What about when the patients are not infected and you can demonstrate the defect?

Dr. Quie: There is, typically, eosinophilia. When the patients are not infected, there appears to be a normal leukocyte response to infection.

Dr. Stossel: If I understand you correctly, the principal infecting organism is *S. aureus.*

Dr. Quie: Correct. Staphylococci first and Candida a distant second.

Dr. Goetzl: We have studied several patients with high serum levels of IgE, eczema, and recurring infections, two of whom were black. In one of these subjects, the predominant clinical manifestation was recurrent corneal infections with staphylococci. In two of the patients, a very profound monocyte chemotactic defect was also found. We could not substantially stimulate either polymorphonuclear leukocyte chemotaxis with ascorbic acid either *in vitro* or after several weeks of oral ascorbic acid therapy at doses of 4 to 6 g per day.

Dr. Gallin: Dr. Quie, have you done HL-A typing on this group of patients?

Dr. Quie: No, we have not and that obviously should be done.

Dr. Hill: I would like to mention a patient that we had with the hyper-IgE syndrome who developed a malignant histiocytic lymphoma with central nervous system involvement, so these patients may also be at an increased risk for developing malignant conditions.

Dr. Wright: I would like to comment about the circumstantial evidence provided by these patients that leukocyte motility and chemotactic responses *in vitro* represent important host defense mechanisms. There was some discussion earlier about various agents that stimulate leukocyte migration responses *in vitro,* and of particular interest to us is the compound levamisole, which Dr. Hill discussed earlier. We have found that this drug stimulates leukocyte migration responses both of monocytes and of neutrophils at a concentration of 0.1 μM, which can be achieved *in vivo*. This stimulation of locomotion is found with cells obtained from hyperimmunoglobulin-E patients and also with cells from normal people but not with cells from Chediak-Higashi patients. Like Dr. Hill, we have been able to show that the abnormal *in vitro* migration responses of cells from patients with hyper-IgE improve after they have taken a 2-day course of levamisole.

Levamisole certainly deserves further attention in these patients, and a clinical trial would be of great interest—particularly in terms of understanding chemotaxis as a host defense mechanism. If one can alter the chemotaxis defect of these patients *in vitro,* and at the same time achieve a clinical benefit *in vivo,* one may conclude that indeed directed leukocyte motility as measured *in vitro* represents an important host defense mechanism *in vivo.*

Dr. Quie: I certainly agree. What is needed in this field now is some method for improving or correcting neutrophil abnormalities. That would certainly be helpful in establishing an association between chemotactic defects and systemic disease.

Dr. Leddy: Dr. Quie what proportion of the patients with the hyper-IgE syndrome have a chemotactic defect initially and then, after antibiotic therapy and drainage, etc., have normal chemotactic function?

Dr. Quie: That may be a fairly typical pattern, Dr. Leddy. It is our general impression that patients that have followed the course of therapy outlined and have been free of infection for a long time demonstrate normal neutrophil chemotactic responsiveness. A recent report (43) describes patients in whom there is a return of neutrophil responsiveness toward normal with control of skin problems and infections.

Dr. Maderazo: Are these defects cells-associated or plasma-associated?

Dr. Quie: The patients I discussed have cell-associated defects. We have not been able to identify an inhibiting factor in their serum or plasma, and neutrophil function is not corrected by incubation in control plasma.

Dr. Jensen: Neutrophils from these patients must have masses of IgE on the surface. Is there loss of IgE during overnight incubation?

Dr. Quie: We have not really looked for cytophilic antibodies on the surface of these cells. I am intrigued by the report of Dr. Dennis Van Epps and Dr. Ralph Williams about IgA chemotaxis inhibitors. Polymeric IgA is very cytophilic for human neutrophils, and depressed chemotaxis has been described in patients with hyper-IgA in a report in the *Journal of Infectious Diseases* in 1976 by Björksén et al. from Sweden (5). These patients reported by Björksén have normal IgE but hyper-IgA. The possibility of a cytophilic material that influences neutrophil responsiveness is a good one.

Dr. Gallin: One other clinical characteristic that I have been struck by is the dental status of these patients. All our patients with chemotactic defects, including patients with Chediak-Higashi syndrome, the hyper-IgE and alpha-mannosidase deficiency, have periodontal disease.

Dr. Quie: Dr. Maderazo has more information on the periodontal disease in these patients than I do. He presented it last fall at the ICAAC meetings in Chicago. It certainly is true that these patients have very serious dental problems, and the findings of severe periodontal disease should be a stimulus for assay of leukocyte function.

Dr. Snyderman: We have looked at IgE myeloma proteins to see if that blocks either neutrophil or monocyte chemotaxis but we have not been able to get inhibitory activity. We are also interested in the possibility that IgA may be contributing to cellular abnormalities.

Leukocyte Chemotaxis, edited by John I. Gallin
and Paul G. Quie. Raven Press, New York
© 1978.

Disorders of Granulocyte Chemotaxis

Robert A. Clark

Department of Medicine, University of Washington, Seattle, Washington 98195

Since the first applications in the late 1960s of the Boyden chamber technique to the study of patients with increased susceptibility to infection, a remarkable proliferation of reports of clinical defects in granulocyte chemotaxis has taken place. The purpose of this chapter is to summarize these accumulated observations. The intention is not to be all inclusive, but rather to emphasize the various types of chemotactic disorders and provide schemes for their classification. Other reviews of this subject have appeared in recent years (57,87,118,134,146).

Methodology is not dealt with here, since the authors of other chapters in this volume have discussed this area extensively and a number of acceptable variations in the *in vitro* chemotactic assays are available. A deficiency in some of the clinical reports has been the failure to provide enough data on variability and number of observations to allow for meaningful statistical analyses. In certain clinical conditions, it is apparent that some affected individuals may have defective chemotaxis while others may be normal; in these instances, rather than lumping all patients together, as has often been done, it seems preferable to consider the two groups separately and to determine whether various clinical or laboratory parameters may distinguish those with abnormal chemotaxis. It is highly desirable to confirm the chemotactic defect by *in vivo* (e.g., skin window) and alternative *in vitro* assays, to assess related granulocyte parameters such as adherence, deformability, and random migration, and to evaluate other biological functions such as phagocytosis, metabolic responses and microbicidal activity. As might be anticipated, the most consistent clinical feature in patients with defective granulocyte chemotaxis is recurrent pyogenic infections.

CLASSIFICATION OF CHEMOTACTIC DISORDERS

The most fundamental division of chemotactic disorders is into cellular defects and chemotactic factor defects. In the former, the patient's leukocytes respond poorly to preformed chemotactic attractants; in the latter, there is a failure in the formation of humoral chemotactic mediators, but the response of the leukocytes remains intact. In addition, a number of examples of defects caused by chemotactic inhibitors have been described; these may be considered as a separate category or, since the inhibitors may be cell-directed or chemotactic factor-directed, they can be included as subheadings under cellular or chemotactic factor defects, respectively. The latter approach is employed in the current discussion. It has become readily apparent that this scheme, while providing an acceptable framework for the classification of chemotactic defects, requires further division in order to deal effectively with the wide variety of disorders described. In the area of chemotactic factor defects, this can be accomplished without great difficulty because a number of these disorders are well-characterized at the molecular level. Unfortunately, this is not true of the cellular defects, and here classification is generally made on the basis of either clinical features or associated leukocytic functional parameters.

CHEMOTACTIC FACTOR DEFECTS

Abnormal generation of chemotactic factors

The outline presented below divides the chemotactic factor defects into those caused by abnormal generation of chemotactic agents derived from the complement system, from the Hageman factor system, and from cells, and those caused by inhibitors of chemotactic factors.

A. Abnormal generation of chemotactic factors
  1. Complement system-derived agents
    a. Complement component deficiencies
       C1r, C4, C2 (rate defect)
       C3, C5
       C3 hypercatabolism
       C5 dysfunction
    b. Immunoglobulin deficiencies
    c. Miscellaneous
       Systemic lupus erythematosus
       Neonates
       Diabetes mellitus
  2. Hageman factor system-derived agents
    a. Hageman factor
    b. Prekallikrein (Fletcher factor)
  3. Cell-derived agents
    a. Chemotactic lymphokine
       Mucocutaneous candidiasis
       Wiskott-Aldrich syndrome
    b. Transfer factor
       Sézary syndrome

B. Inhibitors of chemotactic factors
  1. Excessive chemotactic factor inactivators
    a. Anergic states
       Hodgkin's disease
       Lepromatous leprosy

Sarcoidosis
Other systemic diseases
b. Alcoholic liver disease
2. Deficient chemotactic factor inactivators
a. α_1 antitrypsin deficiency
3. Inhibitors of chemotactic factor generation
a. Uremia
4. Reversible inhibitors of chemotactic factor expression
a. Glomerulonephritis

Complement-derived factors are generally evaluated by measuring chemotactic activity in serum following activation by agents such as immune complexes, endotoxin, or zymosan. The choice of activating agent and the use of more than one agent may be important, since different complement pathways are involved in mediating chemotactic factor generation (33,51). Regardless of which pathway is employed, the bulk of the activity generated in whole serum under the usual experimental conditions is attributable to the low-molecular-weight C5 cleavage product (33,51,119).

Inherited absence of early components of the classic complement pathway is associated with defective generation of chemotactic activity which is manifest as a delayed rate of formation of effector molecules. This was initially demonstrated in the guinea pig model of C4 deficiency (33) and has also been shown in human serum deficient in C2 (51) or C1r (49). We have recently had an opportunity to confirm the findings in the guinea pig model in a patient with inherited absence of C4 (39). The data illustrated in Fig. 1 are typical of the

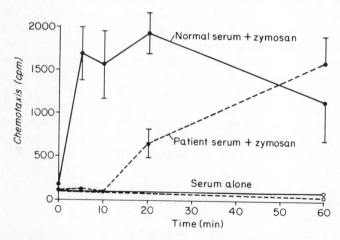

FIG 1. Kinetics of the generation of chemotactic activity in normal and C4-deficient human serum. Serum alone (○) or with the activating agent zymosan (●) was incubated at 37°C for the indicated time, and residual complement was then inactivated by heat (56°C for 30 min). Samples were tested for chemotactic activity in quadruplicate chambers, as described in reference 52. Means ± SE are shown. Solid line, normal serum; dashed line, C4-deficient patient serum.

TABLE 1. *Chemotactic activity generated in C4-deficient human serum*

	Additions		Chemotaxis (cpm)[a]	
Serum (%)	Zymosan	C4[b]	Normal serum	C4-deficient serum
3	—	—	150 ± 18 (21)[c]	79 ± 11 (13)
3	+	—	1,957 ± 201 (16)	106 ± 30 (9)
3	—	+	121 ± 61 (3)	102 ± 22 (3)
3	+	+	1,694 ± 407 (2)	1,244 ± 223 (8)
6	—	—	110 ± 39 (3)	90 ± 15 (2)
6	+	—	1,892 ± 412 (6)	410 ± 281 (6)
50	—	—	76 ± 13 (5)	40 ± 8 (4)
50	+	—	1,305 ± 315 (7)	1,233 ± 204 (9)

[a] Method described in reference 52. The indicated concentrations of serum in gelatin-veronal-buffered saline (GVB) were incubated with additions as shown at 37°C for 60 min and 56°C for 30 min. All samples were then diluted in GVB to the same final serum concentration (3%) and tested in quadruplicate chemotaxis chambers.
[b] Cordis Corp., Miami, Fla; 1000 units/ml of serum.
[c] Mean ± SE, (n) experiments.

findings in all the early component deficiencies. While normal serum shows the very rapid appearance of chemotactic activity within 5 to 10 min, C4-deficient serum shows a prolonged lag period. Nonetheless, the final level of activity is comparable in the two sera. The implication of these studies is that an intact classic pathway is required for an optimal rate of generation of chemotactic activity.

An additional problem which has become apparent in our studies of C4-deficient human serum is a concentration-dependent defect. As the data in Table 1 demonstrate, no chemotactic activity could be generated in C4-deficient serum at a 3% concentration, while normal serum generated substantial activity under the same conditions. At 6% serum, there was partial correction, and at 50% serum, complete correction of this defect. These findings have been duplicated with serum from another C4-deficient patient; this serum was kindly supplied to us by Dr. Georges Hauptmann (60). Also shown in Table 1 is the correction of the abnormality at low serum concentrations by the addition of purified C4. Thus, it appears that an intact classic pathway is required for optimal chemotactic factor generation at limiting concentrations of serum. This concept is supported further by similar results (Table 2) in experiments with serum from a patient with hereditary C2 deficiency and an unusual hereditary angioedema patient with persistently undetectable C4 and C2 (sera generously provided by Dr. John Atkinson and Dr. Michael Frank, respectively). The *in vivo* significance of these observations on the rate-dependent and concentration-dependent serum chemotactic defects in patients with early complement component deficiencies is unknown. Although some of these patients have had a history of frequent infections (2,43,48,102), this is not usually the case. The most common clinical problem encountered in this group is the occurrence of connective

TABLE 2. *Chemotactic activity generated in C2-deficient and hereditary angioedema serum*

Serum (%)	Additions		Chemotaxis (cpm)[a]		
	Zymosan	C2[b]	Normal serum[c]	C2-deficient serum[d]	HAE Serum[d]
3	—	—	150	128	192
3	+	—	1,957	386	165
3	+	+	—	1,910	—
6	+	—	1,892	—	845
50	+	—	1,305	2,135	1,822

[a]Method described in reference 52 and Table 1.
[b]Cordis Corp., Miami, Fla; 1000 units/ml of serum.
[c]Means as in Table 1.
[d]Mean of quadruplicate chambers in a single representative experiment.

tissue disorders such as systemic lupus erythematosus, dermatomyositis, or anaphylactoid purpura (2,39,43,46,60,76,102,123).

Inherited complete absence of C3 has been reported in three patients to date (6,8,16). All have a striking history of severe and recurrent pyogenic infections from early childhood. As might be expected from the pivotal position of C3 in the complement sequence, a variety of functional abnormalities have been detected in C3-deficient serum. Although chemotactic activity has not been extensively studied in these patients, Alper et al. (8) stated that *in vitro* activity was deficient, and Ballow et al. (16) reported an early defect in the *in vivo* skin window response. In our laboratory, serum from the patient of Alper et al. (6) (kindly supplied by Dr. A. R. Rabson) generated no chemotactic activity on activation with either endotoxin or zymosan (Table 3); the defect was corrected by the addition of purified C3.

A single patient with so-called type I hypercatabolism of C3 and frequent infections has been described by Alper et al. (3,4). In a long series of studies, it has been demonstrated that the abnormality in this patient is the genetically

TABLE 3. *Chemotactic activity generated in C3-deficient serum*

Activating agent	Chemotaxis (cpm)[a]	
	Normal serum	C3-deficient serum
None	43 ± 13[b]	40 ± 5
Endotoxin	1,141 ± 385	51 ± 9
Zymosan	2,443 ± 535	75 ± 17
Zymosan (+C3[c])	—	1,920 ± 1

[a]Method described in reference 52 and Table 1.
[b]Mean ± SE, quadruplicate chambers in a single representative experiment.
[c]Cordis Corp., Miami, Fla; 1,000 units/ml of serum.

determined absence of the C3 inactivator or KAF (conglutinogen activating factor) as this agent is otherwise known (1,7,149). Since the C3 inactivator inactivates C3b and inhibits factor $\bar{D}$, it appears to serve as an inhibitor of the alternate pathway (7,96). It is postulated that its absence results in continued *in vivo* activation of this pathway with depletion of C3 substrate. Incubation of the patient's serum with immune complexes resulted in only minimal generation of chemotactic activity (3); this defect could be improved *in vitro* by the addition of normal serum or *in vivo* by the infusion of normal plasma (3,4). A second variety of C3 hypercatabolism (type II) is associated with partial lipodystrophy, mesangiocapillary glomerulonephritis, and, in some instances, increased susceptibility to infection (5,103,113,126), but studies of chemotaxis have not been reported in such patients.

C5 deficiency has been identified by Rosenfeld et al. (108,109) in a single kindred with two homozygous deficient individuals. The propositus had systemic lupus erythematosus and an impressive history of infections, while a C5-deficient sibling was in good health. Sera from both siblings were defective in the generation of chemotactic activity on incubation with either aggregated IgG or endotoxin (108); the defect was substantially corrected by the addition of purified C5. These results parallel earlier studies of chemotactic activity of C5-deficient mouse serum (116,137) and provide further support for the role of C5-derived chemotactic activity.

Two children with a clinical syndrome of dermatitis, diarrhea, wasting, dystrophy, and recurrent pyogenic infections (Leiner's disease) have been characterized by Miller and colleagues (73,89,92) as having C5 dysfunction. This is thought to represent a subtle abnormality in the C5 molecule which reduces opsonization of baker's yeast but leaves most other functional and immunologic features of C5 intact. The yeast opsonization assay has been a controversial point, and normal results have recently been reported with both C5-deficient and C5 dysfunctional sera (108). Chemotactic activity of serum from patients with C5 dysfunction has been reported to be reduced in one kindred (89,97) and normal in the other (73).

Normal generation of chemotactic activity has been reported in the serum of patients with inherited deficiency of C6 (75,78) or C8 (104; R. A. Clark, *unpublished data*). The situation is less clear in inherited C7 deficiency. Serum from a healthy teenage boy with complete absence of C7 showed normal generation of activity using zymosan as the activating agent (145). In contrast, serum from a 42-year-old woman with a scleroderma-like disorder and C7 deficiency had defective generation of activity with immune complexes, an abnormality which was corrected by the addition of C7 (27).

Abnormal generation of chemotactic activity on incubation of serum with endotoxin has been reported in several patients with hypogammaglobulinemia (36,49,122), although the basis for this defect has not been elucidated. Other clinical situations associated with unexplained defects in the generation of complement-derived chemotactic activity include some patients with systemic lupus erythematosus (37,77) or diabetes mellitus (88) and neonates (85).

Abnormalities in the formation of the Hageman factor-dependent chemotactic agents, kallikrein and plasminogen activator, have been demonstrated in the plasma of patients with genetically determined deficiencies of Hageman factor (57) or prekallikrein (144). In each case, the defect was corrected by the addition of the missing protein. Disorders of cell-derived chemotactic factors have been described in relatively few situations. A patient with mucocutaneous candidiasis and a cellular defect in monocyte chemotaxis was found to have decreased *in vitro* production of a chemotactic lymphokine (115). Patients with the Wiskott-Aldrich syndrome had a cellular defect in monocyte chemotaxis and their lymphocytes spontaneously produced excessive amounts of chemotactic lymphokine (10); it was suggested that chemotactic inhibition by the patients' plasma could be a result of deactivation of leukocytes by circulating lymphokine. Dialyzable transfer factor prepared from the leukocytes of patients with the Sézary syndrome was deficient in chemotactic activity (54).

Inhibitors of Chemotactic Factors

Abnormalities related to chemotactic factor-directed inhibitors have been divided into excessive or deficient levels of chemotactic factor inactivators, inhibitors of the generation of chemotactic factors, and reversible inhibitors of chemotactic factor expression (see tabulation above). The chemotactic factor inactivators are present in normal human serum and destroy the biologic activity of a variety of chemotactic factors by enzymatic cleavage (22,127,139). Excessive serum levels of these inactivators have been detected in several disorders associated with cutaneous anergy; these include Hodgkin's disease (136), lepromatous leprosy (138), and sarcoidosis (81). A similar phenomenon has been observed in association with anergy in patients with a wide variety of underlying systemic diseases (128,129,131). Sera from patients with alcoholic liver disease often contain chemotactic inhibitors (11,44,80,130,131). This may be related to excessive levels of chemotactic factor inactivators (80), to cell-directed inhibitors (131), or to both of these mechanisms. Sera from patients with α_1-antitrypsin deficiency have reduced levels of chemotactic factor inactivators (141). Inhibitory activity directed at the generation of chemotactic factor in serum rather than at the factor itself has been described in an animal model of uremia (34). Patients with glomerulonephritis were found to have a serum component which reversibly interfered with the expression of complement-derived chemotactic activity (59).

CELLULAR DEFECTS IN CHEMOTAXIS

The cellular chemotactic defects present some difficulty in classification primarily because of a lack of understanding of their pathophysiologic basis at a biochemical or structural level. These disorders have often been dealt with on purely clinical grounds (87,118,146). A variation is the division into familial and acquired defects (134). Alternatively, Gallin and Wolff (57) proposed a functional classification scheme based on the presence of associated defects in granulocyte adherence, deformability or random migration. This has the appeal of more closely approaching the underlying basis for defective chemotaxis, since these associated functional parameters all appear to be prerequisites for intact directed migration; however, it should be noted that these parameters have not been systematically evaluated in many patients with cellular chemotactic defects. In view of the foregoing considerations, it appears that the rather fragmentary state of our current knowledge about the basis for cellular chemotactic defects precludes the formulation of a classification scheme which is both comprehensive and usable. I propose to deal with these disorders from the point of view of a clinical classification, shown below, and then discuss how they might fit into functional or etiologic schemes.

Clinical Classification of Cellular Chemotactic Defects

A. Primary defects
    1. Chediak-Higashi syndrome
    2. Lazy leukocyte syndrome
    3. Diabetes mellitus
 — 4. Rheumatoid arthritis
    5. Neonates
    6. Hyperimmunoglobulinemia E
    7. Congenital icthyosis
    8. Active infection
    9. Hypophosphatemia
    10. Hypogammaglobulinemia
    11. Thermal injury
    12. Bone marrow transplantation
    13. Down's syndrome
    14. Idiopathic juvenile periodontitis
    15. α-Mannosidase deficiency
    16. Actin dysfunction
    17. Isolated cases

B. Cell-directed inhibitors
    1. Isolated cases
    2. Wiskott-Aldrich syndrome
    3. Neoplasms
    4. IgA myeloma

Primary Cellular Defects

The Chediak-Higashi syndrome (CHS) is one of the most extensively studied examples of a cellular chemotactic defect. Patients with this inherited disorder have recurrent pyogenic infections, partial oculocutaneous albinism, and, in many instances, an accelerated lymphoma-like phase (23). The presence of giant lysosomal granules in all granule-bearing cells, including leukocytes, has been considered to be the hallmark of the disease. Clark and Kimball (36) reported a decreased *in vivo* inflammatory response by the skin window method and an *in vitro* chemotactic defect in three CHS patients. The patients' polymorphonuclear leukocytes (PMNs) responded poorly to several different chemotactic stimuli and their serum contained no chemotactic inhibitors. Subsequent studies confirmed the granulocyte chemotactic defect by another assay (52), extended these findings to animal models of CHS in mink (38) and mice (50), and documented an analogous monocyte chemotactic defect in CHS patients as well as mink and cattle (55). An early defect in bactericidal activity related to delayed degranulation has also been documented in CHS leukocytes (107) and mild granulocytopenia with impaired bone marrow granulocyte reserves is often present (23). On the basis of the exaggeration of the chemotactic defect by the use of smaller pore size filters in the chemotaxis chamber (36,38,50,55), and the finding that random migration is normal in capillary tubes (36) but decreased in Boyden chambers (49), it has been suggested that decreased deformability caused by a membrane defect or by the presence of giant cytoplasmic granules might be the reason for the impaired chemotaxis. More recently abnormal patterns of lectin binding to the surface of granulocytes from CHS mice (100) and humans (101) have been reported. CHS cells showed spontaneous capping of the binding sites and thus behaved similarly to colchicine-treated normal cells, a finding suggestive of a microtubule derangement. Abrogation of this abnormal response by cyclic-GMP or agents which increase cellular levels of cyclic-GMP raised the possibility of a cyclic nucleotide defect resulting in impaired microtubule function. Evidence has also been presented that these defects may be the basis for the bizarre granulogenesis seen in the CHS (99,101). These observations have raised therapeutic possibilities directed at altering cellular cyclic nucleotides. Boxer et al. (26) have, in fact, reported that ascorbate added to CHS leukocytes *in vitro* or administered to a CHS patient resulted in reversal of defects in chemotaxis, degranulation, and bactericidal activity. Parallel measurements of leukocyte cyclic nucleotides showed normal cyclic-GMP, but markedly increased cyclic-AMP, which was decreased by ascorbate.

Miller et al. (91) coined the term "lazy leukocyte syndrome" in reference to two children with recurrent fever, oral lesions, and otitis, and who were shown to have severe neutropenia, impaired release of neutrophils from the bone marrow, decreased random migration in capillary tubes, and a cellular chemotactic defect. Impaired granulocyte chemotactic responses in some patients with diabetes mellitus have been reported by several groups (69,88,93). These defects were at least partially corrected by incubation of the diabetic leukocytes with insulin and glucose. Random migration was reported to be normal (69). A recent preliminary report describes impaired granulocyte adherence in hyperglycemic diabetic subjects (14). In studies of 24 classic rheumatoid arthritis patients and 8 patients with the juvenile form of the disease, Mowat and Baum

(94) observed decreased granulocyte chemotaxis in all adult patients and 3 juvenile patients. Incubation of normal leukocytes with rheumatoid factor positive serum or isolated rheumatoid factor complexes diminished their chemotactic responses, and it was postulated that *in vivo* ingestion of such complexes by leukocytes might be the basis for the poor migration of the patients' cells. A similar effect of rheumatoid arthritis sera on normal granulocytes was subsequently reported (20), although in this study the effect did not correlate with the presence of rheumatoid factor.

Miller (85) found defective granulocyte chemotaxis in apparently healthy neonates when compared to adult controls. It is unclear whether neonatal granulocytes also have a defect in random migration (86,87). Recent studies have demonstrated a decrease in deformability in neonatal PMNs (86,87), and it was suggested that this cellular rigidity might be a reflection of metabolic immaturity which would lead to impaired chemotaxis.

A number of reports have documented an association between markedly elevated serum IgE levels and a cellular chemotactic defect in a clinical setting of recurrent infections and allergic disorders such as eczema, urticaria, or asthma (31,40,42,62,66–68,105,133). The clinical syndrome was first described by Buckley et al. (28) in 1972 and the chemotactic defect was documented by Clark et al. (40) in 1973. No serum inhibitors of granulocyte chemotaxis are present and random migration is normal. This syndrome appears to be familial in some instances (133). In addition to pyogenic infections, some patients have mucocutaneous candidiasis which may be related to defective lymphocyte function (28,-40,133). Particular clinical syndromes with closely related features, high IgE, and the chemotactic defect include Job's syndrome (66), incontinentia pigmenti (42), and an unusual type of icthyosis (105). The basis for the association between hyperimmunoglobulinemia E and impaired chemotaxis is unknown. It has been suggested (67,68) that histamine released by IgE-dependent mechanisms in these allergic subjects might suppress leukocyte migration. *In vitro* improvement of chemotaxis by H_2 receptor antagonists supports a role for histamine (62). Defective chemotaxis in allergic disorders need not be associated with elevated IgE, since patients have recently been described with allergic rhinitis, pyogenic infections, and reduced PMN chemotaxis, but normal IgE (71); the migration defect was present only during periods of active rhinitis and infection and could be induced *in vitro* by incubation of patient's leukocytes with an appropriate allergen.

A familial chemotactic defect associated with congenital icthyosis and infections caused by bacteria and cutaneous fungi has been described (by Miller et al.) [90] in three patients from two families. Random migration and serum chemotactic activity were normal. The possible relationship between these patients and the icthyosis patient of Pincus et al. (105) with high IgE and impaired chemotaxis is not known. IgE levels were not reported in the patients of Miller et al. (90). We have recently studied a 2-year-old boy with congenital icthyosis, tuberculous meningitis, and a prior history of *Haemophilus influenza* meningitis.

The chemotactic response of his PMNs to C5a averaged 30% of the normal control (patient 167 ± 17 cpm, normal 554 ± 26 cpm; mean $\pm$ SE, $n = 4$, $p < 0.001$). Random migration was normal and serum IgE was slightly elevated (364 U/ml, normal < 100).

The status of neutrophil chemotactic responses during the course of active infection is not entirely clear. In patients with acute severe bacterial infections and the morphologic finding of toxic neutrophils, impairments were demonstrated in PMN chemotaxis as well as in random migration and microbicidal activity (84). Other groups have found cellular chemotactic defects in patients having bacterial infections without toxic neutrophils (15,47,95); in general, defects were seen most frequently in acute rather than chronic infections. A transient decrease in granulocyte chemotaxis was observed in experimental endotoxemia (125). Defects in PMN chemotaxis have also been reported during viral infections (12,82), although much of the work in this area has dealt with monocyte migration. In contrast to the foregoing, Hill et al. (64,65,70) have observed augmented PMN chemotactic responsiveness during active bacterial infections. The patients were mostly children and were evaluated early in the course of infection; follow-up studies in some subjects showed a return to normal chemotaxis with resolution of infection. Increased chemotactic responses have also been reported in volunteers with induced *Mycoplasma pneumoniae* infection (83). Although the discrepancies among these studies are not completely resolvable, variations in age and in the type, severity, and duration of infection may be important. It seems likely that PMN chemotaxis may be enhanced in the early phases of acute bacterial infection, especially in children, but with advanced age, increasing severity of infection, toxic neutrophils, or viral infection, chemotaxis may decrease.

Defective PMN chemotaxis and phagocytosis in association with hypophosphatemia have been demonstrated in a dog model and in a patient receiving hyperalimentation (41); depletion of cellular ATP was found and incubation of leukocytes with adenosine and phosphate improved migration. Several patients with severe hypogammaglobulinemia have been found to have cellular defects in PMN chemotaxis, but normal random migration (49,122). Some patients with Down's syndrome have reduced PMN chemotactic responses (74,111). A preliminary report has appeared which describes defective chemotaxis, but normal adherence and random migration in a child with inherited deficiency of α-mannosidase (58). Impaired chemotaxis has been reported in patients with thermal injury (9,142,143); the defect correlated with the extent of the burn and indicated a decreased likelihood of survival. In one study, evidence was presented for a cellular defect correctable by heat-labile factors from normal serum and for dialyzable serum inhibitors related to topical therapeutic agents (143); another report describes heat-stable, nondialyzable, nondrug-related serum chemotactic inhibitory activity (9). Cellular chemotactic defects were observed in 24 of 34 patients following bone marrow transplantation for leukemia or aplastic anemia (35). Depressed neutrophil chemotaxis correlated with the pres-

TABLE 4. *Granulocyte chemotaxis in patients with idiopathic juvenile periodontosis*

Patient	Chemotaxis (% of normal control)[a]	
	PMN response[b]	Serum activity[c]
1	27.5 ± 3.3 (15)[d]	66.9 ± 7.0 (12)
2	45.4 ± 3.8 (15)	83.0 ± 5.2 (12)
3	55.6 ± 6.1 (15)	54.8 ± 6.5 (12)
4	56.2 ± 5.2 (15)	80.1 ± 4.8 (12)
5	59.5 ± 8.7 (15)	83.7 ± 8.6 (12)
6	63.4 ± 4.2 (10)	115.0 ± 16.3 (8)
7	73.3 ± 13.3 (10)	110.7 ± 11.4 (8)
8	82.1 ± 8.8 (15)	108.3 ± 10.6 (12)

[a] Method described in ref. 52.
[b] Response of patient's PMNs to C5a expressed as a percent of response of normal control PMNs.
[c] Activity of the patient's serum following activation with endotoxin or zymosan expressed as a percent of the activity of similarly treated normal control serum
[d] Mean ± SE of (n) observations

ence of graft-vs-host disease and the administration of antithymocyte globulin, an agent which was found to have *in vitro* chemotactic suppressive activity. Patients with impaired chemotaxis experienced significantly more infections than those with normal chemotaxis, and this was predominantly related to bacterial pathogens. Random migration in Boyden chambers was normal (R. A. Clark, *unpublished data*), and although a few patients had serum chemotactic inhibitors, most of the defects could not be explained on this basis.

The frequent association of defective chemotaxis with early and severe periodontal disorders (35,36,61,91,105) has prompted our laboratory to examine chemotactic function in patients with periodontitis. Particular interest has centered on idiopathic juvenile periodontitis, also known as periodontosis, since these patients develop progressive destructive lesions at an early age although they have no indication of systemic illness. The results of studies on eight such patients, all in their teens or early twenties, with well-documented clinical periodontosis, are shown in Table 4 (studied in collaboration with Dr. R. C. Page). Significantly decreased PMN migration in response to C5a was seen in patients one through 6 ($p < 0.001$) and the mean response of the entire group was $57.9 ± 5.9\%$ of normal ($p < 0.001$). In addition, serum chemotactic activity generated by activation with either endotoxin or zymosan was significantly reduced in patients nos. 1 through 4. Normal PMN responses and serum activity were seen in a group of middle-aged adults with ordinary periodontitis. Random migration of PMNs was normal in the periodontosis patients.

Boxer et al. (25) have described a very interesting male infant with repeated infections and a poor *in vivo* inflammatory response in infected tissues. *In vitro* studies demonstrated cellular defects in PMN chemotaxis and phagocytosis but enhanced degranulation (when corrected for the decreased ingestion). The granulocytes spread poorly on glass with small narrow pseudopods and remained relatively immobile, presumably a correlate of impaired random migration. Electron micrographs showed a relative paucity of cortical microfilaments. Isolated actin from the patient's granulocytes showed defective *in vitro* polymerization. It was hypothesized that a defect in the PMN actomyosin system could account for the functional abnormalities observed.

A number of isolated cases warrant discussion, although they cannot be easily fitted into any specific clinical syndrome. Higgins et al. (61) coined the term *granulocytasthenia* in reference to one of the earliest descriptions of a cellular chemotactic defect, although a full report has not appeared. A 4-year-old boy had recurrent infections, lymphadenopathy, hepatosplenomegaly, gingivitis, and nonpurulent skin lesions. Defective PMN chemotaxis was accompanied by decreased adherence to glass beads, but phagocytosis and bactericidal activity were normal. Edelson et al. (45) emphasized the importance of evaluating random migration and adherence in a report of three different patients with recurrent infections. All three had impairment of PMN chemotaxis, random migration, and microbicidal activity, and one of the three had decreased adherence as well. A patient with refractory macrocytic anemia, granulomatous ulcerations, and severe chromosomal alterations was reported to have diminished PMN chemotaxis, metabolic activity, and bacterial killing (112). A teenage boy with recurrent pyogenic infections was found to have decreased PMN chemotaxis and bactericidal activity but normal random migration (32); an interesting feature of this report was the selectivity of the cellular chemotactic defect which was demonstrable with casein but not with activated serum as the attractant. Two siblings with recurrent infections and red hair had cellular defects in PMN chemotaxis, but random migration and IgE were normal (147).

Cell-Directed Inhibitors

Also listed in the tabulation above are disorders associated with cell-directed inhibitors of chemotaxis. These have to date consisted largely of isolated case reports. A young boy described by Ward and Schlegel (140) had severe recurrent infections, neutrophil defects in metabolic and bactericidal activities, and a cell-directed serum inhibitor of chemotaxis; in subsequent studies, this patient was found to have typical x-linked chronic granulomatous disease (21,106,107). Two isolated patients (114,121) were found to have a heat-stable inhibitor in serum but not plasma, and the inhibitory activity was antagonized by normal plasma or serum but not by patient plasma; the interpretation was that the serum inhibitor is a normal constituent which is activated or released during coagulation, but is ordinarily antagonized by a second plasma or serum factor which is absent in these patients. Another patient appeared to have defective PMN microbicidal activity as well as a cell-directed chemotactic inhibitor (124). Impaired chemotaxis of monocytes and PMNs has been described in the Wiskott-

Aldrich syndrome, and this is attributable to a serum inhibitor which may represent a circulating chemotactic lymphokine (10,98; R. A. Clark, *unpublished data*). Cell-directed inhibitors of PMN and monocyte chemotaxis have been detected in the serum of cancer patients (135), although studies in a mouse model disclosed a neoplasm-derived, low-molecular-weight inhibitor specific for macrophage migration (117).

A recent article by Van Epps and Williams (132) demonstrates inhibition of PMN chemotaxis and random migration by IgA myeloma sera; IgG myeloma or macroglobulinemia sera were not inhibitory, and the effect was specifically attributable to an IgA M component. We have evaluated a patient with recurrent furuncles and severe periodontal disease who had a monoclonal gammapathy but no evidence of myeloma. The abnormal protein was an IgA kappa M component. The patient's neutrophils responded poorly to C5a ($56.3 \pm 3.8\%$ of normal control, mean $\pm$ SE of 3 experiments, $p < 0.01$) and his serum contained a heat-stable ($56°C$ for 30 min) factor which inhibited chemotaxis of normal PMNs ($54.0 \pm 10.2\%$ inhibition by 10% patient serum compared to 10% normal serum, mean $\pm$ SE of 4 experiments, $p < 0.02$). Van Epps and Williams (132) hypothesized that IgA M components inhibit chemotactic responses by binding to the neutrophil surface where they may interfere with the interaction of chemotactic factors with receptors or suppress cellular mechanisms essential for chemotaxis.

Functional Classification of Cellular Defects

Table 5 illustrates a suggested classification scheme based on the presence of various functional abnormalities in association with impaired directed migration (adapted from Gallin and Wolff [57]). These categories—adherence, deformability, and random migration—are not mutually exclusive, since abnormal adherence or deformability is generally associated with impaired random migration as well. Disorders listed under random migration are those in which adherence and deformability are either normal or in many instances have not been examined. Likewise, in many of the conditions with no associated abnormality detected, adherence and deformability have not been carefully studied, although the finding of normal random migration in most militates against adherence or deformability defects.

Defective granulocyte adherence may be induced *in vitro* by ethanol and *in vivo* by corticosteroids or salicylates (79). Clinical conditions in which chemotactic defects have been associated with impaired adherence include diabetes mellitus (14), a case reported as "granulocytasthenia" (61), and other isolated cases (45). Decreased adherence has been described in a patient with trimethylaminuria (72) and in acute hypocomplementemic poststreptococcal glomerulonephritis (110), but chemotaxis was not examined in these reports. Diminished deformability is observed in leukocytes exposed to glycolytic inhibitors or trypsin (87) and has been demonstrated in neonatal granulocytes (86,87). The inclusion of the Chediak-Higashi syndrome in the deformability category is uncertain, since

TABLE 5. *Functional classification of cellular chemotactic defects*

Associated functional abnormality	Pharmacologic models	Clinical examples
Adherence	Corticosteroids	Diabetes mellitus
	Salicylates	Granulocytasthenia
	Ethanol	Isolated cases
Deformability	Glycolytic inhibitors	Neonates
	Trypsin	Chediak-Higashi syndrome
Random migration	Cytochalasin B	Lazy leukocyte syndrome
		Toxic neutrophils
		Actin Dysfunction syndrome
		Isolated cases
None detected		
Random migration normal		Hypogammaglobulinemia
		Hyper-IgE syndromes
		Icthyosis
		Bone marrow transplantation
		Idiopathic juvenile periodontitis
		α-Mannosidase deficiency
		Down's syndrome
Random migration not tested		Rheumatoid arthritis
		Thermal injury
		Hypophosphatemia

Adapted from Gallin and Wolff (57).

the evidence for this is very indirect (see above). Cytochalasin B impairs random migration and at some concentrations decreases directed migration as well (18,150). Defective random migration has been demonstrated in the lazy leukocyte syndrome (91), toxic neutrophils (84), the actin dysfunction syndrome (25), and in other isolated cases (45).

Etiologic Classification of Cellular Defects

Although the present dearth of knowledge regarding the basic biochemical or structural aberrations underlying various examples of cellular chemotactic defects precludes a detailed etiologic classification, an attempt has been made (Table 6) to incorporate what is known into such a scheme. Theoretically, abnormalities could occur in any of the structures or processes involved in the cellular chemotactic response. These have been divided into membrane-related and intracellular phenomena. While the pharmacologic models listed are reasonably well-established, the clinical examples suggested are in most instances somewhat speculative, and for several categories there are no suitable candidates for related clinical defects.

Chemotaxis of rabbit PMNs is blocked by protease inhibitors and by hydrolysis products of synthetic chemotactic peptides, and it has been suggested that these effects may relate to blockage of a chemotactic factor receptor (13). Earlier studies had implicated serine esterases in rabbit PMN chemotaxis and demon-

TABLE 6. *Etiologic classification of cellular chemotactic defects*

Defect	Pharmacologic models	Possible clinical examples
Cell membrane		
Receptors	Hydrolysis products of chemo-tactic peptides	IgA myeloma
Esterases	Phosphonate esters	
Ion fluxes	Ca^{++} efflux - cytochalasin B Ca^{++} influx - lanthanum	
Surface charge	Hydrocortisone	
Intracellular elements		
Microtubules	Colchicine, vinblastine, other antitubulins	Chediak-Higashi syndrome
Microfilaments	Cytochalasin B	Actin Dysfunction syndrome
Metabolism	Glycolytic inhibitors	Hypophosphatemia
Cyclic nucleotides	Autonomic agonists, prosta-glandins, cholera toxin, etc.	Chediak-Higashi syndrome

strated inhibition of chemotaxis and esterase activity by phosphonate esters (17). The precise relationship between proteases and receptors is unknown. Although the role of such proteases in human PMN chemotaxis is uncertain and no clinical disorders relating to these enzymes have been identified, it has been suggested that the chemotactic inhibitory activity of IgA M components may be mediated through interference with chemotactic factor receptor sites (132). Ion fluxes across the cell membrane are induced by exposure to chemotactic factors; the chemotactic response as well as Ca^{++} efflux or Ca^{++} influx are blocked by cytochalasin B at high concentrations (56) or lanthanum, respectively (24). The chemotactic factor-induced decrease in negative surface charge of granulocytes is blocked by hydrocortisone, an agent which also inhibits chemotaxis (53). Abnormalities in either ion fluxes or surface charge have not been implicated in clinical chemotactic disorders. Inhibitors of microtubule aggregation block chemotaxis under some circumstances (19), and some evidence suggests that the functional abnormalities in Chediak-Higashi syndrome leukocytes relate to microtubule dysfunction (see above). Impaired microfilament function is the presumed basis for decreased chemotactic activity of cytochalasin B-treated leukocytes (18,150) and of cells from a patient with abnormal leukocyte actin (25). Chemotaxis is blocked by glycolytic inhibitors (29,30; R. A. Clark and S. J. Klebanoff, *unpublished data*) presumably by depletion of ATP; the abnormal chemotactic response seen in hypophosphatemia has similarly been attributed to decreased leukocyte ATP levels (41). Alterations in cyclic nucleotide levels have striking effects on chemotaxis (63), and it has recently been suggested that abnormalities in either cyclic-GMP or cyclic-AMP levels might account for the impaired chemotaxis seen in the Chediak-Higashi syndrome (see above). The categories listed are not mutually exclusive since, for example, the postulated

TABLE 7. *Therapeutic Agents in Patients with Defective Chemotaxis*

Agent	Condition	References
Normal plasma	C3 hypercatabolism	4,149
	C5 dysfunction	73,89,92
	Cell-directed inhibitors	114,121
Transfer factor	Mucocutaneous candidiasis	115
BCG	Neoplasms	120
Agents affecting cyclic nucleotides Autonomic agonists, ascorbate	Chediak-Higashi syndrome	26
H$_2$ receptor antagonists	Hyper-IgE syndromes	62
Levamisole	Hyper-IgE syndromes	148

cyclic nucleotide abnormality in the CHS might limit chemotaxis through an adverse effect on microtubule function.

It is hoped that the classification schemes proposed will serve as a stimulus both for further discussion and for more intensive study of patients with chemotactic defects. Only by the application of careful and sophisticated analytical methods to these problems will the basis for clinical disorders become apparent. This in turn will surely advance our basic understanding of the mechanisms involved in the chemotactic response and lead to useful therapeutic approaches.

THERAPEUTIC CONSIDERATIONS

Unfortunately, therapy in patients with recurrent infections associated with defective chemotaxis has generally been limited to conventional management of individual infections; however, some advances aimed at correction of the functional defect have been made (Table 7). Certain of the humoral defects may be ameliorated by infusion of normal plasma. The use of immunotherapeutic agents such as transfer factor or BCG has proven helpful in other instances. Currently, attention is focusing on pharmacologic agents such as autonomic agonists, ascorbic acid, H$_2$ receptor antagonists, and levamisole.

SUMMARY

Clinical disorders of granulocyte chemotaxis have now been described in a wide range of conditions associated with increased susceptibility to infections. Chemotactic factor defects have been divided into those caused by abnormal generation of agents derived from the complement system, from the Hageman factor system, or from cells, and those caused by inhibitors of chemotactic factors. Cellular chemotactic defects have been divided into those resulting from a primary disorder of the granulocyte and those resulting from the action of cell-directed inhibitors. Subclassification of the primary cellular disorders is difficult because, in most instances, of a lack of knowledge about the pathophysiologic basis for the impaired chemotaxis. Alternatives to the traditional clinical classification of these disorders include a scheme based on associated functional abnormalities in granulocyte adherence, deformability or random migration, and a proposed etiologic classification system. Although some therapeutic modalities currently being evaluated may improve functional defects in granulocyte chemotaxis, a systematic approach to treatment will require more complete understanding of pathophysiology.

ACKNOWLEDGMENTS

The author gratefully acknowledges the excellent technical assistance of Coralie Baker. These studies were supported in part by grants DE02600, AI07763, and CA18354 and Research Career Development Award CA00164 from the National Institutes of Health.

DISCUSSION

Dr. Wilkinson: Methodology, particularly in this field of the clinical study of chemotaxis, really needs attention. Practically everybody is looking at what has happened to a sample of the cell population and not at the detailed movement of single cells. I think this is really the reason for the inadequate information. Unless you carry out checkerboard assays you do not really know, and I do not think that it has really been established in any of these abnormalities, whether the cells are showing defects in locomotion or whether the defect lies in the locomotor or in the sensory apparatus of the cell. It is important, therefore, to distinguish between tactic and kinetic locomotion.

Also, it will be important in clinical studies actually to watch the cells moving about. A lot can be found out that way. There is a whole world of information about what these cells are actually doing and why.

Dr. Robert Clark: You are absolutely right. I don't know of any published clinical applications of the direct observation of cells. Do you have any experience with this, Dr. Wilkinson.

Dr. Wilkinson: We have started to do it but we really have not gotten far enough with anything we have actually seen so far to say anything very much about it. But I am certain it will turn up eventually.

Dr. Robert Clark: Yes, I am sure it will.

Dr. Gallin: We have done some morphologic studies of neutrophils from patients with defects of chemotaxis and some of these are presented elsewhere in this volume. In particular, Dr. Malech and I have performed electron microscopic evaluation of cells oriented on Millipore filters under conditions of chemotaxis. These studies have yielded considerable information regarding the nature of the chemotactic defects.

For example, in a patient with Chediak-Higashi syndrome, fewer pseudopods were seen penetrating the filter than normally. To what extent this reflects a microtubule defect, as suggested by Dr. Oliver (99–101), remains to be determined.

Another patient we looked at this way had leukocyte dysfunction associated with increased microtubule assembly, and her cells did not orient properly in a gradient of chemotactic factor. Interestingly, the cytoplasmic membrane of her cells had blebs or protuberances similar to what is seen in cytochalasin B-treated normal cells. The point I would like to emphasize is that morphologic analysis of cells under conditions of chemotaxis can be very helpful in understanding the basis of the defect, and the analysis should include electron microscope studies.

Dr. Ward: Are you surprised at the findings of the zymosan activation in C4-deficient serum? Does this suggest the possibility that, in fact, the serum may have some additional deficiency, particularly in view of the fact the patient has a leukocyte dysfunction syndrome? How carefully did you look at the alternative pathway or the other complement components to determine if in fact the deficiency is selective in C4?

Second, in your list of the areas of defective chemotactic functions you included patients with a deficiency of Hageman factor and Fletcher factor. I am not aware of any studies that have been done or any clinical observations that in any way suggest that patients with these deficiencies have any problems in mobilization of leukocytes or in their ability to resist the onslaught of infective agents. While theoretically, it is possible that these deficiencies could be associated with a chemotactic defect. I wonder if one can make a global statement of that type.

Dr. Robert Clark: Regarding the latter question, I think I emphasized that in fact such patients do not have problems with infection or anything else for that matter. They are really of interest more in terms of dissecting the intricacies of the various biochemical pathways involved, and there are no clinical problems related to the chemotactic abnormalities.

Dr. Gallin, you have been involved in some of those studies; would you want to comment on that?

Dr. Gallin: I agree with that, but that does not exclude a role of these molecules in inflammatory processes. One could argue that patients with Hageman factor or Fletcher factor deficiency do as well as they do because they have alternative or back-up systems. No one, of course, has challenged these patients to see how they would do under stress.

Dr. Becker: In regard to the C4 findings, these are exactly analogous to the findings with C2 deficiency where the bactericidal test was used as a measure rather than the generation of chemotactic activity. The probable explanation is the concentration of serum used in the tests. The alternative pathway mechanism cannot stand dilution. That fits exactly with both your findings in C4 deficiency and others in C2 deficiency.

Dr. Robert Clark: I agree completely. I want to address Dr. Ward's question about whether there were some other abnormalities in our C4-deficient serum. I can not really rule that out completely. We have measured all the classic pathway components and they are normal or near normal, except for C4, which is completely absent. We have measured Factor B which is normal; properdin is somewhat reduced. We were able to reproduce most of these results with the serum from the French C4-deficient patient; this serum was kindly supplied to us by Dr. Georges Hauptmann. If those findings are related to some other abnormality, it would appear to be present in both of these families.

Dr. Snyderman: I would like to mention two things. One is related to the C4 and C2 deficiencies. I think we very clearly showed, as have other laboratories, that in the absence of early classic complement components, inulin and endotoxin do not kinetically activate C3 normally. And the reason for this may be the requirement for the generation of C3b to fire the alternative pathway optimally. It is not surprising to me that those individuals with a deficiency of classic complement components should be kinetically abnormal. This is not because of dilution, because we could show this in undiluted as well as diluted serum. So I think the classic pathway certainly has a synergistic role in firing the alternative pathway.

I would also like to comment on the patient Dr. Gallin described with leukocyte dysfunction and increased microtubule assembly. We also studied this patient on several occasions. Unfortunately, she died about 2 weeks after we did our last studies; however, it is worth noting that in addition to the abnormalities Dr. Gallin described, her cells had decreased binding of the fMet peptide.

Dr. Stossel: Dr. Gallin, what was the neutrophil count of this patient?

Dr. Gallin: It was not abnormal when I studied her. Her leukocyte count was about 6,000/mm with about 60% neutrophils.

Dr. Stossel: She did not have neutrophilia?

Dr. Gallin: No.

Dr. Stossel: What kind of infections did she have?

Dr. Gallin: Bacterial and viral infections. She died of chicken pox pneumonia.

Dr. Stossel: I am just concerned about this outpouring of syndromes. I would like to try a little of my kind of logic on this. What would we expect if there was a disorder of chemotaxis? What sort of clinical presentations would we expect to get? I think congenital neutropenia is a good model for chemotaxis defects. There are no neutrophils there. One can make certain generalizations. When congenital neutropenics get infected, they tend to get *Staphylococcus aureus* and gram-negative enterics of the skin and lungs. They do not get meningitis or infections with virulent encapsulated pathogens.

So I do not like the idea of C3 deficiency being used as an example of clinical chemotactic defect just because you can demonstrate deficiency of generation of chemotactic factors *in vitro*. The C3-deficient patient gets meningitis, septicemia, pneumonia, with the pneumococcus, meningococcus, streptococcus and *H. influenza*.

To my way of thinking, if you have an invading bug it should, if everything is working, call for an inflammatory response. If the leukocyte cannot respond, that is, if it can not crawl or can not chemotax, either because of an intrinsic locomotion defect or a sensory defect, a signal is going to go out to produce more cells. That is just basically what we know about the kinetics of neutrophil production in response to infection. I think it was Dr. Miller who first made the imaginative suggestion that perhaps if the cell can not crawl, it would not get out of the bone marrow. Is this true?

I would like to present two patients to look at this question.

The first is just a reminder of one that has already been presented. This is that patient with what we call neutrophil-actin dysfunction, whose neutrophils would not migrate at all into inflammatory sites. This patient had a leukocytosis, a tremendous neutrophilic *leukocytosis* all the time, not neutropenia. Histologically, the infections, which were of the skin and the GI tract, consisted of mononuclear cells, lymphocytes, and monocytes, but no neutrophils. I thought that was impressive as was the fact that there seemed to be a compensatory response with leukocytes. So, I have sort of come to think that when you really have a problem of migration this may indeed be what you would expect to happen.

Concerning the other patient, Dr. Edward Sweeney and I investigated a 13-year-old boy with severe juvenile periodontosis, chronic neutrophilia, and hypergammaglobulinemia. He has had relatively little problems with other infections, but because of the neutrophilia, we decided to look further. His phagocytosis was, if anything, hyperactive. His skin window filled up with monocytes but very few neutrophils.

When we looked at his cells directly, they tried to get very much involved with the substrate and would not orient at all.

I thought this was terrific; we have now got a sensory defect. We can go on to pursue the molecular basis of this thing, even though we really do not know what it is. But, again, I was nervous about the "horse-cart problem" that has been discussed in context of these patients with the hyper-IgE and the eczema, etc. So we sat on it. We tried to treat his dental problem, and he did not respond, so his teeth were extracted. Thereafter, he had a decline in his neutrophil count to normal and his cells functioned perfectly. You can no longer demonstrate his abnormality. We examined a number of patients of Dr. Sigmund Socransky with periodontosis, none of whom had the extreme neutrophilia or hypergammaglobulinemia exhibited by this patient and none had similar neutrophil abnormalities. We did not attempt to document subtle chemotactic deficiencies, however.

So I think that a lot of these syndromes are going to turn out to be carts and not horses. I would like to make a plea that maybe we ought not to write so many case reports and try to use a little logic and pin these things down a little more strongly.

Dr. Leddy: There was a paper in *Blood* (24a), of which Harry Jacob was an author, in which they demonstrated abnormal chemotaxis in an individual undergoing a severe immunologic drug reaction, and associated with this was a profound drop in complement. After the disorder ran its course, the complement levels came back to normal and then the neutrophils exhibited normal chemotactic behavior. This, I think is an example of a "cart" phenomenon, rather than "horse." Something in the products of an acute immunologic reaction, no doubt affected neutrophils, so that they were unresponsive. And this happened to be a very acute reaction, so you could observe the "before" and "after" effect. I think this just adds another point along those lines.

REFERENCES

1. Abramson, N., Alper, C. A., Lachmann, P. J., Rosen, F. S., and Jandl, J. H. (1971): Deficiency of C3 inactivator in man. *J. Immunol.,* 107:19–27.
2. Agnello, V., de Bracco, M. M. E., and Kunkel, H. G. (1972): Hereditary C2 deficiency with some manifestations of systemic lupus erythematosus. *J. Immunol.,* 108:837–840.
3. Alper, C. A., Abramson, N., Johnston, R. B., Jandl, J. H., and Rosen, F. S. (1970): Increased susceptibility to infection associated with abnormalities of complement-mediated functions and of the third component of complement. *N. Engl. J. Med.,* 282:349–354.
4. Alper, C. A., Abramson, N., Johnston, R. B., Jandl, J. H., and Rosen, F. S. (1970): Studies *in vivo* and *in vitro* on an abnormality in the metabolism of C3 in a patient with increased susceptibility to infection. *J. Clin. Invest.,* 49:1975–1985.
5. Alper, C. A., Bloch, K. J., and Rosen, F. S. (1973): Increased susceptibility to infection in a patient with type II essential hypercatabolism of C3. *N. Engl. J. Med.,* 288:601–606.
6. Alper, C. A., Colten, H. R., Rosen, F. S., Rabson, A. R., MacNab, G. M., and Gear, J. S. S. (1972): Homozygous deficiency of C3 in a patient with repeated infections. *Lancet,* 2:1179–1181.
7. Alper, C. A., Rosen, F. S., and Lachmann, P. J. (1972): Inactivator of the third component of complement as an inhibitor in the properdin pathway. *Proc. Natl. Acad. Sci. U.S.A.* 69:2910–2913.
8. Alper, C. A., Stossel, T. P., and Rosen, F. S. (1975): Genetic defects affecting complement and host resistance to infection. In: *The Phagocytic Cell in Host Resistance,* edited by J. Bellanti and D. Dayton, pp. 127–141. Raven Press, New York.
9. Altman, L. C., Furukawa, C. T., and Klebanoff, S. J. (1977): Defective polymorphonuclear leukocyte (PMN) function in thermally injured patients. *Clin. Res.,* 25:117A.
10. Altman, L. C., Snyderman, R., and Blaese, R. M. (1974): Abnormalities of chemotactic lymphokine synthesis and mononuclear leukocyte chemotaxis in Wiskott-Aldrich syndrome. *J. Clin. Invest.,* 54:486–493.
11. Andersen, B. R. (1975): Host factors causing increased susceptibility to infection in patients with Laennec's cirrhosis. *Ann. N. Y. Acad. Sci.,* 252:348–352.
12. Anderson, R., Sher, R., Rabson, A. R., and Koornhof, H. J. (1974): Defective chemotaxis in measles patients. *S. Afr. Med. J.,* 7:1819–1820.
13. Aswanikumar, S., Schiffmann, E., Corcoran, B. A., and Wahl, S. M. (1976): Role of a peptidase in phagocyte chemotaxis. *Proc. Natl. Acad. Sci. U.S.A.,* 73:2439–2442.
14. Bagdade, J. D., and Stewart, M. (1976): Host defense in diabetes mellitus: Impaired granulocyte adherence in poorly controlled diabetic patients. *Clin. Res.,* 24:112A.
15. Baisero, M. H. (1973): Chimiotactisme des polynucléaires humains *in vitro:* III. Etude de L'infection aiguë et chronique de L'adulte. *Schweiz. Med. Wochenschr.,* 103:1599–1605.
16. Ballow, M., Shira, J. E., Harden, L., Yang, S. Y., and Day, N. K. (1975): Complete absence of the third component of complement in man. *J. Clin. Invest.,* 56:703–710.
17. Becker, E. L. (1972): The relationship of the chemotactic behavior of the complement-derived factors, C3a, C5a, and $C\overline{567}$, and a bacterial chemotactic factor to their ability to activate the proesterase 1 of rabbit polymorphonuclear leukocytes. *J. Exp. Med.,* 135:376–387.
18. Becker, E. L., Davis, A. T., Estensen, R. D., and Quie, P. G. (1972): Cytochalasin B: IV. Inhibition and stimulation of chemotaxis of rabbit and human polymorphonuclear leukocytes. *J. Immunol.,* 108:396–402.

19. Becker, E. L., and Showell, H. J. (1974): The ability of chemotactic factors to induce lysosomal enzyme release: II. The mechanism of release. *J. Immunol.*, 112:2055–2062.
20. Beeuwkes, H., and Bijlsma, A. (1974): Reduced chemotaxis of polymorphonuclear leukocytes in sera from patients with rheumatoid arthritis. *Antonie Van Leeuwenhoek*, 40:233–239.
21. Bellanti, J. A., Cantz, B. E., and Schlegel, R. J. (1970); Accelerated decay of glucose 6-phosphate dehydrogenase activity in chronic granulomatous disease. *Pediatr. Res.*, 4:405–411.
22. Berenberg, J. L., and Ward, P. A. (1973): Chemotactic factor inactivator in normal human serum. *J. Clin. Invest.*, 52:1200–1206.
23. Blume, R. S., and Wolff, S. M. (1972): The Chediak-Higashi syndrome: Studies in four patients and a review of the literature. *Medicine*, 51:247–280.
24. Boucek, M. M., and Snyderman, R. (1976): Calcium influx requirement for human neutrophil chemotaxis: Inhibition by lanthanum chloride. *Science*, 193:905–907.
24a. Bowers, T. K., Craddock, P. R., and Jacob, H. S. (1977): Acquired granulocyte abnormality during drug allergic reactions. *Blood*, 49:3–8.
25. Boxer, L. A., Hedley-Whyte, E. T., and Stossel, T. P. (1974): Neutrophil actin dysfunction and abnormal neutrophil behavior. *N. Engl. J. Med.*, 291:1093–1099.
26. Boxer, L. A., Watanabe, A. M., Rister, M., Besch, H. R., Jr., Allen, J., and Baehner, R. L. (1976): Correction of leukocyte function in Chediak-Higashi syndrome by ascorbate. *N. Engl. J. Med.*, 295:1041–1045.
27. Boyer, J. T., Gall, E. P., Norman, M. E., Nilsson, U. R., and Zimmerman, T. S. (1975): Hereditary deficiency of the seventh component of complement. *J. Clin. Invest.*, 56:905–913.
28. Buckley, R. H., Wray, B. B., and Belmaker, E. Z. (1972): Extreme hyperimmunoglobulinemia E and undue susceptibility to infection. *Pediatrics*, 49:59–70.
29. Carruthers, B. M. (1966): Leukocyte motility: I. Method of study, normal variation, effect of physical alterations in environment, and effect of iodoacetate. *Can. J. Physiol. Pharmacol.*, 44:475–485.
30. Carruthers, B. M. (1967): Leukocyte motility: II. Effect of absence of glucose in medium; effect of presence of deoxyglucose, dinitrophenol, puromycin, actinomycin D, and trypsin on the response to chemotactic substance; effect of segregation of cells from chemotactic substance. *Can. J. Physiol. Pharmacol.*, 45:269–280.
31. Church, J. A., Frenkel, L. D., Wright, D. G., and Bellanti, J. A. (1976): T-lymphocyte dysfunction, hyperimmunoglobulinemia-E, recurrent bacterial infections, and defective neutrophil chemotaxis in a Negro child. *J. Pediatr.*, 88:982–985.
32. Chusid, M. J., Gallin, J. I., Dale, D. C., Fauci, A. S., and Wolff, S. M. (1976): Defective polymorphonuclear leukocyte chemotaxis and bactericidal capacity in a boy with recurrent pyogenic infections. *Pediatrics*, 58:513–520.
33. Clark, R. A., Frank, M. M., and Kimball, H. R. (1973): Generation of chemotactic factors in guinea pig serum via activation of the classical and alternate complement pathways. *Clin. Immunol. Immunopathol.*, 1:414–426.
34. Clark, R. A., Hamory, B. H., Ford, G. H., and Kimball, H. R. (1972): Chemotaxis in acute renal failure. *J. Infect. Dis.*, 127:460–463.
35. Clark, R. A., Johnson, F. L., Klebanoff, S. J., and Thomas, E. D. (1976): Defective neutrophil chemotaxis in bone marrow transplant patients. *J. Clin. Invest.*, 58:22–31.
36. Clark, R. A., and Kimball, H. R. (1971): Defective granulocyte chemotaxis in the Chediak-Higashi syndrome. *J. Clin. Invest.*, 50:2645–2652.
37. Clark, R. A., Kimball, H. R., and Decker, J. L. (1974): Neutrophil chemotaxis in systemic lupus erythematosus. *Ann. Rheum. Dis.*, 33:167–172.
38. Clark, R. A., Kimball, H. R., and Padgett, G. A. (1972): Granulocyte chemotaxis in the Chediak-Higashi syndrome of mink. *Blood*, 39:644–649.
39. Clark, R., Klebanoff, S., Ochs, H., Gilliland, B., Schaller, J., and Wedgwood, R. (1975): C4 deficient human serum: Opsonic and chemotactic activity. *Clin. Res.*, 23:410A.
40. Clark, R. A., Root, R. K., Kimball, H. R., and Kirkpatrick, C. H. (1973): Defective neutrophil chemotaxis and cellular immunity in a child with recurrent infections. *Ann. Intern. Med.*, 78:515–519.
41. Craddock, P. R., Yawata, Y., Van Santen, L., Gilberstadt, S., Silvis, S., and Jacob, H. S. (1974): Acquired phagocyte dysfunction: A complication of the hypophosphatemia of parenteral hyperalimentation. *N. Engl. J. Med.*, 290:1403–1407.
42. Dahl, M. V., Matula, G., Leonards, R., and Tuffanelli, D. L. (1975): Incontinentia pigmenti and defective neutrophil chemotaxis. *Arch. Dermatol.*, 111:1603–1605.

43. Day, N. K., Geiger, H., McLean, R., Michael, A., and Good, R. A. (1973): C2 deficiency: Development of lupus erythematosus. *J. Clin. Invest.*, 52:1601–1607.
44. DeMeo, A. N., and Andersen, B. R. (1972): Defective chemotaxis associated with a serum inhibitor in cirrhotic patients. *N. Engl. J. Med.*, 286:735–740.
45. Edelson, P. J., Stites, D. P., Gold, S., and Fudenberg, H. H. (1973): Disorders of neutrophil function: Defects in the early stages of the phagocytic process. *Clin. Exp. Immunol.*, 13:21–28.
46. Einstein, L. P., Alper, C. A., Bloch, K. J., Herrin, J. T., Rosen, F. S., David, J. R., and Colten, H. R. (1975): Biosynthetic defect in monocytes from human beings with genetic deficiency of the second component of complement. *N. Engl. J. Med.*, 292:1169–1171.
47. Frei, P. C., Baisero, M. H., and Ochsner, M. (1974): Chemotaxis of human polymorphonuclears *in vitro:* Critical study of clinical interpretations. *Antibiot. Chemother.*, 19:350–361.
48. Friend, P., Repine, J. E., Kim, Y., Clawson, C. C., and Michael, A. F. (1975): Deficiency of the second component of complement (C2) with chronic vasculitis. *Ann. Intern. Med.*, 83:813–816.
49. Gallin, J. I. (1975): Abnormal chemotaxis: Cellular and humoral components. In: *The Phagocytic Cell in Host Resistance*, edited by J. A. Bellanti and D. H. Dayton, pp. 227–248. Raven Press, New York.
50. Gallin, J. I., Bujak, J. S., Patten, E., and Wolff, S. M. (1974): Granulocyte function in the Chediak-Higashi syndrome of mice. *Blood*, 43:201–206.
51. Gallin, J. I., Clark, R. A., and Frank, M. M. (1975): Kinetic analysis of the generation of the chemotactic factor in human serum via activation of the classical and alternate complement pathways. *Clin. Immunol. Immunopathol.*, 3:334–346.
52. Gallin, J. I., Clark, R. A., and Kimball, H. R. (1973): Granulocyte chemotaxis: An improved *in vitro* assay employing ^{51}Cr-labelled granulocytes. *J. Immunol.*, 110:233–240.
53. Gallin, J. I., Durocher, J. R., and Kaplan, A. P. (1975): Interaction of leukocyte chemotactic factors with the cell surface: I. Chemotactic factor-induced changes in human granulocyte surface charge. *J. Clin. Invest.*, 55:967–974.
54. Gallin, J. I., and Kirkpatrick, C. H. (1974): Chemotactic activity in dialyzable transfer factor. *Proc. Natl. Acad. Sci. U.S.A.*, 71:498–502.
55. Gallin, J. I., Klimerman, J. A., Padgett, G. A., and Wolff, S. M. (1975): Defective mononuclear leukocyte chemotaxis in the Chediak-Higashi syndrome of humans, mink, and cattle. *Blood*, 45:863–870.
56. Gallin, J. I., and Rosenthal, A. S. (1974): The regulatory role of divalent cations in human granulocyte chemotaxis: Evidence for an association between calcium exchanges and microtubule assembly. *J. Cell Biol.*, 62:594–609.
57. Gallin, J. I., and Wolff, S. M. (1975): Leucocyte chemotaxis: Physiological considerations and abnormalities. *Clin. Heamatol.*, 4:567–607.
58. Gallin, J. I., Wright, D. G., Fauci, A. S., Rosenwasser, L. J., Chusid, M. J., Taylor, H. A., Thomas, G., Libaers, I., Shapiro, L. J., and Neufeld, E. F. (1976): Defective leukocyte chemotaxis in mannosidosis. *Clin. Res.*, 24:344A.
59. Gewurz, H., Page, A. R., Pickering, R. J., and Good, R. A. (1967): Complement activity and inflammatory neutrophil exudation in man. Studies in patients with glomerulonephritis, essential hypocomplementemia and agammaglobulinemia. *Int. Arch. Allergy Appl. Immunol.*, 32:64–90.
60. Hauptmann, G., Grosshans, E., Heid, E., Mayer, S., and Basset, A. (1974): Lupus érythémateux aigu avec déficit complet de la fraction C4 du complément. *Nouv. Presse Med.*, 3:881–884.
61. Higgins, G. R., Swanson, V., and Yamazaki, J. (1970): Granulocytasthenia: A unique leukocyte dysfunction associated with decreased resistance to infection. *Clin. Res.*, 18:209.
62. Hill, H. R., Estensen, R. D., Hogan, N. A., and Quie, P. G. (1976): Severe staphylococcal disease associated with allergic manifestations, hyperimmunoglobulinemia E and defective neutrophil chemotaxis. *J. Lab. Clin. Med.*, 88:796–806.
63. Hill, H. R., Estensen, R. D., Quie, P. G., Hogan, N. A., and Goldberg, N. D. (1975): Modulation of human neutrophil chemotactic responses by cyclic 3′,5′-guanosine monophosphate and cyclic 3′,5′-adenosine monophosphate. *Metabolism*, 24:447–456.
64. Hill, H. R., Gerrard, J. M., Hogan, N. A., and Quie, P. G. (1974): Hyperactivity of neutrophil leukotactic responses during active bacterial infection. *J. Clin. Invest.*, 53:996–1002.
65. Hill, H. R., Kaplan, E. L., Dajani, A. S., Wannamaker, L. W., and Quie, P. G. (1974):

Leukotactic activity and reduction of nitroblue tetrazolium by neutrophil granulocytes from patients with streptococcal skin infection. *J. Infect. Dis.,* 129:322–326.

66. Hill, H. R., Ochs, H. D., Quie, P. G., Clark, R. A., Pabst, H. F., Klebanoff, S. J., and Wedgwood, R. J. (1974): Defect in neutrophil granulocyte chemotaxis in Job's syndrome of recurrent "cold" staphylococcal abscesses. *Lancet,* 2:617–619.
67. Hill, H. R., and Quie, P. G. (1974): Raised serum-IgE levels and defective neutrophil chemotaxis in three children with eczema and recurrent bacterial infections. *Lancet* 1:183–187.
68. Hill, H. R., and Quie, P. G. (1975): Defective neutrophil chemotaxis associated with hyperimmunoglobulinemia E. In, *The Phagocytic Cell in Host Resistance,* edited by J. A. Bellanti and D. H. Dayton, pp. 249–266. Raven Press, New York.
69. Hill, H. R., Sauls, H. S., Dettloff, J. L., and Quie, P. G. (1974): Impaired leukotactic responsiveness in patients with juvenile diabetes mellitus. *Clin. Immunol. Immunopathol.,* 2:395–403.
70. Hill, H. R., Warwick, W. J., Dettloff, J., and Quie, P. G. (1974): Neutrophil granulocyte function in patients with pulmonary infection. *J. Pediatr.,* 84:55–58.
71. Hill, H. R., Williams, P. B., Krueger, G. G., and Janis, B. (1976): Recurrent staphylococcal abscesses associated with defective neutrophil chemotaxis and allergic rhinitis. *Ann. Intern. Med.,* 85:39–43.
72. Humbert, J. R., Hammond, K. B., Hathaway, W. E., Marcoux, J. G., and O'Brient, D. (1970): Trimethylaminuria: The fish-odour syndrome. *Lancet,* 2:770–771.
73. Jacobs, J. C., and Miller, M. E. (1972): Fatal familial Leiner's disease: A deficiency of the opsonic activity of serum complement. *Pediatrics,* 49:225–232.
74. Khan, A. J., Evans, H. E., Glass, L., Shin, Y. H., and Almonte, D. (1975): Defective neutrophil chemotaxis in patients with Down syndrome. *J. Pediatr.,* 87:87–89.
75. Leddy, J. P., Frank, M., Gaither, T., Baum, J., and Klemperer, M. R. (1974): Hereditary deficiency of the sixth component of complement in man: I. Immunochemical, biologic and family studies. *J. Clin. Invest.,* 53:544–553.
76. Leddy, J. P., Griggs, R. C., Klemperer, M. R., and Frank, M. M. (1975): Hereditary complement (C2) deficiency with dermatomyositis. *Am. J. Med.,* 58:83–91.
77. Leimgruber, A., Frei, P. C., Ochsner, M., Schubert, M., and Saudan, Y. (1975): Chimiotactisme des polynucleaires humains in vitro. Etude dans les maladies rhumatismales inflammatoires. *Schweiz. Med. Wochenschr.,* 105:1730–1732.
78. Lim, D., Gewurz, A., Lint, T. F., Ghaze, M., Sepheri, B., and Gewurz, H. (1976): Absence of the sixth component of complement in a patient with repeated episodes of meningococcal meningitis. *J. Pediatr.,* 89:42–47.
79. MacGregor, R. R., Spagnuolo, P. J., and Lentnek, A. L. (1974): Inhibition of granulocyte adherence by ethanol, prednisone, and aspirin, measured with an assay system. *N. Engl. J. Med.,* 291:642–646.
80. Maderazo, E. G., Ward, P. A., and Quintiliani, R. (1975): Defective regulation of chemotaxis in cirrhosis. *J. Lab. Clin. Med.,* 85:621–630.
81. Maderazo, E. G., Ward, P. A., Woronick, C. L., Kubik, J., DeGraff, A. C., Jr. (1976): Leukotactic dysfunction in sarcoidosis. *Ann. Intern. Med.,* 84:414–419.
82. Magliulo, E., and Benzi-Cipelli, R. (1975): Impaired leukotaxis in viral hepatitis B. *N. Engl. J. Med.,* 293:303–304.
83. Martin, R. R., Warr, A., Couch, R., and Knight, V. (1973): Chemotaxis of human leukocytes: Responsiveness to mycoplasma pneumoniae. *J. Lab. Clin. Med.,* 81:520–529.
84. McCall, C. E., Caves, J., Cooper, R., and DeChatelet, L. (1971): Functional characteristics of human toxic neutrophils. *J. Infect. Dis.* 124:68–75.
85. Miller, M. E. (1971): Chemotactic function in the human neonate: Humoral and cellular aspects. *Pediatr. Res.,* 5:487–492.
86. Miller, M. E. (1975): Developmental maturation of human neutrophil motility and its relationship to membrane deformability. In: *The Phagocytic Cell in Host Resistance,* edited by J. A. Bellanti and D. H. Dayton, pp. 295–307. Raven Press, New York.
87. Miller, M. E. (1975): Pathology of chemotaxis and random motility. *Semin. Hematol.,* 12:59–82.
88. Miller, M. E., and Baker, L. (1972): Leukocyte functions in juvenile diabetes mellitus: Humoral and cellular aspects. *J. Pediatr.,* 81:979–982.
89. Miller, M. E., and Nilsson, U. R. (1970): A familial deficiency of the phagocytosis-enhancing activity of serum related to a dysfunction of the fifth component of complement (C5). *N. Engl. J. Med.,* 282:354–358.

90. Miller, M. E., Norman, M. E., Koblenzer, P. J., and Schonauer, T. (1973): A new familial defect of neutrophil movement. *J. Lab. Clin. Med.*, 82:1–8.

91. Miller, M. E., Oski, F. A., and Harris, M. B. (1971): Lazy-leukocyte syndrome: A new disorder of neutrophil function. *Lancet,* 1:665–669.

92. Miller, M. E., Seals, J., Kaye, R., and Levitsky, L. C. (1968): A familial, plasma-associated defect of phagocytosis. *Lancet,* 2:60–63.

93. Mowat, A. G., and Baum, J. (1971): Chemotaxis of polymorphonuclear leukocytes from patients with diabetes mellitus. *N. Engl. J. Med.*, 284:621–627.

94. Mowat, A. G., and Baum, J. (1971): Chemotaxis of polymorphonuclear leukocytes from patients with rheumatoid arthritis. *J. Clin. Invest.*, 50:2541–2549.

95. Mowat, A. G., and Baum, J. (1971): Polymorphonuclear leucocyte chemotaxis in patients with bacterial infections. *Br. Med. J.,* 3:617–619.

96. Nicol, P. A. E., and Lachmann, P. J. (1973): The alternate pathway of complement activation: The role of C3 and its inactivator (KAF). *Immunology,* 24:259–275.

97. Nilsson, U. R., Miller, M. E., and Wyman, S. (1974): A functional abnormality of the fifth component of complement (C5) from human serum of individuals with a familial opsonic defect. *J. Immunol.,* 112:1164–1176.

98. Ochs, H. D., Clark, R. A., Klebanoff, S. J., and Wedgwood, R. J. (1974): Impaired host defense mechanisms in the Wiskott-Aldrich syndrome. Program and abstracts, 14th Interscience Conference on Antimicrobial Agents and Chemotherapy, No. 142.

99. Oliver, J. M., Krawiec, J. A., and Berlin, R. D. (1976): Carbamylcholine prevents giant granule formation in cultured fibroblasts from beige (Chediak-Higashi) mice. *J. Cell Biol.,* 69:205–210.

100. Oliver, J. M., Zurier, R. B., and Berlin, R. D. (1975): Concanavalin A cap formation on polymorphonuclear leukocytes of normal and beige (Chediak-Higashi) mice. *Nature,* 253:471–473.

101. Oliver, J. M., and Zurier, R. B. (1976): Correction of characteristic abnormalities of microtubule function and granule morphology in Chediak-Higashi syndrome with cholinergic agonists. *J. Clin. Invest.,* 57:1239–1247.

102. Osterland, C. K., Espinoza, L., Parker, L. P., and Schur, P. H. (1975): Inherited C2 deficiency and systemic lupus erythematosus: Studies on a family. *Ann. Intern. Med.,* 82:323–328.

103. Peters, D. K., Williams, D. G., Charlesworth, J. A., Boulton-Jones, J. M., Sissons, J. G. P., Evans, D. J., Kourilsky, O., and Morel-Maroger, L. (1973): Mesangiocapillary nephritis, partial lipodystrophy, and hypocomplementaemia. *Lancet,* 2:535–538.

104. Petersen, B. H., Graham, J. A., and Brooks, G. F. (1976): Human deficiency of 8th component of complement: The requirement of C8 for serum *Neisseria gonorrhoeae* bactericidal activity. *J. Clin. Invest.,* 57:283–290.

105. Pincus, S. H., Thomas, I. T., Clark, R. A., and Ochs, H. D. (1975): Defective neutrophil chemotaxis with variant icthyosis, hyperimmunoglobulinemia E and recurrent infections. *J. Pediatr.* 87:908–911.

106. Root, R. K. (1975): Comparison of other defects of granulocyte oxidative killing mechanisms with chronic granulomatous disease. In: *The Phagocytic Cell in Host Resistance,* edited by J. A. Bellanti and D. H. Dayton, pp. 201–226. Raven Press, New York.

107. Root, R. K., Rosenthal, A. S., and Balestra, D. J. (1972): Abnormal bactericidal, metabolic, and lysosomal functions of Chediak-Higashi syndrome leukocytes. *J. Clin. Invest.,* 51:649–665.

108. Rosenfeld, S. I., Baum, J., Steigbigel, R. T., and Leddy, J. P. (1976): Hereditary deficiency of 5th component of complement in man: II. Biological properties of C5-deficient human serum. *J. Clin. Invest.,* 57:1635–1643.

109. Rosenfeld, S. I., Kelly, M. E., and Leddy, J. P. (1976): Hereditary deficiency of 5th component of complement in man: I. Clinical, immunochemical, and family studies. *J. Clin. Invest.,* 57:1626–1634.

110. Ruby, E. J., Huang, S.-W., Plant, J., and Morris, N. (1976): Defective phagocytic adherence in acute poststreptococcal glomerulonephritis: Clinical and laboratory observations. *J. Pediatr.,* 89:758–754.

111. Seger, R., Wildfeuer, A., Buchinger, G., Romen, W., Catty, D., Dybas, L., Haferkamp, O., and Stroder, J. (1976): Defects in granulocyte function in various chromosome abnormalities. *Klin. Wochenschr.,* 54:177–183.

112. Singh, H., Boyd, E., Hutton, M. M., Wilkinson, P. C., Brown, D. A. P., and Ferguson-

Smith, M. A. (1972): Chromosomal mutation in bone-marrow as cause of acquired granulomatous disease and refractory macrocytic anemia. *Lancet* 1:873–879.

113. Sissons, J. G., West, R. J., Fallows, J., Williams, D. G., Boucher, B. J., Amos, N., and Peters, D. K. (1976): The complement abnormalities of lipodystrophy. *N. Engl. J. Med.,* 294:461–465.

114. Smith, C. W., Hollers, J. C., Dupree, E., Goldman, A. S., and Lord, R. A. (1972): A serum inhibitor of leukotaxis in a child with recurrent infections. *J. Lab. Clin. Med.,* 79:878–885.

115. Snyderman, R., Altman, L. C., Frankel, A., and Blaese, R. M. (1973): Defective mononuclear leukocyte chemotaxis: A previously unrecognized immune dysfunction; studies in a patient with chronic mucocutaneous candidiasis. *Ann. Intern. Med.,* 78:509–513.

116. Snyderman, R., Gewurz, H., and Mergenhagen, S. E. (1968): Interactions of the complement system with endotoxic lipopolysaccharide: Generation of a factor chemotactic for polymorphonuclear leukocytes. *J. Exp. Med.,* 128:259–275.

117. Snyderman, R., and Pike, M. C. (1976): An inhibitor of macrophage chemotaxis produced by neoplasms. *Science,* 192:370–372.

118. Snyderman, R., Pike, M. C., and Altman, L. C. (1975): Abnormalities of leukocyte chemotaxis in human disease. *Ann. N. Y. Acad. Sci.,* 256:386–401.

119. Snyderman, R., Shin, H. S., Phillips, J. K., Gewurz, H., and Mergenhagen, S. E. (1969): A neutrophil chemotactic factor derived from C′5 upon interaction of guinea pig serum with endotoxin. *J. Immunol.,* 103:413–422.

120. Snyderman, R., and Stahl, C. (1975): Defective immune effector function in patients with neoplastic and immune deficiency diseases. In: *The Phagocytic Cell in Host Resistance,* edited by J. A. Bellanti and D. H. Dayton, pp. 267–281. Raven Press, New York.

121. Soriano, R. B., South, M. A., Goldman, A. S., and Smith, C. W. (1973): Defect of neutrophil motility in a child with recurrent bacterial infections and disseminated cytomegalovirus infection. *J. Pediatr.,* 83:951–958.

122. Steerman, R. L., Snyderman, R., Leiken, S. L., and Colten, H. R. (1971): Intrinsic defect of the polymorphonuclear leucocyte resulting in impaired chemotaxis and phagocytosis. *Clin. Exp. Immunol.,* 9:939–946.

123. Sussman, M., Jones, J. H., Almeida, J. D., and Lachmann, P. J. (1973): Deficiency of the second component of complement associated with anaphylactoid purpura and presence of mycoplasma in the serum. *Clin. Exp. Immunol.,* 14:531–539.

124. Tan, J. S., Strauss, R. G., Akabutu, J., Kauffman, C. A., Mauer, A. M., and Phair, J. P. (1974): Persistent neutrophil dysfunction in an adult; combined defect in chemotaxis, phagocytosis and intracellular killing. *Am. J. Med.,* 57:251–258.

125. Territo, M. C., and Golde, D. W. (1976): Granulocyte function in experimental human endotoxemia. *Blood,* 47:539–544.

126. Thompson, R. A., and White, R. H. R. (1973): Partial lipodystrophy and hypocomplementaemic nephritis. *Lancet,* 2:679.

127. Till, G., and Ward, P. A. (1975): Two distinct chemotactic factor inactivators in human serum. *J. Immunol.,* 114:843–847.

128. Van Epps, D. E., Frierson, J. A., and Williams, R. C., Jr. (1974): Immunological studies of anergic patients. *Infect. Immun.,* 10:1003–1009.

129. Van Epps, D. E., Palmer, D. L., and Williams, R. C. (1974): Characterization of serum inhibitors of neutrophil chemotaxis associated with anergy. *J. Immunol.,* 113:189–200.

130. Van Epps, D. E., Strickland, R. G., and Williams, R. C., Jr. (1975): Inhibitors of leukocyte chemotaxis in alcoholic liver disease. *Am. J. Med.,* 59:200–207.

131. Van Epps, D. E., and Williams, R. C., Jr. (1976): Serum chemotactic inhibitory activity: Heat activation of chemotactic inhibition. *Infect. Immun.,* 13:741–749.

132. Van Epps, D. E., Williams, R. C., Jr. (1976): Suppression of leukocyte chemotaxis by human IgA myeloma components. *J. Exp. Med.,* 144:1227–1242.

133. Van Scoy, R. E., Hill, H. R., Ritts, R. E., and Quie, P. G. (1975): Familial neutrophil chemotaxis defect, recurrent bacterial infections, mucocutaneous candidiasis, and hyperimmunoglobulinemia E. *Ann. Intern. Med.,* 82:766–771.

134. Ward, P. A. (1974): Leukotaxis and leukotactic disorders: A review. *Am. J. Pathol.,* 77:520–538.

135. Ward, P. A., Anton, T., and Maderazo, E. (1976): Defective leukotaxis in cancer patients. *Clin. Res.,* 24:463A.

136. Ward, P. A., and Berenberg, J. L. (1974): Defective regulation of inflammatory mediators

in Hodgkin's disease: Supernormal levels of chemotactic-factor inactivator. *N. Engl. J. Med.,* 290:76–80.

137. Ward, P. A., Cochrane, C. G., and Müller-Eberhard, H. J. (1965): The role of serum complement in chemotaxis of leukocytes *in vitro. J. Exp. Med.,* 122:327–347.

138. Ward, P. A., Goralnick, S., and Bullock, W. E. (1976): Defective leukotaxis in patients with lepromatous leprosy. *J. Lab. Clin. Med.,* 87:1025–1032.

139. Ward, P. A., and Ozols, J. (1976): Characterization of protease activity in chemotactic factor inactivator. *J. Clin. Invest.,* 58:123–129.

140. Ward, P. A., and Schlegel, R. A. (1969): Impaired leucotactic responsiveness in a child with recurrent infections. *Lancet,* 2:344–347.

141. Ward, P. A., and Talamo, R. C. (1973): Deficiency of the chemotactic factor inactivator in human sera with α_1-antitrypsin deficiency. *J. Clin. Invest.,* 52:516–519.

142. Warden, G. D., Mason, A. D., and Pruitt, B. A. (1974): Evaluation of leukocyte chemotaxis *in vitro* in thermally injured patients. *J. Clin. Invest.,* 54:1001–1004.

143. Warden, G. D., Mason, A. D., Jr., and Pruitt, B. A., Jr. (1975): Suppression of leukocyte chemotaxis *in vitro* by chemotherapeutic agents used in the management of thermal injuries. *Ann. Surg.,* 181:363–369.

144. Weiss, A. S., Gallin, J. I., and Kaplan, A. P. (1974): Fletcher factor deficiency: A diminished rate of Hageman factor activation caused by absence of prekallikrein with abnormalities of coagulation, fibrinolysis, chemotactic activity, and kinin generation. *J. Clin. Invest.,* 53:622–633.

145. Wellek, B., and Opferkuch, W. (1975): A case of deficiency of the seventh component of complement in man: Biological properties of a C7-deficient serum and description of a C7-inactivating principle. *Clin. Exp. Immunol.,* 19:223–235.

146. Wilkinson, P. C. (1974): *Chemotaxis and Inflammation.* Churchill-Livingstone, Edinburgh.

147. Witemeyer, S., and Van Epps, D. E. (1976): Familial defect in cellular chemotaxis associated with redheadedness and recurrent infection. *J. Pediatr.,* 89:33–37.

148. Wright, D. G., Kirkpatrick, C. H., and Gallin, J. I. (1976): Effects of levamisole on normal and abnormal leukocyte locomotion. *Clin. Res.,* 24:455A.

149. Ziegler, J. B., Alper, C. A., Rosen, F. S., Lachmann, P. J., and Sherington, L. (1975): Restoration by purified C3b inactivator of complement-mediated function *in vivo* in a patient with C3b inactivator deficiency. *J. Clin. Invest.,* 55:668–672.

150. Zigmond, S. H., and Hirsch, J. G. (1972): Effects of cytochalasin B on polymorphonuclear leucocyte locomotion, phagocytosis and glycolysis. *Exp. Cell. Res.,* 73:383–393.

Leukocyte Chemotaxis, edited by John I. Gallin
and Paul G. Quie. Raven Press, New York
© 1978.

Pathophysiologic Aspects of Leukocyte Chemotaxis: Identification of a Specific Chemotactic Factor Binding Site on Human Granulocytes and Defects of Macrophage Function Associated with Neoplasia

Ralph Snyderman and Marilyn C. Pike

Division of Rheumatic and Genetic Diseases, Departments of Medicine and Microbiology and Immunology, Duke University Medical Center, Durham, North Carolina 27710

Degradation of antigens by leukocytes is the final link in a chain of events by which the immune system protects the complex biochemical integrity of the host against microbial invasion and probably the development of neoplasms. The rapid accumulation of phagocytic wandering cells at sites of antigenic penetration or neoplastic transformation appears to be essential for normal immune function. One mechanism which can lead to the local accumulation of motile cells is chemotaxis, the unidirectional migration of cells along a concentration gradient of a chemoattractant. It is quite clear that immune effector cells such as polymorphonuclear leukocytes and macrophages can migrate along certain chemical gradients (32,33). The directed migration of leukocytes in response to chemotactic gradients is a complex series of biochemical phenomena requiring recognition of chemical signals by the cell membrane, the triggering of energy-forming processes within the cell, and the translation of this energy by cytostructural elements into movement. The events which result in the directed migration of motile cells, as a consequence of their exposure to chemotactic gradients, are obscure at this time; however, several lines of evidence suggest that chemotactic factor binding to leukocytes, divalent cation fluxes, activation of certain metabolic pathways, and polymerization of actomyosin-like molecules within the cells are required for cell movement (1,3,6,10–12,44). In the following material, we will review the evidence available from this laboratory pertaining to certain recognition and translation phenomena associated with chemotaxis. We will describe the effects of several pharmacologic and infectious agents on the directed migration of leukocytes. Finally, we will demonstrate how methodology for studying leukotaxis can be applied to clinical investigation and demonstrate that neoplasia is associated with cell specific defects of monocyte-macrophage migration *in vitro* and *in vivo.*

RECOGNITION OF CHEMOTACTIC GRADIENTS

The exact mechanisms by which chemotactic gradients are recognized by leukocytes is as yet unknown; however, there is evidence to suggest that specific binding of chemotactic molecules to the cells is required (1,44). In addition, data suggest that chemotactic molecules which are relatively hydrophobic may impart to the cell membrane the energy needed for the initiation of a chemotactic response.

Schiffmann et al. have demonstrated that blocked *N*-formyl-methionyl peptides are potent chemotactic factors for polymorphonuclear leukocytes and macrophages (26). Since bacteria initiate protein synthesis with *N*-formyl-methionine, mammalian leukocytes may have evolved binding sites to detect *N*-formyl-methionyl peptides and thereby direct the migration of phagocytic cells toward microorganisms which have entered the internal milieu. The availability of these peptides with greater than 95% purity has allowed the determination of whether specific binding sites for these substances are present on human PMNs (44). Tritiated *N*-formyl-methionyl-leucyl-phenylalanine([³H]FMLP) of high specific radioactivity (40 Ci/mmol) and chemotactic activity enabled the identification of specific binding sites for the peptide on isolated human PMNs. The binding of [³H] FMLP was rapid, with the time for half maximal binding less than 2 minutes at 37°C (Fig. 1). The [³H] FMLP binding, which reached equilibrium in 12 min, was readily reversed by adding a large excess (10 μm) of unlabeled FMLP to an equilibriated mixture of [³H] FMLP and PMNs (Fig. 1). [³H] FMLP binding was saturable approaching a concentration of 70 to 80 fMol per milligram of protein, which corresponded to approximately 2,000 binding sites per PMN. The equilibrium dissociation constant for the interaction of FMLP with the PMN binding sites was 12 to 14 nM. It should be noted that

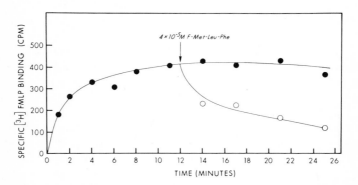

FIG. 1. Time course of [³H] FMLP binding to PMNs. [³H] FMLP (6 nM) was incubated with human PMNs for the indicated time intervals at 37°C and specific binding was assayed. (-●-) To some incubation mixtures (-○-) a large excess of unlabeled FMLP (4 × 10⁻⁵ M) was added after 12 min of incubation and [³H] FMLP binding was assayed at subsequent time intervals as indicated. Each value shown represents the mean of determinations from two separate incubation mixtures. (From Williams et al., ref. 44, with permission.)

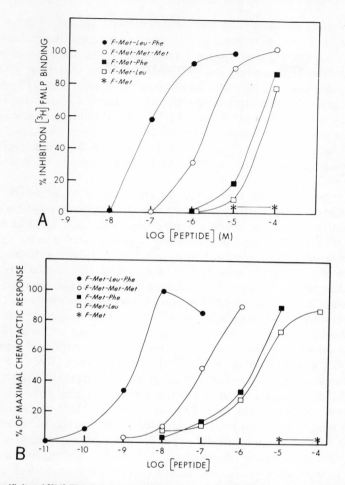

FIG. 2. Specificity of [³H] FMLP binding sites toward chemotactically active peptides. **A:** Effects of *N*-formyl-methionyl peptides on [³H] FMLP binding. [³H] FMLP was incubated with human PMNs in the presence of the indicated concentrations of f-met-leu-phe (-●-), f-met-met-met (-0-), f-met-phe (-■-), f-met-leu (-□-), or f-met (-*-). Specific binding was determined and the percent inhibition of [³H] FMLP binding caused by each concentration of unlabeled peptides was computed. Each value represents the mean of duplicate determinations from 2 to 4 separate experiments. **B:** Chemotactic activity of *N*-formyl-methionyl peptides. Legend for peptides is that as indicated in **A**. The maximal response to 10^{-8} M FMLP was 102 cells per high-power field. Each value represents the mean of triplicate determinations. (From Williams et al., ref. 44, with permission.)

the binding studies using [³H] FMLP are performed in protein-free medium using extensively washed cells. Neither chemotaxis nor binding requires protein in the medium.

We next determined whether the specificity of the [³H] FMLP binding sites correlated with the specificity of the chemotactic response to a series of *N*-

formyl-methionyl peptides. The relative potencies of several of these peptides as chemotactic agents were compared to their relative abilities to compete for the [³H] FMLP binding sites. Figure 2 demonstrates that the order of potencies of these peptides in competing for [³H] FMLP binding sites (Fig. 2A) exactly paralleled their order of potencies as chemotactic agents (Fig. 2B). A plot of the correlation of concentrations giving half-maximal chemotactic responses and causing half-maximal inhibition of [³H] FMLP binding is shown in Fig. 3. Excellent correlation between binding data and the chemotactic response ($r = 0.998$) indicates that the [³H] FMLP binding sites have the specificity expected of receptor sites which mediate the PMN response to chemotactic peptides (44).

Several substances were then tested for their ability to inhibit or compete with [³H] FMLP binding. Neither sodium azide (0.01 M), nor tosyl-L-phenylalanyl chloromethane, an irreversible inhibitor of protease activity, had any effect on [³H] FMLP binding. C5a, a structurally dissimilar chemotactic agent from the *N*-formyl-methionyl peptides, had no effect on [³H] FMLP binding at concentrations of C5a which were 10-fold higher than that which gave a half-maximal chemotactic response. This finding indicates that there may be different cellular sites of interaction for different types of chemotactic substances. Alternatively, it is possible that some substances may not require specific binding sites to exert their chemotactic activity. The positional isomer of f-met-phe, f-phe-met, which inhibits the chemotactic response to formyl-methionyl peptides, behaved as a competitive antagonist of [³H] FMLP binding ($K_D = 9 \times 10^{-5}$ M). Erythrocytes and column-purified lymphocytes demonstrated little or no binding of [³H] FMLP. A mononuclear cell preparation containing 81% lymphocytes and 19% monocytes bound only 29% as much as PMN preparations; this amount of binding might be largely accounted for by binding to the monocytes which also respond chemotactically to the formyl-methionyl peptides.

In summary, these studies demonstrate that specific binding sites for peptide chemotactic factors are present on human polymorphonuclear leukocytes and

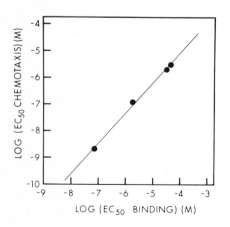

FIG. 3. Correlation of affinity for [³H] FMLP binding sites with chemotactic potency of *N*-formyl-methionyl peptides. The concentrations of each peptide causing half-maximal inhibition of [³H] FMLP binding (EC$_{50}$ binding) or chemotactic response (EC$_{50}$ chemotaxis) were computed from data in Fig. 2A and B, respectively. No values could be computed for the compound f-met, since it neither inhibited binding nor stimulated chemotaxis over the concentration range tested. (From Williams et al., ref. 44, with permission.)

are in agreement with the work of Schiffmann's group (1), who have demonstrated specific binding sites for N-formylated peptides on rabbit neutrophils. Our studies, moreover, show that binding of a peptide to the PMN is of itself not sufficient to trigger a chemotactic response, since a positional isomer of f-met-phe is a competitive antagonist for chemotaxis. The translation of receptor binding to a chemotactic response, therefore, requires at least one additional component. Transmission of sufficient free energy from the ligand to the membrane or binding of an additional proximally related site may be necessary for chemotaxis to occur. There are currently no data concerning the role of specific receptors for other chemotactic factors such as C5a, oxidized lipids, or denatured proteins. It seems reasonable to hypothesize that high-potency chemotactic peptides such as C5a would bind to specific receptor sites. Low-potency chemotactic materials such as denatured proteins could conceivably trigger chemotaxis upon interacting with the cell membrane via relatively weak attractive forces (i.e., hydrophobic effects). The possibility that some substances could initiate chemotaxis without direct binding to the membrane but via altering the polar forces of water around the membrane remains an interesting but unproven hypothesis. The recognition by PMNs of N-formyl-methionyl peptides as chemotactic agents via specific binding sites may be analogous to the recognition of specific hormones by hormonally responsive tissues. The availability of chemotactic radioligands should prove to be a most useful tool in further delineating the most sophisticated of cell movements, chemotaxis.

PHYSIOLOGY OF THE CHEMOTACTIC RESPONSE

The finding that neutrophils from several species contain contractile proteins such as actin and myosin (6,27,42) has raised the question of whether divalent cation exchange, and Ca^{2+} in particular, is involved in the directed migration of leukocytes. Lanthanum ion (La^{3+}), which inhibits transmembrane calcium movement, was employed in this laboratory to determine the role of calcium fluctuation in chemotaxis (3). Human neutrophils were placed in modified Boyden chambers in the presence of varying concentrations of La^{3+} and tested for their chemotactic responsiveness (30,32) to endotoxin-activated human serum (AHS) containing equal amounts of La^{3+}. Almost complete inhibition of the chemotactic response occurred at 10^{-3} M La^{3+} and the concentration of La^{3+} which resulted in half-maximal inhibition (ED_{50}) was 5×10^{-4} M. Increasing the external Ca^{2+} concentration decreased the inhibitory effects of La^{3+}. Random motility, as measured by the migration of cells in the absence of chemotactic factor, was also depressed by La^{3+} at doses greater than 10^{-3} M. The chemotactic response of human monocytes was equally depressed by La^{3+} (3). In an attempt to correlate Ca^{2+} flux with chemotaxis, human PMNs were incubated with ^{45}Ca until equilibrium was attained. After such time, incubation was continued in the presence of various concentrations of medium alone or containing various concentrations of La^{3+} and AHS or heated normal serum ($\overline{AHS}$) which served as a nonchemotactic control substance. At various times after the addition of AHS or $\overline{\text{AHS}}$, incubation was terminated by filtration, followed by washing, and the ^{45}Ca content in the cells determined. These experiments indicated that there was a fourfold increase in Ca^{2+} influx in cells incubated in the presence of AHS when compared to cells incubated with $\overline{\text{AHS}}$. The addition of various concentrations of La^{3+} to the incubation mixture resulted in a dose-dependent inhibition of AHS-induced Ca^{2+} influx, $(ED_{50} = 6 \times 10^{-4}$ M) which correlated well with the inhibition of PMN chemotactic responsiveness by La^{3+}. The chemotactically active peptide f-met-phe (26) and the purified chemotactic peptide derived from the fifth component of complement, C5a, also induced Ca^{2+} influx in human neutrophils (3).

These studies suggest that calcium influx is correlated with chemotaxis, and the amount of calcium that enters the cells is sufficient to activate a contractile process. Since the Ca^{2+} influx studies are performed in the absence of a chemotactic factor gradient, it appears that these agents exert their effects in the absence of a gradient. To induce chemotaxis, the gradient may provide a polarized contraction of the leukocytes which results in directed cell movement.

MODULATION OF CHEMOTAXIS BY PHARMACOLOGIC AND INFECTIOUS AGENTS

Reproducible quantitative methods for the study of human monocyte chemotaxis were recently developed (29). The method employs modified Boyden chambers and 5.0 μ pore size polycarbonate (Nuclepore) filters for separation of cell preparations from chemotactic stimuli or control substances. Figure 4 shows that studies carried out using this method can distinguish between chemokinesis and chemotaxis. Cells incubated in the presence of increasing chemotactic factor gradients exhibit increased migration, whereas cells incubated in the presence of increasingly negative chemotactic gradients exhibit less migration through the filter.

Using these methods, this laboratory has studied the effects of several pharmacologic and infectious agents on human monocyte and PMN migratory functions. These agents include prostaglandins, levamisole and its analogs, and several types of common viruses which infect man. The role of prostaglandins (Pg) in inflammation has not been clearly defined, although they have been implicated as being modulators of the inflammatory response (5,15,25). Specifically, it has been demonstrated that some Pg stimulate cAMP levels (4) and inhibit the intracellular killing of candida by PMNs (5) and the PHA-induced blastogenesis of lymphocytes (25). In light of these findings, this laboratory investigated the effect of Pg on the chemotactic responsiveness of human monocytes (19). These studies showed that of the Pg tested, including PGA, PGA_2, PGB, PGB_2, PGE, PGE_2, $PGF_{1\alpha}$, or $PGF_{2\alpha}$, none had direct chemotactic activity in doses ranging from 1.0 pg/ml to 0.1 mg/ml. The incubation of normal monocytes with PGE_2 for 1 hr, however, resulted in a 200% increase in their chemotactic responsiveness to AHS. Cells treated similarly with $PGF_{2\alpha}$ exhibited no such

PERCENTAGE LDCF (v/v) ON BOTTOM OF CHAMBER

		0	10	20	30	40	50
	0	2.8 ± 1.2	28.9 ± 0.5	34.2 ± 1.4	37.8 ± 0.8	33.2 ± 1 7	36.9 ± 1.3
PERCENTAGE LDCF (v/v) IN CELL COMPARTMENT	10	3.7 ± 1.9	12.5 ± 2.2	22.1 ± 1.3	24.5 ± 0.2	26.9 ± 1.3	25.9 ± 0.4
	20	3.2 ± 0.3	12.8 ± 1.3	18.4 ± 1.1	20.9 ± 2.4	23.9 ± 3.3	23.3 ± 2.0
	30	3.6 ± 0.4	12.1 ± 1.0	16.0 ± 1.3	17.6 ± 1.0	16.5 ± 0.8	14.7 ± 1.1
	40	4.6 ± 0.2	10.8 ± 1.9	14.2 ± 1.5	13.5 ± 0.9	17.4 ± 0.4	15.8 ± 0.8
	50	3.8 ± 0.6	9.9 ± 2.1	11.8 ± 0.4	14.9 ± 0.1	14.5 ± 0.7	15.4 ± 1.1

FIG. 4. Chemotaxis and chemokinesis of human blood monocytes to lymphocyte-derived chemotactic factor (LDCF). Isolated monocytes were placed in the upper compartment of a modified Boyden chamber in the presence of medium alone or medium containing the indicated percent (v/v) LDCF and tested for chemotactic responsiveness to medium alone or medium containing the indicated amount of LDCF in the bottom of the chamber. Polycarbonate filters (5 μ) separated the cell compartment from the bottom chamber. Chemotaxis is scored as the average number of monocytes migrating completely through the filter per oil immersion (1,000 X) grid ± SEM. The diagonal line indicates those values obtained when the concentration of chemoattractant on both sides of the filter is identical.

increase of chemotactic responsiveness. The enhancement of chemotaxis produced by PGE_2 could not be correlated directly with increased cAMP levels, and other agents which augment cAMP in leukocytes did not exert stimulatory effects on monocyte chemotaxis (19). These findings implicate some role for PGE_2 in the amplification of monocyte accumulation at inflammatory sites.

Another agent capable of enhancing human monocyte chemotaxis is levamisole (22). Doses of levamisole ranging from 10^{-5} to 10^{-3}M incubated with monocytes prior to deposition into modified Boyden chambers enhanced the chemotactic responsiveness of these cells to AHS, f-met-phe and lymphocyte-derived-chemotactic-factor (LDCF). The parabromo derivative of levamisole, p-Br(−) tetramisole, also exerted an enhancing effect on chemotaxis, while the dextroisomer, (+) tetramisole, was not active. These results demonstrated that levamisole's enhancing effect was stereospecific. Kinetic studies in the presence of levamisole indicated that the drug increased both the rate of migration of the monocytes and the total number of cells capable of responding chemotactically. To determine whether binding of the drug to the monocytes was necessary for its enhancing effect, cells were incubated with various concentrations of levamisole alone or in the presence of 10^{-3} or 10^{-4}M (+) tetramisole (Fig. 5). The addition of the inactive dextroisomer decreased levamisole's enhancing effect, resulting in a downward shift in the dose-response curve. The parallel nature of the curves suggested that (+) tetramisole behaved as a competitive antagonist of the enhancing effect produced by levamisole. (K_D for levamisole = 1×10^{-4}M; K_D for (+) tetramisole = 0.8×10^{-4}M). Doses of levamisole ranging from 10^{-6} to 10^{-3}M

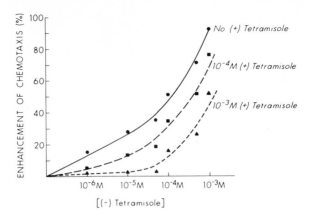

FIG. 5. Competitive inhibition of the enhancing effect of levamisole on monocyte chemotaxis by (+) tetramisole. Isolated monocytes were incubated (37°C for 30 min) with medium containing 10^{-3} to 10^{-6} M levamisole alone or with 10^{-3} to 10^{-6} M levamisole plus 10^{-3} M or 10^{-4} M (+) tetramisole and tested for chemotactic responsiveness to LDCF (15% v/v). K_D for levamisole = 10^{-4} M; K_D for (+) tetramisole = 0.8×10^{-4} M.

% enhancement =

$$\left(\frac{\text{Chemotactic responsiveness of cells incubated with drugs}}{\text{Chemotactic responsiveness of cells incubated with medium alone}} - 1 \right) \times 100$$

(From Pike et al., ref. 22, with permission.)

had no effect on PMN chemotaxis in response to AHS or f-met-phe. The stereospecificity, as well as cell-type specificity of the effect of levamisole, indicates that this drug has differential cell membrane effects on chemotactically responsive cells. This drug and its isomers can therefore be useful tools in delineating mechanisms of unidirectional cell migration.

The ability of certain viruses to alter an infected host's immune response is well recognized; however, the exact mechanism of this action remains unclear. An attempt to delineate the effect of viruses on monocyte function was undertaken in this laboratory. Isolated human monocytes were incubated *in vitro* with various concentrations of herpes simplex, influenza, vaccinia, reovirus, or polio viruses; they were washed and tested for chemotactic responsiveness to LDCF (16). Herpes simplex and influenza viruses depressed monocyte chemotaxis, while comparable doses of vaccinia, polio, and reoviruses had no such effect. UV-irradiated herpes simplex virus lost the ability to depress monocyte chemotaxis despite the fact that it is still capable of absorbing to the monocyte. To determine whether depression of monocyte chemotaxis also occurred during an acute viral illness *in vivo,* the monocytes from fifteen patients with serologically proven influenza were tested for chemotactic responsiveness in modified Boyden chambers (17). All patients with documented influenza had depressed monocyte chemotaxis when compared to normal individuals or to a febrile hospitalized patient control group (Fig. 6). Three weeks following the acute illness, the

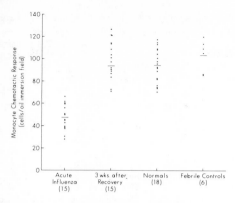

FIG. 6. Monocyte chemotactic response of influenza patients, normal subjects, and febrile controls. The horizontal line represents the mean of the group. The patients with influenza were tested during the acute illness and 3 weeks after recovery. (From Kleinerman et al., ref. 17, with permission.)

monocyte chemotactic responsiveness of all influenza patients tested returned to normal. The monocyte defect observed in these studies could not be attributed to a circulating inhibitor of chemotaxis. Depression of monocyte chemotaxis by influenza is one mechanism by which the virus could depress the host's cellular immunity and resistance to subsequent microbial challenges. Since levamisole was shown to enhance normal monocyte chemotaxis *in vitro,* we performed studies to determine whether this drug could reverse the defect of monocyte chemotaxis in influenza patients (21). Isolated monocytes from four patients with serologically proven acute influenza and from two normal individuals were incubated in medium alone or containing various concentrations of levamisole and tested for chemotactic responsiveness to a maximal or less than maximal dose of LDCF. Table 1 indicates that the chemotactic responsiveness of monocytes from three of four patients with influenza was significantly ($p < 0.0025$) depressed, confirming the previous findings of depressed chemotactic responsiveness in influenza patients (17). The response of the patients' monocytes to a maximal dose of chemotactic factor was restored to normal by $10^{-3}M$ levamisole and to just below normal when incubated with $10^{-4}M$ levamisole. The response of the patients' monocytes to less than a maximal dose of chemotactic factor also was markedly improved by levamisole treatment, but not restored to the maximum potential value. The depression of chemotaxis produced by incubation of monocytes with preparations of influenza virus *in vitro* could also be reversed by subsequent incubation of the cells with levamisole. The ability of levamisole to enhance the chemotactic function of monocytes from patients with influenza and to prevent virus-induced depression of chemotaxis *in vitro* suggests that the drug may be useful in restoring or preventing the depressed cell-mediated immunity in debilitated patients who contract influenza.

TABLE 1. *Effect of levamisole on the monocyte chemotaxis of patients with acute influenza*

Monocytes isolated from	Clinical and laboratory diagnosis[c]	Dose of chemotactic factor (%)[d]	Chemotactic activity[a] of cells incubated with[b]		
			Medium alone	10^{-4} M levamisole	10^{-3} M levamisole
M.P.	Healthy	15	67.3 ± 5.0	80.9 ± 5.6	91.1 ± 1.0
		30	96.7 ± 3.0	92.4 ± 5.6	91.1 ± 2.0
M.N.	Healthy	15	60.4 ± 2.0	—	86.5 ± 3.3
		30	92.7 ± 1.3	90.8 ± 4.0	91.1 ± 5.6
K.H.	Influenza	15	41.3 ± 7.9	61.7 ± 7.9	67.7 ± 7.3
		30	57.1 ± 5.0	81.2 ± 1.0	93.4 ± 2.6
T.W.	Influenza	15	37.6 ± 1.3	65.0 ± 7.9	63.4 ± 9.6
		30	52.8 ± 5.9	83.2 ± 4.3	94.7 ± 3.6
W.R.	Influenza	15	39.9 ± 3.3	55.4 ± 0.7	64.4 ± 1.0
		30	75.2 ± 2.0	85.8 ± 2.0	95.4 ± 3.6
G.P.	Influenza	15	60.1 ± 2.6	66.3 ± 2.0	84.2 ± 7.9
		30	86.5 ± 5.3	87.8 ± 2.6	91.7 ± 2.3

[a] Chemotactic activity is expressed as the average number of cells per oil immersion field ($\times$ 1,540) of triplicate samples ± SEM migrating completely through the filter in a 90-min incubation period.

[b] The isolated MNL from patients and normal subjects were incubated with either medium alone or with medium containing 10^{-3} or 10^{-4} M levamisole and tested for chemotactic responsiveness.

[c] All patients had a fourfold or greater increase in complement fixation of H.A.I. titer to influenza A/England/864/75 or A/Port Chalmers/1/73.

[d] LDCF was diluted to be a maximal (30% v/v) or less than maximal (15% v/v) chemotactic stimulus.

From Pike et al. (21), with permission.

CHEMOTAXIS AND NEOPLASTIC DISEASE

The role of immunologic surveillance in preventing the spontaneous development and spread of neoplasms has not yet been defined; however, it has been repeatedly demonstrated that cellular immune inflammatory responses occurring within tumors can produce their destruction (7,18,28,45). In addition, the increased incidence of cancer in patients with immunodeficiencies or undergoing immunosuppressive therapy suggests some role for immune surveillance in human subjects (43). Arguments against the surveillance hypothesis have cited that T-cell deficient humans and mice do not have an increased incidence of nonlymphomatous neoplasms (24); however, these observations do not preclude the concept that macrophages are instrumental for surveillance. Indeed, it has been observed that the influx of macrophages to a tumor site can result in its destruction (9,14) and that tumors containing the largest numbers of macrophages within them are the least likely to metastasize (8).

In light of these observations, this laboratory has undertaken the study of monocyte chemotactic responsiveness in more than 200 patients with various

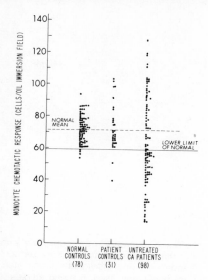

FIG. 7. Monocyte chemotactic responsiveness of normal subjects, hospitalized patients with nonneoplastic disease, and patients with neoplasms. The lower limit of normal indicates the level below which only 5% of the normal responses fall. The responses of approximately 60% of the patients with cancer fall below this level. (From Snyderman et al., ref. 33, with permission.)

types of neoplasms. Greater than 50% of the cancer patients studied had depressed monocyte chemotaxis when compared to a large group of normal individuals or hospitalized controls (Fig. 7) (33,40). Similar results have been found during the course of other studies (2,13). The extended duration of our investigation has allowed the assessment of the possible prognostic significance of abnormal monocyte migratory function in cancer patients. In a longitudinal study of 56 patients with melanoma, abnormal chemotaxis was found in 36 (64%) patients prior to immunotherapy (39). Seventy percent of the abnormal responders had decreased chemotaxis, while 30% had elevated responsiveness. Immunotherapy with BCG, sensitized autologous lymphocytes, and X-irradiated neuraminidase-treated melanoma cells or surgical removal of the neoplasms both reduced the percentage of patients with abnormal responses, but the best prognosis was found in those patients who had normal chemotaxis prior to therapy (39). Mortality in the elevated and depressed patient groups was significantly higher than in the patient group with normal monocyte chemotaxis. Over 44% of those with initially abnormal responses have died of their disease compared to 5% in those whose initial responses were normal. It appeared that normal monocyte chemotactic responsiveness was associated with a better prognosis and abnormal chemotaxis with the presence of clinically detectable disease (39).

An additional provocative finding was encountered during the study of patients with cancer of the breast, benign breast masses, and patients with a history of

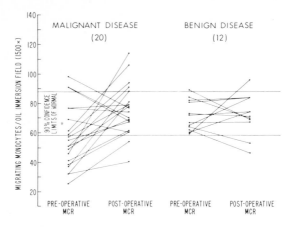

FIG. 8. Monocyte chemotactic responsiveness in a group of patients with malignant disease (left) and benign disease (right) tested just prior to and approximately 4 weeks after surgery. Each point represents the response of one individual's monocytes. Confidence limits were calculated in the normal control population used in these studies. (From Snyderman et al., ref. 31, with permission.)

breast cancer but clinically free of disease at the time of testing (31). These studies showed that 68% of patients with breast cancer *in situ* had abnormal monocyte chemotactic responsiveness, while patients with benign breast masses, or with a history of breast cancer, but free of disease, had chemotactic responses comparable to a normal control population. It was also found that the monocyte chemotactic responsiveness of patients with malignant but not benign masses was normalized following surgical removal of the neoplasm (Fig. 8). These findings, together with the data that chemotaxis was normal in patients who had a history of breast cancer but who were clinically free of disease at the time of testing, indicated that abnormal chemotaxis in cancer patients is an acquired defect which is dependent upon the presence of the tumor itself. To test this hypothesis, a method of assessing delayed hypersensitivity in normal mice and mice with transplantable neoplasms was developed (37,38). Injection of PHA into the peritoneal cavities of mice results in an inflammatory reaction characterized by the accumulation of macrophages, the peak influx of which occurs by 24 hours after infection (37). The maximum PMN response occurs at 6 hours and contrasts markedly with endotoxin-evoked inflammatory reactions in which PMN are found in far greater numbers and persist as the predominant cell type for at least 48 hr (34). To determine the effect of tumor implantation on macrophage accumulation *in vivo* and the chemotactic responsiveness of the recovered cells *in vitro,* groups of five mice were injected subcutaneously (S.C.) with 2.5×10^6 BP8 sarcoma or hepatoma 129 cells and at various times thereafter given an intraperitoneal (I.P.) injection of PHA. Two days later, the mice were sacrificed and the total and differential leukocyte counts determined for individual mice. There was a dramatic depression of both macrophage accumulation in response to PHA and the *in vitro* chemotactic responsiveness

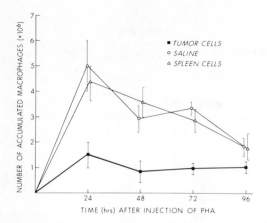

FIG. 9. Effect of implantation of BP8 sarcoma cells on the kinetics of macrophage accumulation in response to i.p. injection of PHA. Mice were injected with either 2.5×10^6 tumor cells, syngeneic spleen cells, or saline S.C. in the thigh and 7 days later were injected with 35 μg of PHA i.p. At the indicated times thereafter, groups of five mice were sacrificed, the peritoneal cavities lavaged, and the total and differential leukocyte counts determined for each animal. The indicated values represent the mean ± SEM of each group minus the number of macrophages in groups of mice identically treated but not injected with PHA I.P. (From Snyderman et al., ref. 37, with permission.)

of the recovered macrophages by as early as 6 days following tumor implantation. The depression was still present at 12 days (37). To determine whether this depression was a consequence of delayed kinetics of macrophage accumulation or a depressed response to the inflammatory stimulus, mice were injected S.C. with saline, spleen cells, or tumor cells and 7 days later, given an I.P. challenge of PHA. At various times thereafter, mice were sacrificed and the total number of macrophages migrating into the peritoneal cavity quantified. Figure 9 shows that the number of accumulated macrophages was highest at 24 hr and declined thereafter. The tumor animals, however, had markedly depressed macrophage accumulation which never approached the maximal response of the normal mice.

No depression of polymorphonuclear leukocyte accumulation in response to either PHA or endotoxin was noted in tumor-bearing animals (37). Depressed macrophage chemotaxis in tumor-bearing animals has also been noted by others (20,41). The foregoing results demonstrate that tumor implantation itself directly depresses macrophage accumulation. To elucidate the mechanism of this depression, three types of syngeneic C3H tumors—hepatoma 129, lymphoma 6C3HED, and sarcoma BP8—and an allogeneic teratocarcinoma which originated in 129 mice as well as normal liver and spleen cells were sonicated, centrifuged, and the cell-free supernatants dialyzed against RPMI 1640 overnight. The dialysates (0.2 ml) or whole tumor cells were injected S.C. in the thighs of mice, and the number of accumulated macrophages in response to I.P. PHA was determined (23,35,36). Table 2 shows that the three types of syngeneic tumor cells

TABLE 2. *Inhibition of macrophage accumulation* in vivo *by neoplastic cells and their soluble products*

| Source of cells | Number of macrophages[a] ($\times 10^6$) in the peritoneal cavities of mice given: | | | |
	Intact cells[b]	Inhibition[c] (%)	Dialysate[d]	Inhibition (%)
Hepatoma 129	3.2 ± 0.3	54	2.3 ± 0.3	66
Lymphoma 6C3HED	3.5 ± 0.3	49	1.8 ± 0.3	73
Sarcoma BP8	3.4 ± 0.4	51	3.8 ± 0.3	43
Teratocarcinoma	5.9 ± 0.5	14	2.4 ± 0.3	64
Liver	7.1 ± 0.7	0	6.6 ± 0.3	1
Spleen	6.2 ± 0.4	10	6.7 ± 0.6	0
No cells	6.9 ± 0.6	—	6.7 ± 0.4	—

[a] The values represent the mean (± SEM) number of macrophages recovered from the peritoneal cavities 2 days after i.p. injection of 35 μg of PHA into five normal mice or five mice previously injected in the thigh with the indicated cells or dialysates.

[b] Mice were injected subcutaneously with 2.5×10^6 of the indicated cells 7 days prior to sacrifice.

[c] Percent inhibition =

$$(1 - \frac{\text{Values obtained from mice injected with cells or dialysates}}{\text{Values obtained from mice not injected with cells or dialysates}}) \times 100$$

[d] The indicated tissues (5×10^7 cells/ml PBS) were sonicated, centrifuged ($1,800 \times g$ for 10 min) and 2.5 ml of the supernatant dialyzed overnight against 5 ml RPMI 1640 and 0.2 ml of the indicated dialysate injected in the thighs of groups of five C3H mice 3 days prior to sacrifice.

From Snyderman et al. (36), with permission.

depressed macrophage accumulation by 49 to 54%. The allogeneic cells did not depress macrophage accumulation, perhaps because of rapid destruction by the host's cells. The injection of the dialysates derived from neoplastic cells but not from normal tissues depressed macrophage accumulation, indicating that the tumor cells contained a dialyzable inhibitor(s) of macrophage accumulation. The effect of the various tumor and control dialysates on *in vitro* macrophage chemotaxis also has been determined (23,35,36). PHA-induced macrophages from normal mice were incubated with dilutions of the tumor or control dialysates and tested for chemotactic responsiveness to activated mouse serum in modified Boyden chambers (Table 3). The dialysates derived from the four murine tumors depressed macrophage chemotaxis in a dose-dependent fashion, while dialysates derived from normal tissues had no effect on this function. Experiments were also performed to test whether the tumor dialysates affected PMN chemotaxis *in vitro*. Table 3 also shows that neither the tumor nor control dialysates had any effect on PMN chemotaxis, indicating some specificity of the inhibitor(s) for macrophages.

The inhibitor derived from hepatoma 129 cells was found to have an apparent molecular weight of between 8,000 and 12,000 daltons and was heat-stable for 30 min at 56°C and for 10 min at boiling (23). To evaluate the biologic significance

TABLE 3. *Inhibition of macrophage chemotaxis* in vitro *by dialysates of sonicated neoplastic cells*

| | | Dialysate incubated with | | | |
| | | Macrophages[b] | | PMNs[c] | |
Dialysate of	(%)[a]	Response[d]	Inhibition[e] (%)	Response[f]	Inhibition (%)
Lymphoma 6C3HED	50	5.0 ± 1.4	93	356.7 ± 34.4	0
	30	18.8 ± 3.1	72		
	10	38.3 ± 0.9	44		
Hepatoma 129	50	39.0 ± 3.8	42	349.8 ± 10.4	0
	30	48.5 ± 5.9	27		
	10	62.4 ± 1.9	9		
Teratocarcinoma	50	36.0 ± 2.1	47	371.9 ± 12.3	0
	30	47.5 ± 2.1	28		
	10	61.4 ± 3.6	10		
Sarcoma BP8	50	31.0 ± 7.8	54	372.6 ± 14.1	0
	30	31.4 ± 3.3	52		
	10	44.9 ± 0.5	34		
Spleen	50	70.3 ± 3.6	0	361.7 ± 32.8	0
	30	65.0 ± 4.2	2		
	10	68.0 ± 1.6	0		
Liver	50	64.7 ± 1.2	4		
	30	68.6 ± 4.7	0		
	10	68.0 ± 1.4	0		
Medium alone	50	67.7 ± 4.7	—	373.2 ± 6.8	—
	30	66.0 ± 2.9	—		
	10	68.3 ± 5.9	—		
No dialysate[g]		63.7 ± 3.1		334.0 ± 22.9	
Negative control[h]		8.9 ± 2.1		5.3 ± 0.5	

[a] 2.5 ml of the indicated tumor cell supernatant, control cell supernatant, or medium alone was dialyzed overnight against 5 ml RPMI 1640. The amount of dialysate used in the chemotaxis assay is indicated by its final v/v percent concentration in medium containing leukocytes.

[b] Peritoneal macrophages (2.2 × 10^6/ml) from normal mice injected 2 days earlier with PHA were incubated for 30 min and tested for chemotactic responsiveness to endotoxin-activated mouse serum (AMS).

[c] Peritoneal polymorphonuclear leukocytes (PMNs) (3 × 10^6/ml) from normal mice injected 18 hr prior to sacrifice with 75 µg *Salmonella typhosa* endotoxin were incubated for 30 min at 37° C with RPMI 1640 containing the indicated amount of the appropriate dialysate and tested for chemotactic responsiveness to AMS.

[d] Chemotactic response is expressed as the average number of migrating macrophages per oil immersion field (× 1,540) ± SEM.

[e] % Inhibition = $(1 - \dfrac{\text{chemotactic activity of cells or AMS incubated with experimental dialysates}}{\text{chemotactic activity of cells or AMS incubated with the dialysate of medium alone}}) \times 100$

[f] Chemotactic response is expressed as the average number of migrating PMNs per high-power field (× 780) ± SEM.

[g] Macrophages or PMNs incubated with undialyzed RPMI 1640 and tested for chemotactic responsiveness to AMS.

[h] Macrophages or PMNs incubated with undialyzed RPMI 1640 and tested for response to RPMI 1640 medium alone.

From Snyderman et al. (36), with permission.

of the inhibitor of macrophage migration in tumorigenesis, mice were given S.C. injections of 10^3 hepatoma 129 cells contained in medium alone or medium containing the dialysate from 3×10^6 hepatoma cells. Mice receiving the cells plus dialysate received subsequent S.C. injections of the dialysate every 3 days at a site distant from tumor implantation. The results of these experiments indicated that animals receiving cells plus inhibitor had markedly enhanced tumor growth when compared to animals receiving tumor cells alone (23).

In more recent studies, we have found that following approximately 14 days of tumor growth, macrophage accumulation to PHA *in vivo* returns to normal levels. Examination of the serum of tumor-bearing mice disclosed that inhibitory activity for macrophage accumulation to PHA in normal mice was present by 24 hr after tumor implantation and persisted for at least 4 weeks (Snyderman et al., *unpublished observations*). Thus, stimulated macrophage accumulation into the peritoneal cavity normalizes despite continued tumor growth and the persistence of inhibitory activity in the circulation. Whether these findings indicate that a tumor-bearing animal's macrophages acquire a resistance to the inhibitor(s) with time or that there is an expansion of a resistant subpopulation of macrophages remains to be determined. Depressed macrophage migratory function during early rapid tumor growth may prevent rapid mobilization of sufficient numbers of macrophages to prevent the establishment of the neoplasm.

SUMMARY

The availability of reproducible quantitative methods for the study of cellular migration *in vitro* has allowed rapid advances in our understanding of the biochemistry, physiology, and pathology of leukocyte chemotaxis. It is now clear that polymorphonuclear leukocytes (PMNs) have specific membrane binding sites for certain peptide chemotactic factors. The interaction of chemotactic factors with PMNs produces a rapid influx of sufficient Ca^{+2} to trigger the response of contractile elements. The metabolic pathways which supply the energy required to sustain cellular migration are currently being elucidated. The clinical application of chemotaxis methodology has disclosed that abnormalities of leukocyte motility are associated with numerous human diseases. Of particular interest to us has been the finding of abnormal monocyte chemotaxis in patients with cancer. Such abnormalities were shown to be correlated with extent of disease and prognosis, and were reversed by surgical removal of the neoplasm. Studies in animals support the hypothesis that neoplasms themselves may produce factors which subvert monocyte-macrophage function. The implication of these findings is that clinically apparent neoplasms may arise from dedifferentiated replicating cells which acquire the ability to prevent their rapid destruction by normal host surveillance mechanisms.

Although our understanding of the pathophysiology of leukocyte chemotaxis is still in its infancy, the continued rapid development of this field can be expected to provide new insight into the basic mechanisms of cellular recognition as well as novel approaches to the treatment of some human diseases.

ACKNOWLEDGMENTS

Supported in part by a grant from the National Institutes of Dental Research 2 R01 DEO3738–04 and a contract from the National Institutes for Cancer Research NO1 CP 33313.

Ralph Snyderman is an investigator of the Howard Hughes Medical Institute.

REFERENCES

1. Aswanikumar, S., Corcoran, B., Schiffmann, E., Day, A. R., Freer, R. J., Showell, H. J., Becker, E. L., and Pert, C. B. (1977): Demonstration of a receptor on rabbit neutrophils for chemotactic peptides. *Biochem. Biophys. Res. Commun.,* 74:810.
2. Boetcher, D. A., and Leonard, E. (1974): Abnormal monocyte chemotaxis in cancer patients. *J. Natl. Cancer Inst.,* 52:1091–1099.
3. Boucek, M. M., and Snyderman, R. (1976): Calcium influx requirement for human neutrophil chemotaxis: Inhibition by lanthanum chloride. *Science,* 193:905–907.
4. Bourne, H. R., Lichtenstein, L. M., and Melmon, K. L. (1972): Pharmacologic control of allergic histamine release in vitro: Evidence for an inhibitory role of 3', 5' adenosine monophosphate in human leukocytes. *J. Immunol.,* 108:695–705.
5. Bourne, H. R., Zehrer, R. J., Cline, M. J. and Melmon, K. L. (1971): Cyclic 3',5' adenosine monophosphate in the human leukocyte: Synthesis, degradation and effects on neutrophil candidicidal activity. *J. Clin. Invest.,* 50:920–929.
6. Boxer, L. A., Hedley-Whyte, E. T., and Stossel, T. (1974): Neutrophil actin dysfunction and abnormal neutrophil behavior. *N. Engl. J. Med.,* 291:1093–1099.
7. Cerrottini, J. C., and Brunner, K. T. (1974): Cell mediated cytotoxicity, allograft rejection, and tumor immunity. *Adv. Immunol.,* 18:57–132.
8. Evans, R. (1972): Macrophages in syngeneic animal tumors. *Transplantation,* 14:468–473.
9. Evans, R., and Alexander, P. (1972): Mechanism of immunologically specific killing of tumor cells by macrophages. *Nature,* 236:168–170.
10. Gallin, J. I., and Rosenthal, A. S. (1974): The regulatory role of divalent cations in human granulocyte chemotaxis: Evidence for an association between calcium exchanges and microtubule assembly. *J. Cell. Biol.,* 62:594–609.
11. Gallin, J. I., and Wolff, S. M. (1975): Leukocyte chemotaxis: Physiological considerations and abnormalities. *Clin. Haematology,* 4:567–607.
12. Goetzl, E. J., and Austen, K. F. (1974): Stimulation of human neutrophil leukocyte aerobic glucose metabolism by purified chemotactic factors. *J. Clin. Invest.,* 53:591–599.
13. Hausman, M. S., Brosman, S., Snyderman, R., Mickey, M. R., and Fahey, J. (1975): Defective monocyte function in patients with genitourinary carcinoma. *J. Natl. Cancer Inst.,* 55:1047–1054.
14. Hibbs, J. B., Lambert, L. H., and Remington, J. S. (1972): Possible role of macrophage mediated nonspecific cytotoxicity tumor killing. *Nature,* 235:48–50.
15. Kaley, G., and Weiner, R. (1971): Effect of prostaglandin E_1 on leukocyte migration. *Nature* [*New Biol.*], 234:114–115.
16. Kleinerman, E. K., Snyderman, R., and Daniels, C. A. (1974): Depression of human monocyte chemotaxis by herpes simplex and influenza viruses. *J. Immunol.,* 113:1562–1567.
17. Kleinerman, E. K., Snyderman, R., and Daniels, C. A. (1975): Depression of human monocyte chemotaxis during acute influenza infection. *Lancet,* 2:1063–1064.
18. Levy, M. H., and Wheelock, E. F. (1974): The role of macrophages in defense against neoplastic disease. *Adv. Cancer Res.,* 20:131–145.
19. McClatchey, W., and Snyderman, R. (1976): Prostaglandins and inflammation: Enhancement of monocyte chemotactic responsiveness by prostaglandin E_2. *Prostaglandins,* 12:415–426.

20. Norman, S. J., and Sorkin, E. (1976): Cell specific defect in monocyte function during tumor growth. *J. Natl. Cancer Inst.*, 57:135–140.
21. Pike, M. C., Daniels, C. A., and Snyderman, R. (1977): Influenza induced depression of monocyte chemotaxis: Reversal by levamisole. *Cell. Immunol.*, 32:234–238.
22. Pike, M. C., and Snyderman, R. (1976): Augmentation of human monocyte chemotactic responsiveness by levamisole. *Nature*, 261:136–137.
23. Pike, M. C., and Snyderman, R. (1976): Depression of macrophage function by a factor produced by neoplasms: A mechanism for abrogation of immune surveillance. *J. Immunol.*, 117:1243–1249.
24. Prehn, R. T., and Prehn, L. V. (1975): Pathobiology of neoplasia. *Am. J. Pathol.*, 80:525–550.
25. Ramwell, P. W., editor (1972): *Prostaglandins in Cellular Biology.* Plenum Press, New York.
26. Schiffman, E., Corcoran, B. A., and Wahl, S. M. (1975): N-formylmethionyl peptides are chemotactic for polymorphonuclear leukocytes., *Proc. Natl. Acad. Sci. U.S.A.*, 72:1059–1062.
27. Sends, N., Shibata, N., Tatsumi, N., Kondo, K., and Hamada, K. (1969): A contractile protein from leukocytes: Its extraction and some of its properties. *Biochim. Biophys. Acta*, 181:191–200.
28. Shin, H. S., Hayden, M., Langley, S., Kaliss, N., and Smith, M. R. (1975): Antibody mediated suppression of grafted lymphoma: III. Evaluation of the role of thymic function, non-thymus derived lymphocytes, macrophages, platelets and human polymorphonuclear leukocytes in syngeneic and allogeneic hosts. *J. Immunol.*, 114:1255–1263.
29. Snyderman, R., Altman, L. C., Hausman, M. S., and Mergenhagen, S. E. (1972): Human mononuclear leukocyte chemotaxis: A quantitative assay for humoral and cellular chemotactic factors. *J. Immunol.*, 108:857–860.
30. Snyderman, R., Gewurz, H., and Mergenhagen, S. E. (1968): Interaction of the complement system with endotoxic lipopolysaccharide: Generation of a chemotactic factor for polymorphonuclear leukocytes. *J. Exp. Med.*, 128:259–275.
31. Snyderman, R., Meadows, L., Holder, W., and Wells, S. (1977): Abnormality of monocyte chemotaxis in patients with breast cancer: Evidence for a tumor mediated effect. *Submitted for publication.*
32. Snyderman, R., and Mergenhagen, S. E. (1972): Characterization of polymorphonuclear leukocyte chemotactic activity in serums activated by various inflammatory agents. In: *Biological Activities of Complement,* edited by D. G. Ingram, pp. 117–132. Karger, Basel.
33. Snyderman, R., and Mergenhagen, S. E. (1976): Chemotaxis of macrophages. In: *Immunobiology of the Macrophage,* edited by D. S. Nelson, pp. 323–348. Academic Press, New York.
34. Snyderman, R., Phillips, J. K., and Mergenhagen, S. E. (1971): Biological activity of complement in vivo: Role of C5 in the accumulation of polymorphonuclear leukocytes in inflammatory exudates. *J. Exp. Med.*, 134:1131–1143.
35. Snyderman, R., and Pike, M. C. (1976): Defective macrophage migration produced by neoplasms: Identification of an inhibitor of macrophage chemotaxis. In: *The Macrophage in Neoplasia,* edited by M. A. Fink, pp. 49–65. Academic Press, New York.
36. Snyderman, R., and Pike, M. C. (1976): An inhibitor of macrophage function produced by neoplasms. *Science,* 192:370–372.
37. Snyderman, R., Pike, M. C., Blaylock, B. L., and Weinstein, P. (1976): Effects of neoplasms on inflammation: Depression of macrophage accumulation after tumor implantation, *J. Immunol.*, 116:585–589.
38. Snyderman, R., Pike, M. C., McCarley, D., and Lang, L. (1975): Quantification of mouse macrophage chemotaxis in vitro: Role of C5 for the production of chemotactic activity. *Infect. Immun.*, 11:488–492.
39. Snyderman, R., Seigler, H. F., and Meadows, L. (1977): Abnormalities of monocyte chemotaxis in patients with melanoma: Effects of immunotherapy and tumor removal. *J. Natl. Cancer Inst.*, 58:37–41.
40. Snyderman, R., and Stahl, C. (1975): Defective immune effector function in patients with neoplastic and immune deficiency diseases. In: *The Phagocytic Cell in Host Resistance,* edited by J. A. Bellanti and D. H. Dayton, pp. 267–281, Raven Press, New York.
41. Stevenson, M. M., and Meltzer, M. S. (1975): Defective macrophage chemotaxis in tumor bearing mice. *Fed. Proc.*, 34:991.
42. Stossel, T. P., and Pollard, T. D. (1973): Myosin in polymorphonuclear leukocytes. *J. Biol. Chem.*, 218:8288–8294.

43. Waldman, T. A., Strober, W., and Blaese, R. M. (1972): Immunodeficiency disease and malignancy: Various immunologic deficiencies in man and the role of immune processes in the control of malignant disease. *Ann. Intern. Med.*, 77:606–628.
44. Williams, L. T., Snyderman, R., Pike. M. C., and Lefkowitz, R. J. (1977): Specific receptor sites for chemotactic peptides on human polymorphonuclear leukocytes. *Proc. Natl. Acad. Sci. U.S.A.*, 74:1204–1208.
45. Zbar, B., Wepsic, H. T., Rapp, H. J., Stewart, L. C., and Borsos, T. (1970): Two step mechanism of tumor graft rejection in syngeneic guinea pigs. *J. Natl. Cancer Inst.*, 44:710–713.

DISCUSSION

Dr. Ward: Have you looked at serum from patients with malignant conditions to see if in fact they have a circulating chemotactic inhibitor? Do you have any evidence that your inhibitor has an effect on any other leukocyte functions?

Dr. Snyderman: We have had a lot of difficulties looking at inhibitors in serum. This has been the least pleasant thing that I have ever done because we find that the variation in effects of normal serum is very, very wide, much wider than the chemotactic response. So when we wanted to look for an inhibitor of cell function, we did experiments adding the stimulus to the upper compartment or the cell side of our chambers. We had to be sure any observed inhibitor was not a result of the presence of a chemotactic activity in the upper compartment. We also put serum on both sides of the chamber to determine if any inhibitory activity was cell-directed or chemotactic factor-directed. We sometimes found inhibitors in cancer patients' serum but it was not a uniform finding. If we fractionated the serum on Sephadex G200, we did not see anything striking. What we have seen is that with the usual kind of G200 pattern, inhibitory activity is similar to what you described and what Dr. Van Epps talked about; that is, there are essentially two areas that are somewhat variable from individual to individual. In the tumor patients, we occasionally see inhibitory activity just at the trailing edge of the albumin. In one experiment, which we are going to have to do again, we have done this at pH 6.8 in addition to 7.2, and we found more lower-molecular-weight activity. We think that if there is inhibitory activity, it is probably different from what has already been described and very much hidden by all the other things that are in serum.

We have also looked at pleural effusions of a few patients with malignant conditions. We have not done nearly as many controls as we should. We have seen a lot more of the inhibitor activity but this needs more work.

Dr. Ward: What about the effect on lymphocyte function?

Dr. Snyderman: I can tell you it suppresses lymphocyte transformation, in addition to everything else. The problem that I have with interpreting that is that there is a macrophage-dependence for lymphocyte transformation. We have not separated whether it is affecting the lymphocyte or the small number of macrophages that are necessary for normal transformation.

Dr. Williams: Would it be practical to try to make antibodies to this material and give it to patients?

Dr. Snyderman: We are trying to raise antibody in rabbits. We are using the mouse material. I am not sure that we have antibody yet, because it is a fairly low-molecular-weight material. But we are injecting whatever there is with complete Freud's adjuvant and we are up to about 3 months worth of immunization. It looks as though we are starting to get something. In order to test our antibodies we have been taking the inhibitor plus the serum, preimmune versus immune serum, putting it in a dialysis bag, and seeing what we get back. It looks as though we are losing some of the inhibitory activity with immune serum; we may be getting antibody, but we cannot see anything that approaches a precipitating line and I do not think we ever will.

Dr. Williams: Have you tried conjugating it to albumin or some other carrier protein?

Dr. Snyderman: That is a good point. No, we did not.

Dr. Schiffmann: During the supernormal phase, when you get macrophages, did you test to see whether or not there's a chemotactic factor in the peritoneal fluid, which might account for some of the influx of these cells?

Dr. Snyderman: These are stimulated exudates. So, we are putting PHA in to draw the cells in. Essentially, it is an active response.

Dr. Schiffmann: Do you know whether or not the macrophages have less killing power later on during the supernormal phase?

Dr. Snyderman: No, I do not know that. We are just in the process of developing this assay and we are using Monty Meltzer's technique. I know he is very interested in doing this, as well. If I understand what he has told me, and I really should not speak for him, I do not think they have a depressed cytotoxic activity at that late point.

Dr. Jensen: Have you looked for the inhibitor in the urine of patients or mice?

Dr. Snyderman: No, we have not. But this is the area that we expect to put most of our emphasis on. Because, if it is low-molecular-weight, it should be in the urine. And if it is not broken down, it could be there.

Dr. Jensen: Since this is a tumor product, it might be that the animal actually makes antibody against it; that could be what accounts for the disappearance of the factor with time.

Dr. Snyderman: But in these studies, we still find inhibitory activity. I am not sure how long it persists. It may eventually go down.

Dr. Van Epps: Have you looked for antibody in your rebound sera, to see if there were any activity against the inhibitor?

Dr. Snyderman: No. We did not really quantify how much material is present. We could have lost 90% of the activity and not have detected this since we did not do a great many dilutions to see whether we are losing some of this inhibitory activity. We just did one dose. And I think Dr. North was also overwhelmed with the biologic potency of the material in the serum. He transferred his susceptibility to Listeria with 50-μl quantities of serum.

Dr. Van Epps: Have you ever had a chance to look at the monocytes or macrophages in the rebound period with respect to enzyme content or surface receptors to see if they represent a different population of cells?

Dr. Snyderman: Yes, although we have not looked at them carefully enough. We measured monocyte or macrophage adherence. And they seem to adhere quite well. We have assayed phagocytosis which is supernormal while chemotaxis is depressed. These data may be indicating that we are losing a particular type of cell population.

Dr. Wilkinson: There is a colleague in Glasgow (A. Otu) who uses as a model the metastatic Lewis lung carcinoma in mice. He gets curves very similar to yours but not quite the same. He, like you, gets inhibition very early after the tumor begins to grow for 2 or 3 days. Later, the tumors start metastasizing and the mice die. At the terminal stage (3 to 4 weeks) there is again a profound drop in chemotactic and other activities of the mouse macrophages. I think from his work that the important stage in getting the tumor started is the depression of macrophage function in the early days.

Dr. Snyderman: That is very exciting. We have not looked at our animals just prior to death.

Dr. Leddy: Dr. Snyderman, in your mouse model, are the tumors sufficiently localized that you could surgically remove them and test whether you have a parallel to the human situation presented in the beginning of your talk?

Dr. Snyderman: The way we do it, probably not. But if we implanted tumors in the footpad, we probably could. We had thought about doing that but just have not gotten around to it. In our studies, the tumor is grown in the thigh, and eventually as it grows bigger, it grows up in the thigh and dissects into the subcutaneous area. If one did the studies entirely in the footpad, I think one could amputate the foot and look at the effects of tumor removal.

Dr. Lynn: There seems to be a lot of this material produced. It would not surprise me if there were another biological function for it. Do you have any thoughts in this regard?

Dr. Snyderman: I think the obvious thing that we have considered is that the neoplastic cell has not acquired anything new but rather lost some functions of specialization. So I suspect we might find evidence for what it is by looking for precedents in normal biology. The obvious thing would be to look at the trophoblast, in terms of maternal-fetal relationships. What we have done is really circuitous. We have looked at amniotic fluid, and we find in normal human amniotic fluid there is a substance that inhibits human monocyte chemotactic responsiveness.

Dr. Turner: Dr. Snyderman, your model would seem to suggest there is more to immunosurveillance or cellular surveillance and tumor growth than just chemotactic function of the monocyte. When you have this supernormal chemotactic function you are still getting metastases. Does that make you modify your thinking?

Dr. Snyderman: No, because what we are really doing is looking at a functional state of the circulating cell. We are not looking at anything in terms of the local conditions. I think that people who work with tumors are impressed that tumors often contain macrophages and frequently, somebody in the audience will say, how could the work presented here have any meaning if there are macrophages within the tumor. Macrophages are obviously getting to the tumor site. We have to think of mammalian or biologic functions in terms of gaussian types of distributions rather than quantitative mechanics, where there is the all-or-none phenomenon. I think the kinetics of the cells getting there at the time that the numbers of tumor cells are low is the critical thing, not whether or not they ever get there. In all the patients that Dr. Quie mentioned and every patient we see, with infection, there are always some inflammatory cells. The problem is that the inflammatory cells did not get there fast enough to do what they were supposed to do.

The fact that chemotaxis becomes supernormal systemically does not bother me very much. The fact that macrophages even get to the tumor does not bother me very much either. The important factor may be how many arrive at what time and with what functional capacity. Shin (28) has shown, that with increasing numbers, tumors build up a resistance to an immune destruction which is caused by a shortage of macrophages at the tumor site.

Dr. Turner: That speaks to the primary tumor, but how about new metastases just starting out with small numbers of cells?

Dr. Snyderman: Well Dr. Wilkinson just addressed that question. I do not know about the metastatic problem, but I think that that is a very important observation.

Dr. Williams: You anticipated my question a little, but, it seems likely that you can show *in vitro* production of the inhibitor by tumor culture. Have you tried culturing any fetal tissues? You do not necessarily have to use human fetal tissues; mouse fetal tissues might produce undesirable amounts.

Dr. Snyderman: Yes, I think those are superb experiments and we hopefully will start to do them.

Dr. Altman: Dr. Snyderman, in your experimental mouse model have you used a tumor that the animals are capable of rejecting to see if your findings are different in this experimental situation?

Dr. Snyderman: Yes. Using a teratocarcinoma, which is an allogeneic tumor and is rejected, we do not see the depression in the animal. In other words, if you look at it 6 days after implantation, you do not see that depression. And the other thing that I might mention is that Shin essentially had two C3H, 6C3HED lymphosarcomas, one which he attenuated by multiple passes *in vitro,* and the other which grew well *in vivo.* The attenuated one grew normally in an irradiated animal, but did not grow normally in a normal animal. He sent it to us blind, and we tested them for the presence of the inhibitor. What we found is that the attenuated tumor did not make inhibitor; the normal grown tumor did, in experiments where he put the attenuated tumor in one thigh, and the virulent tumor in the other thigh. Without the growing tumor, the attenuated tumor would not grow, but if the virulent tumor was present, the attenuated tumor grew.

Leukocyte Chemotaxis, edited by John I. Gallin
and Paul G. Quie. Raven Press, New York
© 1978.

Cell Elastimetry in the Characterization of Normal and Abnormal PMN Movement

Michael E. Miller

Department of Pediatrics, Harbor General Hospital, Torrance, California 90509

For the past 4 years, we have utilized the method of cell elastimetry in the dissection of mechanisms which control human polymorphonuclear leukocyte (PMN) movement and in the characterization of disorders of that movement. Our impetus to develop this assay for the study of peripheral blood PMNs was provided by Lichtman, who, in 1970 (4), successfully employed elastimetry in the study of deformability of maturing human bone marrow granulocytes. Lichtman demonstrated a progressive increase in deformability of granulocytes during maturation and suggested that this was a controlling factor in marrow egress of mature PMNs. These studies suggested to us that elastimetry might offer a valuable probe in the study of movement of human peripheral blood PMNs. Previous data from our laboratory, and material now to be summarized, have supported this suggestion.

METHOD AND PREVIOUS DATA

The technique of cell elastimetry is modified from the original descriptions of Mitchison and Swann (9). In principle, the negative pressure required to aspirate a cell into the orifice of a micropipette is measured. For the study of PMNs, pipettes are drawn from 75 mm × 1.2 mm (internal diameter) borosilicate glass capillary tubing (Kimble Products, Toledo, Ohio) with a glass microelectrode puller (Narishige Scientific Instruments, Model PN-3 Labtron Scientific Corp., Farmingdale, N.Y.). After drawing, each pipette tip is examined microscopically for splintered edges, and the internal diameter measured using a micrometer eyepiece. Pipettes with rough edges or internal diameters outside the acceptable range (3 to 5 μ) are discarded.

PMN suspensions are prepared from heparinized, venous blood following sedimentation with 6% dextran. The PMNs are washed twice in medium CMRL 1066 (GIBCO, Grand Island, N.Y.) and resuspended to a final concentration of 5×10^6 PMNs/cc 1066. Several drops of the PMN suspension are placed in a 3-mm moist chamber. A PMN is manipulated into the orifice of a suitably mounted micropipette with a micromanipulator. Microscopic examination is performed with a 2-mm working distance objective (E. Leitz, Inc.). The micropipette is connected to a negative pressure source controlled by a sensitive needle valve and read on a mercury column. Negative pressures required to aspirate either a hemispherical bulge of cytoplasm or an entire PMN into the micropipette are then recorded.

We have previously characterized a number of the physical and chemical parameters influencing deformability (8). A summary of these studies follows: (a) Mean deformability of PMNs, as determined on a pool of 100 normal PMNs from 10 donors, was 11.4 cm Hg $\pm$ 1.8 (SD). The frequency distribution was small and the vast majority of observations were close to the mean value. Little if any observer subjectivity was involved in these measurements. The PMNs entered the pipettes slowly and ample time was, therefore, afforded for reading. Three separate observers consistently agreed upon recorded data.

(b) pH effects—Deformability is normal within a pH range of 6.9 to 7.5. Alkaline or acid pH outside this range was associated with decreased deformability—i.e., cells were more rigid.

(c) Temperature effects—PMNs at 4°C showed markedly decreased deformability, i.e., were more rigid. Deformability of PMNs at 37°C was slightly increased.

(d) Effect of chelating agents—Each of four chelators (EDTA, EGTA, sodium oxalate, and sodium citrate) significantly decreased deformability. Ca^{2+}, but not Co^{2+}, Mn^{2+}, or Mg^{2+}, completely restored deformability to normal when added in equimolar amounts with EDTA or EGTA. When added following incubation with EDTA or EGTA, however, Ca^{2+} had no effect, suggesting that chelator effects upon deformability are exerted through their effects upon Ca^{2+}, and not through direct interaction with the cell.

(e) Effect of metabolic inhibitors—Deoxyglucose, sodium fluoride, and iodoacetate each markedly decreased deformability. Potassium cyanide and dinitrophenol, however, had no significant effect upon deformability. These results suggested a relationship between normal cell glycolysis and deformability.

(f) Limiting factor of the assay—Of the potential structures influencing the assay, the observations suggested that the cell membrane, rather than the cytoplasm, nucleus, or cell adhesiveness, was the limiting factor. It is for this reason that the assay was considered one of "membrane deformability."

(g) Relationship to chemotaxis—The above data are completely consistent with the effects of pH, chelators, and metabolic inhibitors upon chemotaxis. The correlation of deformability with chemotaxis is further emphasized by previous observations from our laboratory of decreased deformability in chemotactically deficient PMNs from normal, human neonates (5). Based upon these findings, we have pursued the study of membrane deformability in the characterization of intracellular and extracellular determinants of chemotaxis and the further dissection of human disorders of PMN movement. The following findings not only demonstrate the major utility of the assay in definition of basic biology of PMN movement, but provide substantial data to indicate that disorders of PMN movement represent a far more heterogeneous group than previously recognized.

Deformability in the Study of Disorders of Human PMN Movement

A number of disorders of human PMN movement have been described (6). In many of these, we have presented preliminary data utilizing several functional assays, which suggests heterogeneity among disorders of PMN movement. When studied in phagocytosis (Baker's yeast assay), chemotaxis (Boyden chamber assay), capillary tube migration, and *in vivo* inflammatory cycle (Rebuck-Crowley skin window), a number of different patterns have emerged which are not revealed with the use of the Boyden chamber alone. In the further characterization of these functional PMN disorders, we have utilized the study of membrane deformability. PMNS from subjects with "lazy leukocyte syndrome," a familial chemotactic defect, a sporadic chemotactic defect (abnormal Boyden chamber but normal capillary tube migration), diabetes mellitus, and from normal newborn infants were studied. In each of these conditions, we have previously shown abnormal Boyden chamber chemotaxis, but varying profiles of abnormality with one or more of the other functional assays. When studied in deformability, each PMN group demonstrated markedly decreased deformability from normal. The only consistent correlation was with Boyden chamber migration, and not with capillary tube movement, phagocytosis, peripheral neutrophil counts, or "skin window." These data, thus, suggest that: (a) cell elastimetry will consistently detect disorders of PMN movement discernible in the Boyden chamber; (b) a variety of functional abnormalities of PMN movement are reflected by abnormal membrane function; (c) phagocytosis, Boyden chamber migration, and deformability do *not* show a consistent correlation, thereby suggesting that movement and ingestion may not depend upon identical mechanisms; and, (d) membrane deformability appears to be a more sensitive and reproducible probe of cell movement than Boyden chamber chemotaxis. In addition, it offers the advantage of studying individual cells and the effects of modifying agents upon them.

Cell Elastimetry in the Detection of Immune Neutropenia

Antineutrophil antibodies have been demonstrated in the serums of recipients of multiple transfusions, mothers of infants with transient neonatal neutropenia, and in some patients with idiopathic neutropenia. Direct evidence of membrane alteration of PMNs by antineutrophil antibodies has, however, been limited. Boxer and co-workers (2) have demonstrated ingestion of sensitized neutrophils by other phagocytic cells and Cline and co-workers (3) have recently described a patient whose serum contained a circulating cytotoxin that injured primitive myeloid cells as well as differentiated granulocytes and mononuclear cells. While working in collaboration with Dr. Laurence Boxer (7), we have evaluated with cell elastimetry serums from a number of patients with previously demonstrated antineutrophil antibody activities. Normal PMNs were incubated with one of the various sera and then tested for deformability. In order to ensure objectivity, the study was conducted in an entirely blind fashion. Randomly coded serums from patients and controls were studied for deformability by observers unaware of the code. When incubated with normal PMNs, eight of nine serums with known antineutrophil antibodies significantly decreased membrane deformability. PMNs incubated in the various antineutrophil antibody-positive serums showed deformabilities ranging from 25.9 to > 43 cm Hg as compared with deformabilities of 11.4 ± 3.6 (2 SD) for PMNs incubated in antibody-negative serums. The data suggest that elastimetry is a reliable and sensitive probe for the detection of antineutrophil antibodies, and demonstrate a primary effect of antineutrophil antibodies upon PMN membranes.

Cell Elastimetry in the Study of "Benign Neutropenia" of Childhood

Chronic benign granulocytopenia of childhood is generally accepted as a homogeneous, self-limited entity of variable duration, characterized by absolute peripheral blood PMN counts of less than 1,500/mm³, relative depletion of band and mature granulocytes in bone marrow, and absent in mild infections. Our previous observations of heteregeneity among the group of disorders of PMN movement suggested that diversity might also exist in this clinical entity. Accordingly, we have actively studied this problem in some twenty children over the past 2 years. We summarize data here on eleven of these children with absolute PMN counts less than 1,000 PMNs/mm³. Six of the group had absolute PMN counts less than 500/mm³. Four functional PMN assays were performed: chemotaxis (Boyden chamber); capillary tube migration; phagocytosis (Baker's yeast ingestion), and membrane deformability. The data showed marked heterogeneity in functional PMN profiles. One of the children had decreased capillary tube migration, one was deficient in all functions tested, six showed various combinations of functional abnormalities, and only three children had normal PMN activities in each assay. Of the assays employed, membrane deformability was the most consistently abnormal.

Through the use of these profiles, it is, therefore, demonstrated that chronic benign neutropenia of childhood is not a distinct clinical entity. The spectrum of abnormal functional PMN profiles observed strongly suggests that abnormalities of a number of individual steps of normal PMN function may produce a common clinical phenotype. This is further supported by our clinical observations upon this large group of children. There is marked variability of the frequency and severity of infections, ranging from an entirely benign course to, occasionally, life-threatening infections. The correlations between clinical course and functional PMN profile are not yet sufficiently clear to provide predictive values, but it is obvious that the entity represents a common clinical phenotype of multiple levels of functional PMN abnormalities.

Membrane Deformability in the Study of Cell Movement

The above data establish the unique value of cell elastimetry in the characterization of mechanisms of PMN movement. We have applied the technique to the study of Ca^{2+} requirement in the initiation of PMN movement. Our initial findings, summarized above, suggested that chelator effects resulting in decreased deformability were mediated through specific binding of Ca^{2+}. An identical effect was noted upon Boyden chamber chemotaxis, resulting in decreased filter migration. We have further explored the role of Ca^{2+} in deformability of human PMNs by several approaches. Utilizing calcium-specific ionophore, we have found that the addition of Ca^{2+} and ionophore decreases deformability of PMNs. This effect requires the administration of both Ca^{2+} and ionophore, and occurs regardless of order of addition. Other divalent cations, such as Mg^{2+}, Mn^{2+}, or Co^{2+} have no such effect. If PMNs treated with Ca^{2+} and ionophore are allowed to remain in the incubation mixture, recovery occurs with deformability returning to normal values. Decreased deformability can again be induced by the addition of more Ca^{2+} *and* ionophore (not ionophore alone). These findings are identical to those reported for inhibition and recovery of ciliary movement of lamellibranch mollusk gills (10).

Lanthanum ion (La^{3+}) specifically inhibits transmembrane calcium movement. Addition of La^{3+} (as lanthanum chloride) completely inhibits the recovery phase of normal deformability in PMNs rendered rigid by the addition of Ca^{2+} and ionophore. If, as suggested by Satir (10), the recovery phase is related to specific activity of a Ca^{2+} pump, the effect of La^{3+} is consistent. The induction phase of decreased deformability by Ca^{2+} and ionophore is blocked by La^{3+} to a degree. If enough Ca^{2+} and ionophore are added, reduced deformability occurs.

These results are entirely consistent with the recent data of Boucek and Snyderman (1) demonstrating a calcium influx requirement for human PMN chemotaxis and inhibition of the calcium flux and chemotactic response following addition of lanthanum.

Cell Elastimetry in the Study of Other Cell Types

Cell elastimetry has utility in the study of many other cell types. The limiting factor in adaptation of the technique is the glass adhesiveness of the cell. Thus, in erythrocytes, the technique has been used extensively. Since erythrocytes adhere poorly to glass, it is possible to utilize a single micropipette in the study of large numbers of cells. A single observer can easily study several hundred erythrocytes on a given day. Glass-adherent cells, such as PMNs, present a more difficult problem. The size and fragility of the pipettes make it impractical to reuse the same pipette and it is, therefore, necessary to use a new pipette for each PMN studied. Although undesirable, this is by no means an insurmountable obstacle. With experience, one can perform deformability studies on upward of 20 individual PMNs/day.

We have recently modified the technique to the study of rabbit peritoneal macrophages. These cells are so glass-adherent that it is necessary to pretreat them with 0.1% xylocaine. Although preliminary data indicate that this does not alter functional parameters of the cells, further studies will be necessary before concluding that xylocaine treatment has not introduced undesirable artifacts into the interpretation of data obtained on macrophage deformability.

Other cells which might be profitably studied with cell elastimetry include a wide variety of malignant cells. If it is assumed that a reasonably pure suspension of such cells can be obtained, the assay should be readily adapted to their measurement.

REFERENCES

1. Boucek, M. M., and Snyderman, R. (1976): Calcium influx requirement for human neutrophil chemotaxis: Inhibition by lanthanum chloride. *Science,* 193:905.
2. Boxer, L. A., Greenberg, M. S., Boxer, G. J. et al. (1975): Autoimmune neutropenia. *N. Engl. J. Med.,* 293:748.
3. Cline, M. J., Opelz, G., Saxon, A. et al. (1976): Autoimmune panleukopenia. *N. Engl. J. Med.,* 295:1489.
4. Lichtman, M. A. (1970): Cellular deformability during maturation of the myeloblast: Possible role in marrow egress. *N. Engl. J. Med.,* 283:943.
5. Miller, M. E. (1975): Developmental maturation of human neutrophil motility and its relationship to membrane deformability. In: *The Phagocytic Cell in Host Resistance,* edited by J. A. Bellanti and D. H. Dayton, pp. 295–307. Raven Press, New York.
6. Miller, M. E. (1975): Pathology of chemotaxis and random mobility. *Semin. Hematol.,* 12:59.
7. Miller, M. E., and Boxer, L. A. (1977): Cell elastimetry in the detection of immune neutropenia: Demonstration of a membrane perturbation. *Pediatr Res. (in press).*
8. Miller, M. E., and Myers, K. A. (1975): Cellular deformability of the human peripheral blood polymorphonuclear leukocyte: Method of study, normal variation, and effects of physical and chemical alterations. *J. Reticuloendothel. Soc.,* 18:337.
9 Mitchison, J. M., and Swann, M. M. (1954): The mechanical properties of the cell surface: I. The cell elastimeter. *J. Exp. Biol.,* 31:443.
10. Satir, P. (1975): Ionophore-mediated calcium entry induces mussel gill ciliary arrest. *Science,* 190:586.

DISCUSSION

Dr. Gallin: On your data with EGTA, you had 100 mM of EGTA. If it is really a calcium phenomenon, 10 mM EGTA certainly should have been adequate. Did you try lower concentrations?

Dr. Miller: No, and I do not have an explanation. The equimolar additions to which I referred were all done with EDTA.

Dr. Gallin: The data, then, do not enable one to conclude that calcium is the critical ion?

Dr. Miller: Not from the EGTA experiments, but the lanthanum data are highly suggestive.

Dr. Gallin: Dr. Marshall Lichtman, as you know, has made some correlations between deformability of cells during development, and he has related these observations to changes in electrophoretic mobility (surface charge). We have noted that incubation of cells with chemotactic factors decreases the surface charge. Have you looked at the effect of chemotactic factors on the deformability of your cells? Also, most of the agents you studied increased the deformability. With regard to your data with A23187, some yet to be published observations we have made might not fit with your findings in that we find that treating leukocytes with calcium-ionophore A23187 ($10^{-8} - 10^{-6}$ M) results in a calcium-dependent decrease in the surface charge. If Dr. Lichtman's suggestions are correct, and my prejudice is they are, then I am surprised you did not observe increased deformability with A23187.

Dr. Miller: Let me deal with that last question first and then go back to the other. The relationships between surface charge and deformability are not well understood. Lichtman has presented some data which suggest a relationship, but the precise nature of this relationship, particularly upon peripheral blood cells, remains to be characterized. We have not performed measurements of surface charge so I cannot comment further on this point. With regard to your question about the chemotactic factors, this is obviously a major application, upon which we are currently embarking. We have, at the present time, worked only with chemotactically active mixtures. If you take material that has chemotactic activity and incubate it for 5 to 10 min with cells, you observe a marked increase in the deformability of the cells; however, if you let the cells remain there long enough, say 20 to 25 min, they revert and become very rigid. This would support to some degree the overall concept of deactivation.

With cytochalasin B, we find a similar kind of relationship. Concentrations that increase movement in a filter assay give markedly increased deformability, and vice versa.

Dr. Jensen: How many individuals and how many cells from each do you use in getting your normal values?

Dr. Miller: At least ten individual cell measurements from each of 100 different normal donors. If you test the same individual on different days, there is little variability.

Dr. Jensen: Can you do it with lymphocytes?

Dr. Miller: Yes, it works very well with lymphocytes.

Dr. Jensen: Is there a difference between T and B lymphocytes?

Dr. Miller: We have not studied that.

Dr. Snyderman: Can you tell us anything about deformability as it relates to maturation of the neutrophil series? Have you been able to look at different gradations of maturation?

Dr. Miller: In terms of blast cells to mature forms, we have done nothing. The only work on that is Marshall Lichtman's, which, of course, clearly showed a progressive increase in the deformability of the cells. The problem with these studies, however, is the relationship of the cell size to the size of the pipette. This is not easily corrected for. In individual populations of maturing cells, it is difficult to be sure that each cell studied bears a consistent relationship to pipette size.

At the same time, Lichtman's data are really very dramatic in terms of changes through different stages of maturation of cells, so it probably is valid. If you look at PMNs from premature infants, they are far more rigid than cells from normal newborns. If you look at things such as low counts and relative band populations versus relative mature polymorphonuclear leukocyte populations, at the present time, there does not seem to be much difference. We have not performed many of those studies, but there is no apparent difference between a population of polymorphonuclear leukocytes that is full of bands and a population that is full of mature looking cells. More such studies are, however, necessary to clarify this issue.

Dr. Zigmond: Dr. Trinkaus has done some studies on fiberblasts attached to glass. Using a given negative pressure, he measured how long a piece of cytoplasm can be drawn into a pipette on the side of a cell versus the front. Have you tried anything in the leukocytes of front and side deformability?

Dr. Miller: No, because our technique needs improvement. We have not worked hard enough on it. I do not think the current optics really lend themselves well to looking at that type of subtle difference anyway.

Dr. Lynn: Have you any data on the effect of fatty acids? If you coat the glass of your capillary with substances such as fatty acids or silicone does it change the deformability measurement?

Dr. Miller: We have no data on that.

Dr. Becker: I would like to go back to the A23187 data. In our hands, testing for secretion of lysosomal enzymes from rabbit peritoneal cells, we found that 10^{-5} M A23187 causes LDH release. Therefore, we had to go to lower concentrations in order to get our lysosomal enzyme release without any evidence of LDH leakage. Have you tested this concentration on the peripheral blood cells to see whether there is LDH leakage?

Dr. Miller: No.

Dr. Stossel: I think it is a nice assay in the tradition of looking at the cell, but l am not sure I am ready to let you off the hook, as to what it actually measures. I have talked to Marshall Lichtman about this and I think that everyone will agree that when you suck an erythrocyte into the pipette, you really are measuring membrane deformability. What bothers me is when the cell is being assaulted by this vacuum cleaner at one of its surfaces, are you simply activating that cell? And essentially, is it crawling into the pipette? Because you have such a nice correlation between everything that turns off motility, I am suspicious. Are you really sure this is a deformability assay? You would have to go to ghosts, should such a thing be possible, in order really to decide that point.

Dr. Miller: I agree with you fully. The ghosts are one idea, but for leukocytes they are difficult to prepare. The other thing that I think is limiting here is the mechanical apparatus as it now exists. And there are other factors involved, which would help to answer that: the angle the cell comes up to the pipette and all sorts of considerations in terms of the pressure dynamics. What we need is a consistent kind of pipette, which is always the same size and for which we can consider these kinds of factors. There is no way to do that with these capillaries.

But I quite agree with you. Right now the one statement that can be made is that the assay's correlation with all these conditions and its ability to detect chemotactically deficient cells is very good. Whether that means that they are reflected only through the membrane, I do not know.

Dr. Quie: You could test that, could you not? By having a small amount of negative pressure and having your pipettes positioned so that oriented cells would come up to the tip, you could measure response to a little bit of negative pressure. This would help answer the question if there is a difference in the deformability of cells that are capable of orientation.

Dr. Miller: We have done some of that. They do not crawl in. If you actually put some chemotactically reactant material in the pipette and then put the pipette near the cell—so you actually have a chemotactic gradient in the pipette—they still do not crawl in. But I do not think that proves that the mechanical boost they are getting from the negative pressure may be what's necessary actually to get them in.

Dr. Gallin: It seems to me that if you have a cell that has markedly increased deformability or elasticity of the membrane, and you start to suck it into the pipette and its gets a little held up, say, by the nucleus, you might get a tremendous increase in the length of the pseudopod or whatever you are creating. And you might think because it took longer or more pressure actually to pull the whole cell into the pipette you had decreased deformability. Don't you really need to look at the amount of pressure, the amount of time, and the length of the "pseudopod" in the capillary to get meaningful measurements?

Dr. Miller: Yes and no. Those considerations are important, dependent upon the kind of pipette you use, in these systems. And when you get down to pipettes that are small enough to reflect such things as mechanical hang-ups, it is extremely difficult to get those cells into the capillary. If you go down to the 2-μ pipette, it is really very difficult ever to get hold of the cells. These problems do not seem to occur with the pipettes we use.

Dr. Schiffmann: I am trying to get a picture of what elements are involved in this deformability process. There might be some sort of charge neutralization, perhaps. This might be accomplished by a change in volume. Have you looked at that?

Dr. Miller: No, we have not. Again, just inferentially. In terms of that volume change, with the range of the pipettes seeming to give the same data, we would surmise that the volume expansion, if it exists, would not be sufficient to give a mechanical effect in this assay.

Dr. Schiffmann: How about a volume decrease perhaps by a collapse of negative charges strung out on the inner membrane by cations coming in? That might also cause change in rigidity.

Dr. Miller: Yes, that certainly is a possibility.

Leukocyte Chemotaxis, edited by John I. Gallin
and Paul G. Quie. Raven Press, New York
© 1978.

Genetic Deficiencies of Complement-Derived Chemotactic Factors

John P. Leddy, John Baum, and Stephen I. Rosenfeld

*Clinical Immunology Unit, Departments of Medicine and Microbiology, University of
Rochester School of Medicine and Dentistry, Rochester, New York 14642*

Among the promising accomplishments in the study of inflammation and host defense in recent years has been the identification of particular plasma proteins or, more correctly, systems of proteins which, through their activation products, have the capacity to stimulate directed migration of leukocytes (15). Such advances have largely depended upon (a) isolation of these plasma proteins and clarification of their mechanisms of reaction, and (b) the availability of animal or human serum (or plasma) selectively lacking an individual factor by virtue of a genetic defect. Systematic observations of genetically deficient humans (or laboratory animals), moreover, have the added potential for aiding interpretation of the relative importance, in the overall physiology of host defense, of the growing number of chemotactically active substances demonstrable in Boyden chambers.

The complement (C) system is the most extensively studied of the plasma protein systems contributing to chemotaxis, particularly with respect to neutrophil chemotaxis, which will be emphasized in this report. The C activation products which have been found to possess chemotactic activity are, in order of discovery, the macromolecular $\overline{C567}$ complex (21,41–43), the C3a (7,39) and C5a (35,41,45) peptides, and, most recently, fluid-phase $\overline{C3B}$ from the properdin pathway (33).

Even though each of the foregoing C-activation products unquestionably possesses chemotactic activity under laboratory conditions, their respective physiologic roles are not yet clear. C5-deficient (C5D) mouse serum was found to have impaired capacity to generate chemotactic activity *in vitro* (36,42), and these animals also exhibited depressed neutrophil exudation *in vivo* (36). This suggested that C3a was quantitatively not as important as other products involving C5 or requiring C5 for their formation. The original finding that C6-deficient (C6D) rabbit serum was unable to develop normal chemotactic activity focused attention on the $\overline{C567}$ complex (42). Other workers, however, later reported normal chemotactic function in C6D rabbit serum (35,37). Subsequently, by coupling chromatographic analysis of activated serum with inactivation by specific anti-C5, compelling evidence has been obtained that C5a is the major neutrophil chemotactic factor identifiable in whole serum of man, rabbit, or guinea pig activated by immune complexes or endotoxin *in vitro* (14,34,35). Further observations on peritoneal exudates in guinea pigs and mice corroborate the importance of C5a *in vivo* (36,49). C5a or both C5a and $\overline{C567}$ have been identified in inflammatory joint fluids in man (46) and in tissue lesions in animals with immunologic vasculitis (40,44) or arthritis (11).

In this setting, my colleagues and I have had the privilege of studying the first recognized examples of hereditary C6 deficiency (22) and C5 deficiency (30,31) in man. The C5D kindred contains two homozygotes. The proband (L.H.), age 21, has <0.01% normal C5, systemic lupus erythematosus (SLE) since age 11, requiring daily or alternate-day corticosteroid therapy, and a very impressive history of bacterial infections (31). The homozygous C5D half-sister,[1] age 11, has 1 to 2% of normal C5, and is currently healthy, although she did have frequent upper respiratory infections and two episodes of pneumonia in early childhood.

We recognize that it is difficult to evaluate susceptibility to infection in the proband because of the corticosteroid therapy and possibly the SLE itself, and in the sibling because her C5 deficiency is not complete. We proposed (30,31) that C5 deficiency in man, while not as serious as C3 deficiency (3,5), may prove to carry a relative risk to the host, depending on the nature of the microbial challenge and/or the presence of other compromises in host defense. This would be analogous to the situation in C5D mice (reviewed in 31). Observations on additional human cases are clearly needed, however, and comments from Dr. Ralph Snyderman about his newly recognized C5D kindred will be of great interest.

Generation of neutrophil chemotactic activity[2] was markedly impaired in the sera of both of our C5D homozygotes (Fig. 1). The differences between either C5D serum and normal sera are highly significant ($p \leq 0.005$ by Wilcoxon rank sum test) using either activation protocol (Fig. 1). Using protocol 1, the serum of sibling D. H., possessing 1 to 2% of normal C5, consistently yielded higher chemotactic scores than did the proband's serum. These differences were only marginally significant using protocol 2 (Fig. 1). The basis for this difference between protocols is not yet clear. Since Ward has reported that only the high-molecular-weight factor ($\overline{C567}$) is formed detectably at low concentrations of C5 (41), we speculated that small amounts of $\overline{C567}$ may be formed in the sibling's serum in protocol 1 and that protocol 2 may be less favorable for the formation or stability of the $\overline{C567}$ complex (30).

Initially, the superior chemotactic function of the C5D sibling's serum suggested to us that quite small additions of purified C5 might produce measurable improvement in chemotactic performance. Our first studies of this aspect, using

---

[1] The complexities of this pedigree have been discussed elsewhere (31). The data from the family indicate that the two homozygotes have different fathers, implying that each father should be a heterozygote. Neither father was available for testing, however. More recent evidence on HL-A haplotypes suggests that the two homozygotes did indeed have different fathers (32).

[2] The technical aspects of our chemotactic assay procedure have been presented elsewhere (6,30).

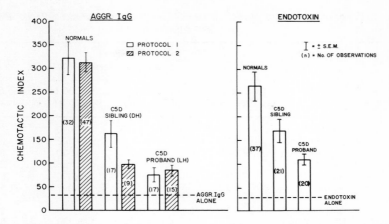

FIG. 1. Generation of chemotactic activity for human neutrophils in C5D and normal human sera in the presence of aggregated human IgG (1 mg/ml) or *Escherichia coli* endotoxin (1 μg/ml). Values shown are means ± SEM based on many observations (indicated by numbers within bars). Two activation protocols were employed. In protocol 1, the activating agent and test serum were mixed at room temperature and placed in the chambers (without heat inactivation). Protocol 2 followed the standard procedure of incubating the activating agent-test serum mixture at 37°C for 30 min, followed by 56°C for 30 min. In both protocols, leukocyte chemotaxis proceeded over 3 hr at 37°C. (From Rosenfeld et al., ref. 30, with permission.)

highly purified human C5 generously supplied by Dr. Ulf Nilsson, are shown in Table 1. In experiment I (using protocol 1), no change in chemotactic score was achieved when the hemolytic C5 titer in the proband's serum was raised to 28% of the normal mean (269,600 U/ml) and nearly half of the lowest range of normal. A larger addition of C5 to both C5D sera, sufficient to normalize fully the CH50 titers and to produce a C5 titer of 46 to 50% of the normal mean, produced only a partial correction of the chemotactic defect (Table 1, expt. II, using protocol 2). Thus, it appeared that full correction would require a normal C5 concentration.[3]

At this point, we paused to prepare a larger quantity of human C5, according to Nilsson et al. (25). We decided that it might be instructive to examine heterozygous C5D sera for their chemotactic potential (Table 2). The chemotactic scores in the various family members show a broad spread, not related to C5 level, with heterozygous and normal sera overlapping. Of interest, in respect to our efforts to reconstitute the homozygous C5D sera, was the finding that heterozygous sera possessing as little as 32 to 35% of the mean normal hemolytic C5 titer yielded excellent chemotactic activity.

---

[3] It must be emphasized that for all these studies, the proband's serum had been carefully chosen from two dates when her SLE was quiescent by clinical and laboratory criteria (ref. 31). Other than C5, hemolytic assays of all components of the classic C pathway were normal in both sera, as were screening assays for properdin pathway activity, except that inulin-induced C3 conversion was somewhat reduced or delayed in the proband's serum (31).

TABLE 1. *Effect of addition of purified human C5 on generation of chemotactic activity in C5-deficient sera*

Experiment	Assay mixtures[a]		Resulting complement levels (U/ml)		Chemotactic index[c]
	Serum source	C5 added (μg/ml serum)	CH50 (80 to 160)[b]	(159,000 to 400,000)[b]	
I	C5d proband	0		0	20
	C5d proband	12		13,000	28
	C5d proband	60		76,500	26
	Normal (A)	0		n.d.[d]	120
	Normal (B)	0		320,000	159
	Medium	60		n.d.	12
II	C5D proband	0	0	0	33
	C5D proband	147	110	125,300	62
	C5D sibling	0	40	$\sim$3000	48
	C5D sibling	147	136	134,200	79
	Normal (A)	0	n.d.	n.d.	135
	Normal (C)	0	160	353,000	138
	Medium alone				18

[a] Activated by addition of heat-aggregated human IgG (1 mg/ml) to all test samples.
[b] Normal ranges for CH50 titer (based on 100 sera) and C5 titer (based on 22 sera).
[c] Mean values based on scores of three chambers. Normal sera are from individuals A, B, and C.
[d] n.d. = not determined.

As shown in Table 3, addition of highly purified C5 sufficient to produce high normal hemolytic C5 levels finally did allow formation of normal chemotactic activity in the homozygous C5D sera. Lower C5 levels ($\sim$60% of the normal mean) were again associated with substantially lower chemotactic scores (Table 3).

We conclude that the chemotactic defect in these sera can be corrected by addition of human C5; however, a high C5 concentration is required, higher than would be expected from the studies of heterozygous C5D sera. Several explanations for this observation appear possible. First, the C5D subjects could have a high level of a chemotactic factor inactivator (38). We are currently testing the effect of C5D serum on chemotactically active normal serum. Second, some aspect of C5 activation may be relatively inefficient in the C5D sera. We have previously reported the finding, in low dilutions of both C5D sera, of an inhibitory effect which appears to interfere with classic pathway C5 convertase (EAC1423b) function (31). More recent work by Dr. Rosenfeld and me indicates that an analogous inhibitory effect is also demonstrable in lesser quantity in C5-depleted normal serum. Quite an analogous activity, i.e., interference with the generation of active C5 sites on EAC1423b, had been described earlier in guinea pig serum (27). Gel filtration analysis of our C5D serum reveals this inhibitory activity in two areas, one of high molecular weight corresponding

TABLE 2. Serum chemotactic activity[a] in kindred of C5-deficient proband

Serum tested[b]	C5 protein (as percent of normal mean)[c]	Hemolytic C5 (as percent of normal mean)[d]	Chemotactic activity (% of concurrently tested normal sera)[e]
Proband III-11 (homozygote)	0	0	0 to 6
Proposed heterozygotes			
II-2	69	61	55
III-4	50	35	96
III-9	50	37	88
III-12	50	32	113
III-13	52	39	99
III-15	47	32	75
Proposed normals			
II-1	96	97	26; 111; 51
II-11	99	93	89
III-1	96	89	34; 44; 41
III-2	97	95	33; 46; 29
III-3	88	82	72
III-10	88	83	90
III-17	101	107	107
III-18	94	93	61; 113; 73
III-20	73	67	96
III-21	76	68	101

[a] Activated by heat-aggregated human IgG (1 mg/ml). Protocol 2 was followed.
[b] Pedigree numbers refer to published pedigree (31).
[c] Mean for 20 normal donors is 113 μg/ml (range 90 to 130).
[d] Mean ± SD for 22 normal donors is 269,600 ± 79,900 U/ml (range 159,000 to 400,000).
[e] Chemotactic indices were corrected for random migration (activating medium without serum) and expressed as percent of mean values for two normal sera included in all experiments. All sera were tested in triplicate; each value shown above is the mean of 3 scores.

closely to the position of β1H (C3b inactivator accelerator)(48), the other of lower molecular weight corresponding closely to the position of C3b inactivator itself. Dr. Shaun Ruddy has found elevated C3b inactivator and high normal β1H levels in both C5D sera. Finally, we have no information on alternative pathway C5 convertase function in these C5D sera. Some contribution of this mechanism may be necessary for optimal formation of C5a.

Dr. Snyderman's two C5D homozygotes also have severely depressed serum chemotactic function, as he will relate in the discussion.

In 1974, we reported that C6D human serum developed normal levels of neutrophil chemotactic activity after incubation with aggregated IgG or Escherichia coli endotoxin (22) (Fig. 2). We concluded that the C$\overline{567}$ complex could not be a major contributor to the overall chemotactic activity formed under these conditions. Subsequently, normal generation of chemotactic activity for neutrophils (24) and for both neutrophils and monocytes (R. Snyderman, personal communication) has been observed in two additional C6D probands.

TABLE 3. *Effect of purified human C5 on generation of chemotactic activity in C5D sera*

	Assay mixtures[a]		Resulting complement levels[b]		Chemotactic index[c]
	Serum source	C5 added (µg/ml serum)	Hemolytic C5 (U/ml)		
Expt. A	Patient L.H.	0	0		182
	Patient L.H.	165	300,900		535
	Patient D.H.	0	~3,000		290
	Patient D.H.	165	307,400		883
	Normal (A)	0	257,100		1,008
	Normal (A)	165	614,800		1,092
	Normal (B)	0	—[d]		922
	HBSS	165	—[d]		200
			Hemolytic C5 (U/ml)	CH_{50} (U/ml)	
Expt. B	Patient L.H.	0	0	0	128
	Patient L.H.	73	170,300	120	428
	Patient L.H.	165	315,400	145	690
	Patient D.H.	0	~3,000	45	247
	Patient D.H.	73	167,000	122	381
	Patient D.H.	175	370,200	136	885
	Normal (A)	0	315,400	148	986
	Normal (A)	165	740,500	—[d]	998
	Normal (B)	0	—[d]	119	944
	HBSS	165	315,400	—	187

[a] Include aggregated human IgG, 1 mg/ml.
[b] Assays on serum:C5 mixtures or untreated sera were performed immediately after serum:C5 mixtures had been made.
[c] Mean values based on scores of 3 chambers. Protocol 2 was followed.
[d] — = not done.
(From ref. 30, with permission.)

The report (8) that C7D human serum exhibited a moderately reduced capacity to generate neutrophil chemotactic activity, and was corrected by addition of small amounts of C7, reopened the question concerning the quantitative importance of C567. Independently, however, another C7D proband discovered in Europe possessed normal serum chemotactic function in the laboratories of Wellek and Opferkuch in Germany (47) and of Hannema et al. in the Netherlands (17). Because this discrepancy between C7D sera was puzzling and because we felt that the C567 question was important, we sought to test both C7D sera concurrently. Drs. John Boyer and A. J. Hannema generously furnished the respective sera. Our results, using both activation protocols (Fig. 1), are shown in Tables 4 and 5. Both C7D sera are normal in our assay. Analysis

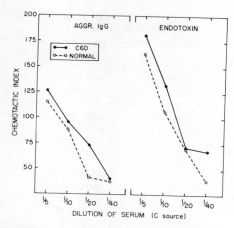

FIG. 2. Effect of increasing dilution of normal and C6-deficient human serum on generation of chemotactic activity in the presence of constant concentrations of aggregated IgG (1 mg/ml) or endotoxin (1 µg/ml). Each point is the mean of triplicate determinations within the experiment. ●——●, C6-deficient; ○···○, normal. Serum activation was according to protocol 1 (see legend to Fig. 1). (From Leddy et al., ref. 22, with permission.)

TABLE 4. *Generation of neutrophil chemotactic activity in C7-deficient human serum (protocol 1)*[a]

Expt.	Serum (complement source)	Activating agent	Chemotactic index (Mean of 3 chambers)
I	C7D (Europe)	aggr. IgG[b]	373
	C7D (Tucson)	aggr. IgG[b]	405
	Normals (2)	aggr. IgG[b]	596, 523
	Buffer	aggr. IgG[b]	66
II	C7D (Europe)	aggr. IgG[b]	1,338
	C7D (Tucson)	aggr. IgG[b]	1,048
	Normals (4)	aggr. IgG[b]	819 ± 181 (SD)
	Buffer		98
III	C7D (Tucson)	aggr. IgG[b]	232
	Normals (3)	aggr. Igg[b]	186 ± 51
	C5D (Rochester)	aggr. IgG[b]	25
	Buffer	aggr. IgG[b]	16
	C7D (Tucson)	endotoxin[c]	226
	Normals (3)	endotoxin[c]	241 ± 67
	Buffer	endotoxin[c]	21

[a] See legend to Fig. 1.
[b] Heat-aggregated human IgG, 1 mg/ml.
[c] *Escherichia coli* 0111 B4 endotoxin (Difco), 1 µg/ml.

TABLE 5. *Generation of neutrophil chemotactic activity in C7-deficient human serum (protocol 2)[a]*

Exp.	Serum (complement source)	Activating agent	Chemotactic index (mean of 3 chambers)
I	C7D (Europe)	aggr. IgG[b]	639
	C7D (Tucson)	aggr. IgG[b]	1,081
	Normals (4)	aggr. IgG[b]	907 ± 88 (SD)
	Buffer	aggr. IgG[b]	212
II	C7D (Europe)	endotoxin[c]	315
	C7D (Tucson)	endotoxin[c]	101
	Normals (4)	endotoxin[c]	115 ± 34
	Buffer	endotoxin[c]	43
III	C7D (Tucson)	none	44
	C7D (Tucson)	aggr. IgG[b]	242
	Normals (2)	aggr. IgG[b]	138, 205
	C5D (Rochester)	aggr. IgG[b]	31
	Buffer	aggr. IgG[b]	15

[a] See legend to Fig. 1.
[b] Heat-aggregated human IgG, 1 mg/ml
[c] *E. coli* 0111 B4 endotoxin (Difco), 1 µg/ml

of the methods used by the various investigators has not revealed an explanation for the apparently discrepant results originally reported for the American C7D serum (8).[4] The question is still under study.

Two C8D human homozygotes have, not surprisingly, demonstrated normal serum chemotactic function (19,29).

Elsewhere in this volume, Dr. Robert Clark has reviewed the chemotactic performance of C1rD, C4D, C2D, C3D, and C3b inactivator-deficient human sera (Chap. 24). Therefore, in this chapter, these deficiencies are simply listed in the overall state-of-the-art summary presented in Table 6. The entries in the tables are based on references already cited plus the following additional reports: one C1rD serum (10), studied for chemotaxis by Gallin (13); two C4D sera (18,26) studied by Clark (Chap. 24); two C2D sera[5] (20,23) studied for Rebuck skin window response by Klemperer et al. (20) and by Gewurz et al. (16), and for *in vitro* chemotaxis by Gewurz et al. (16), Leddy et al. (23), Gallin et al. (14), and Clark (Chap. 24); three C3D sera (3,5,28) studied for *in vitro* chemotaxis by Alper et al. (4), Osofski et al. (28), and Clark (Chap.

---

[4] The C7D donor from Tucson (J. A.) sometimes exhibits small but measurable amounts of C7 (8). Therefore, with the kind cooperation of Dr. Boyer, two dates of bleeding which lacked measurable hemolytic C activity (CH50) were selected for chemotactic study. In our laboratory, serum from both of these dates, as well as the European C7D serum (J. R.), lacked detectable C7 in a hemolytic assay which could have detected 0.01% of normal activity.

[5] A third C2D serum has also been studied for chemotactic activity by Dr. Robert A. Clark (see Chap. 24, ref. 102).

TABLE 6. *Serum chemotactic capacity in genetic complement-deficiency states in man*

Deficiency (number of individuals studied)	Generation of serum chemotactic activity for human neutrophils *in vitro*		Comment
	Activating agent	Result	
C1r (1)	Endotoxin	Kinetic lag but ultimately normal	
C4 (2)	Zymosan, endotoxin, aggr. IgG	Same as above, plus serum concentration effect	Corrected by added C4
C2 (3)	Aggr. IgG, endotoxin, immune complexes	Similar to above	Corrected by C2; Rebuck skin window data conflicting
C3 (3)	Endotoxin, zymosan	Severely impaired	Corrected by C3; Rebuck window: delayed neutrophil response
C5 (4)	Aggr. IgG, endotoxin, cobra venom factor	Severely impaired	Corrected by addition of C5 to normal levels
C6 (3)	Aggr. IgG, endotoxin	Normal[a]	
C7 (2)	Immune complexes, zymosan, aggr. IgG, endotoxin	Probably normal	One study found moderately reduced activity, corrected by small addition of C7
C8 (2)	Immune complexes, aggr. IgG, zymosan	Normal	
C3b INA (1)	Immune complexes	Severely impaired	Improved by normal serum *in vitro* or plasma *in vivo*

[a]Monocyte chemotaxis also normal in the one case tested.

24), and for Rebuck window response by Ballow et al. (5); and, one C3b INA-deficient serum studied by Alper et al. (1,2).

The major lessons learned from the study of C-deficient sera are (a) that generation of chemotactic activity in sera having only the alternative C pathway available is slower and less efficient than in normal serum (9,14); and (b) that C3 and C5 are critical but C6 and probably C7 are not. The latter findings strengthen the evidence from other studies cited earlier that the chemotactic activity in complement-activated serum is principally associated with the C5a peptide (or a related C5 fragment).

This dominance of C5a certainly does not imply that the other C-derived chemotactic factors are not formed. C5a may just be the hardiest survivor. The $C\overline{3B}$ factor is clearly labile (33). There is preliminary evidence that C5a is chemotactically active at lower molar concentrations than C3a (12) and that C5a retains some chemotactic function after exposure to carboxypeptidase B, whereas C3a does not (12). Whatever the basis, this dominant chemotactic role of C5a *in activated whole serum* does not negate other evidence that $C\overline{567}$ may be relevant in certain pathological fluids or tissue lesions (40,46) in which C activation may proceed by other mechanisms and under quite different conditions.

ACKNOWLEDGMENTS

The excellent technical assistance of Charlene Winney, Patricia A. Thiem, and Jill Countryman, and the valuable secretarial help of Sally Ann Hart, are acknowledged with gratitude. This work was supported by U.S.P.H.S. research grant AI-12568; a grant from the National Foundation—March of Dimes; a grant from the Rochester, New York, Chapter of the Arthritis Foundation; and by the David Welk Memorial Fund.

REFERENCES

1. Alper, C. A., Abramson, N., Johnston, R. B., Jandl, J. H., and Rosen, F. S. (1970): Increased susceptibility to infection associated with abnormalities of complement-mediated functions of the third component of complement. *N. Engl. J. Med.*, 282:349–354.
2. Alper, C. A., Abramson, N., Johnston, R. B., Jandl, J. H., and Rosen, F. S. (1970): Studies in vivo and in vitro on an abnormality in the metabolism of C3 in a patient with increased susceptibility to infection. *J. Clin. Invest.*, 49:1975–1985.
3. Alper, C. A., and Rosen, F. S., (1975): Increased susceptibility to infection in patients with defects affecting C3. In: *Immunodeficiency in Man and Animals. Birth Defects: Original Article Series*, edited by D. Bergsma, pp. 301–305. The National Foundation—March of Dimes, Sinauer Associates, Inc., Sunderland, Mass.
4. Alper, C. A., Stossel, T. P., and Rosen, F. S. (1975): Genetic defects affecting complement and host resistance to infection. In: *The Phagocytic Cell in Host Resistance*, edited by J. A. Bellanti and D. H. Dayton, pp. 127–141. Raven Press, New York.
5. Ballow, M., Shira, J. E., Harden, L., Yang, S. Y., and Day, N. K. (1975): Complete absence of the third component of complement in man. *J. Clin. Invest.*, 56:703–710.
6. Baum, J. (1975): Chemotaxis in human disease. In: *The Phagocytic Cell in Host Resistance*, edited by J. A. Bellanti and D. H. Dayton, pp. 282–290. Raven Press, New York.
7. Bokisch, V. R., Müller-Eberhard, H. J., and Cochrane, C. G. (1969): Isolation of a fragment (C3a) of the third component of complement containing anaphylatoxin and chemotactic activity and description of an anaphylatoxin inactivator of human serum. *J. Exp. Med.*, 129:1109–1130.
8. Boyer, J. T., Gall, E. P., Norman, M. E., Nilsson, U. R., and Zimmerman, T. S. (1975): Hereditary deficiency of the seventh component of complement. *J. Clin. Invest.*, 56:905–913.
9. Clark, R. A., Frank, M. M., and Kimball, H. R. (1973): Generation of chemotactic factors in guinea pig serum via activation of the classical and alternate complement pathways. *Clin. Immunol. Immunopathol.*, 1:414–426.
10. Day, N. K., Geiger, R. S., deBracco, M., Mancado, B., Windhorst, D., and Good, R. A. (1972): Clr deficiency: An inborn error associated with cutaneous and renal disease. *J. Clin. Invest.*, 51:1102–1108.
11. DeShazo, C. V., McGrade, M. T., Henson, P. M., and Cochrane, C. G. (1972): The effect of complement depletion on neutrophil migration in acute immunologic arthritis. *J. Immunol.*, 108:1414–1419.
12. Fernandez, H., Henson, P., and Hugli, T. E. (1976): A single scheme for C3a and C5a isolation and characterization of chemotactic behavior (Abstract). *J. Immunol.*, 116:1732.
13. Gallin, J. I. (1975): Abnormal chemotaxis: Cellular and humoral components. In: *The Phagocytic Cell in Host Resistance*, edited by J. A. Bellanti and D. H. Dayton, pp. 227–243. Raven Press, New York.
14. Gallin, J. I., Clark, R. A., and Frank, M. M. (1975): Kinetic analysis of chemotactic factor generation in human serum via activation of the classical and alternate complement pathways. *Clin. Immunol. Immunopathol.*, 3:334–346.
15. Gallin, J. I., and Wolff, S. M. (1975): Leucocyte chemotaxis: Physiological considerations and abnormalities. *Clin. Haematol.*, 4:567–607.
16. Gewurz, H., Page, A. R., Pickering, R. J., and Good, R. A. (1967): Complement activity

and inflammatory neutrophil exudation in man: Studies in patients with glomerulonephritis, essential hypocomplementemia and agammaglobulinemia. *Int. Arch. Allergy,* 32:64–90.
17. Hannema, A. J., Pondman, K. W., Döhmann, U., Gadner, H., and Dooren, L. J. (1975): C7 Deficiency in man. In: Protides Biol. Fluids, 22nd Colloq. (Brugge, 1974), edited by H. Peeters, pp. 581–584. Pergamon Press, New York.
18. Hauptmann, G., Grosshans, E., Heid, E., Mayer, S., and Basset, A. (1974): Lupus erythemateux aigu avec déficit complet de la fraction C4 du complément. *Nouv. Presse Med.,* 3:881–884.
19. Jasin, H. E. (1976): Absence of the eighth component of complement (C8) and systemic lupus erythematosus-like disease (Abstract). *Arthritis Rheum.,* 19:803.
20. Klemperer, M. R., Austen, K. F., and Rosen, F. S. (1967): Hereditary deficiency of the second component of complement (C'2) in man: Further observations on a second kindred. *J. Immunol.,* 98:72–78.
21. Lachmann, P. J., Kay, A. B., and Thompson, R. A. (1970): The chemotactic activity for neutrophil and eosinophil leukocytes of the trimolecular complex of the fifth, sixth, and seventh components of human complement (C567) prepared in free solution by the "reactive lysis" procedure. *Immunology,* 19:895–899.
22. Leddy, J. P., Frank, M. M., Gaither, T., Baum, J., and Klemperer, M. R. (1974): Hereditary deficiency of the sixth component of complement in man: I. Immunochemical, biologic, and family studies. *J. Clin. Invest.,* 53:544–553.
23. Leddy, J. P., Griggs, R. C., Klemperer, M. R., and Frank, M. M. (1975): Hereditary complement (C2) deficiency with dermatomyositis. *Am. J. Med.,* 58:83–91.
24. Lim, D., Gewurz, A., Lint, T. F., Ghaze, M., Sepheri, B., and Gewurz, H. (1976): Absence of the sixth component of complement in a patient with repeated episodes of meningococcal meningitis. *J. Pediatr.,* 89:42–47.
25. Nilsson, U. R., Tomar, R. H., and Taylor, F. B., Jr. (1972): Additional studies on human C5: Development of a modified purification method and characterization of the purified product by polyacrilamide gel electrophoresis. *Immunochemistry,* 9:709–723.
26. Ochs, H. D., Rosenfeld, S. I., Thomas, E. D., Giblett, E. R., Alper, C. A., Dupont, B., Schaller, J. G., Gilliland, B. C., Hansen, J. A., and Wedgwood, R. J. (1977): Linkage between the gene(s) controlling synthesis of the fourth component of complement (C4) and the major histocompatibility loci. *N. Engl. J. Med., (in press).*
27. Okada, H., Kawachi, S., and Nishioka, K. (1969): A new complement inhibitor in guinea pig serum. *Jpn. J. Exp. Med.,* 39:527–531.
28. Osofski, S. G., Thompson, B. H., Lint, T. F., and Gewurz, H. (1977): Hereditary deficiency of the third component of complement in a child with fever, skin rash, and arthralgias: Response to transfusion of whole blood. *J. Pediatr.,* 90:180–185.
29. Petersen, B. H., Graham, J. A., and Brooks, G. F. (1976): Human deficiency of the eighth component of complement: The requirement of C8 for serum *Neisseria gonorrhoeae* bactericidal activity. *J. Clin. Invest.,* 57:283–290.
30. Rosenfeld, S. I., Baum, J., Steigbigel, R. T., and Leddy, J. P. (1976): Hereditary deficiency of the fifth component of complement in man: II. Biological properties of C5-deficient human serum. *J. Clin. Invest.,* 57:1635–1643.
31. Rosenfeld, S. I., Kelly, M. E., and Leddy, J. P. (1976): Hereditary deficiency of the fifth component of complement in man: I. Clinical, immunochemical and family studies. *J. Clin. Invest.,* 57:1626–1634.
32. Rosenfeld, S. I., Weitkamp, L. R., and Ward, F. (1977): Hereditary deficiency of the fifth component of complement in man: IV. Genetic linkage studies. *J. Immunol. (in press).*
33. Ruddy, S., Austen, K. F., and Goetzl, E. J. (1975): Chemotactic activity derived from interaction of factors D and B of the properdin pathway with cobra venom factor or C3b. *J. Clin. Invest.,* 55:587–592.
34. Snyderman, R., and Mergenhagen, S. E. (1972): Characterization of polymorphonuclear leukocyte chemotactic activity in serums activated by various inflammatory agents. In: *Biological Activities of Complement,* edited by D. G. Ingram, pp. 117–132. A. G. Karger, Basel.
35. Snyderman, R., Phillips, J., and Mergenhagen, S. E. (1969): Polymorphonuclear leukocyte chemotactic activity in rabbit serum and guinea pig serum treated with immune complexes: Evidence for C5a as the major chemotactic factor. *Infect. Immun.,* 1:521–525.
36. Snyderman, R., Phillips, J. K., and Mergenhagen, S. E. (1971): Biological activity of complement in vivo: Role of C5 in the accumulation of polymorphonuclear leukocytes in inflammatory exudates. *J. Exp. Med.,* 134:1131–1143.

37. Stecher, V., and Sorkin, E. (1969): Studies on chemotaxis: XII. Generation of chemotactic activity for polymorphonuclear leukocytes in sera with complement deficiencies. *Immunology,* 16:231–240.

38. Till, G., and Ward, P. A. (1975): Two distinct chemotactic factor inactivators in human serum. *J. Immunol.,* 114:843–847.

39. Ward, P. A. (1967): A plasmin split product of C'3 as a new chemotactic factor. *J. Exp. Med.,* 126:189–206.

40. Ward, P. A. (1971): Chemotactic factors for neutrophils, eosinophils, mononuclear cells and lymphocytes. In: *Biochemistry of the Acute Allergic Reactions, Second International Symposium,* edited by K. F. Austen and E. L. Becker, pp. 229–242. Blackwell Scientific Publications, Oxford.

41. Ward, P. A. (1972): Complement-derived chemotactic factors and their interactions with neutrophilic granulocytes. In: *Biological Activities of Complement,* edited by D. G. Ingram, pp. 108–116. A. G. Karger, Basel.

42. Ward, P. A., Cochrane, C. G., and Müller-Eberhard, H. J. (1965): The role of serum complement in chemotaxis of leukocytes *in vitro. J. Exp. Med.,* 122:327–346.

43. Ward, P. A., Cochrane, C. G., and Müller-Eberhard, H. J. (1966): Further studies on the chemotactic factor of complement and its formation in vivo. *Immunology,* 11:141–154.

44. Ward, P. A., and Hill, J. H. (1972): Biologic role of complement products: Complement derived leukotactic activity extractable from lesions of immunologic vasculitis. *J. Immunol.,* 108:1137–1145.

45. Ward, P. A., and Newman, L. J. (1969): A neutrophilic chemotactic factor from human C5. *J. Immunol.,* 102:93–99.

46. Ward, P. A., and Zvaifler, N. J. (1971): Complement-derived leukotactic factors in inflammatory synovial fluids of humans. *J. Clin. Invest.,* 50:606–616.

47. Wellek, B., and Opferkuch, W. (1975): A case of deficiency of the seventh component of complement in man: Biological properties of a C7-deficient serum and description of a C7-inactivating principle. *Clin. Exp. Immunol.,* 19:223–235.

48. Whaley, K., and Ruddy, S. (1976): Modulation of C3b hemolytic activity by a plasma protein distinct from C3b inactivator. *Science,* 193:1011–1013.

49. Wilkinson, P. C., O'Neill, G. J., and Wapshaw, K. G. (1973): Role of anaerobic corneforms in specific and nonspecific immunological reactions: II. Production of a chemotactic factor specific for macrophages. *Immunology,* 24:997–1006.

DISCUSSION

Dr. Snyderman: This is an extremely valuable presentation in that it brings to the study of human serum an understanding of the biological relevance of chemotactic activity *in vitro.* I am pleased to see that C5 fragments are getting some attention.

We recently found a patient with a C5 deficiency. I happened to be the attending on rounds in Rheumatology. A 21-year-old black woman was readmitted with gonococcal arthritis, having been treated adequately with penicillin and ampicillin in Duke Hospital about 10 days to 2 weeks before. She had a whole complement titer of zero and we found that her hemolytic C5 titer, done as an end-point determination, was less than normal. She also has a sister who is probably an identical twin and whose hemolytic complement C5 titer is approximately 0.5% of normal.

Since I saw the patient in the hospital, she has had another bout of gonococcal sepsis with multiple skin lesions of gonococcemia. The sister, who had been completely healthy and never had had any problem with infections whatsoever, recently also developed disseminated gonococcal disease. We found, just as you have, disequilibrium between the C5 deficiency, major histocompatibility loci A or B, and no linkage. We have tested the generation of chemotactic activity with aggregated gammaglobulin and cobra venom factor on five occasions. On three of those times, the patients' sera generated chemotactic activity either equal to or less than background.

In other words, there was no generation of chemotactic activity. A couple of times there was some activity above background, but only a few percent of normal. As Dr. Leddy mentioned, we had a C6-deficient patient with primary biliary cirrhosis who had completely normal chemotactic activity generation.

I would like to mention a few more points about this C5D family. First, I asked them if they had any relatives in Rochester, and they said no. We studied three other family members who were heterozygotes, and had hemolytic activity ranging from about 38 to 42% of normal. They all generated chemotactic activity normally, which was somewhat surprising. There was something that I did not understand until Dr. Leddy gave his presentation. That is, in our hemolytic assay which we do as an end-point determination, their C5 titers were about 0.2 to 0.5% of normal. I sent some serum to Dr. John Curd who is working with Dr. H. J. Muller-Eberhard, and he said that in doing a kinetic assay, he found their values were similar to those you presented. He assumed that it was because of the C3b inactivator. I think that probably our patient is similar to yours and I would be happy to send you some of their serum. Also, there was no C5 protein as determined in our laboratory or in Dr. Muller-Eberhard's laboratory.

Dr. Quie: Have you taken washed neutrophils and/or monocytes from these patients with C5 deficiency, and measured chemotactic activity? Do the cells function normally when normal serum is the source of chemotactic attractant?

Dr. Leddy: Yes, neutrophils from these patients demonstrate normal chemotactic activity and phagocytic activity in the presence of normal serum.

The gonococcal infections in Dr. Snyderman's C5D patient may be similar to those occurring in C6-, C7-, and C8-deficient subjects. All these patients lack serum bactericidal activity.

Dr. Jensen: I am puzzled about the reconstitution with C5. Have you observed any evidence of C5 inhibitory activity on these patients' sera?

Dr. Leddy: As we have reported, there was no true inhibitor of C5 itself, and the C5D serum did not abnormally degrade added C5 at 37°C; however, we did encounter, *in lower dilutions* of C5D serum, an activity which reduced the apparent hemolytic titer of C5. We believe that C5 convertase function is being affected and that the interfering substance(s) in C5D serum may be C3b inactivator with or without the B1H cofactor. One important thing we have not done yet is to generate chemotactic activity in normal serum and then add the C5-deficient patient's serum to see if preformed chemotactic activity is inhibited.

Dr. Gallin: Although the patients with C5 deficiency are obviously sick and have infections, they are not seriously compromised. Did either you or Dr. Snyderman look at any inflammatory sites in these patients, or in mice with C5-deficiency, to see what kind of mediators are present?

Dr. Leddy: Rebuck window studies have not been done because the proband is always on some form of steroid therapy, and such results would be difficult to interpret. I hope Dr. Snyderman does that with his patients. I believe you are already familiar with his study on the C5 dependence on peritoneal exudation in mice (36).

When C5D serum was activated and tested without prior heating at 56°C, a small amount of chemotactic activity was generated, particularly in the C5D sibling's serum. The nature of this chemotactic activity has not been determined. It may possibly relate to Dr. Ward's earlier suggestion (41) that in the presence of very limiting amounts of C5, $\overline{C567}$ may be formed preferentially. Possibly this $\overline{C567}$ is at least partially inactivated by heating, since we did not observe it when the activated serum was heated before being placed in the chambers.

Would you comment on that, Dr. Ward?

Dr. Ward: The ratios of the complement components are important in the cleavage of C5. The amount of C6 and of C7 can effect the amounts of C5 fragments, but I think it is terribly difficult to translate observations based on hemolytic interactions to chemotactic models.

Dr. Hill: Have any opsonin studies been done with the serum from either one of these patients?

Dr. Leddy: We found normal opsonic function for baker's yeast and for staphylococci in the C5-deficient serum. Both of these girls have so much heat-stable opsonic activity against Candida, it was not possible to study heat-labile Candida opsonic function.

Dr. Michael Miller's studies were done on young infants who had what he called C5 dysfunction. He found a serum opsonic defect for the phagocytosis of baker's yeast. My colleagues and I are well aware of what I think is an excellent study by Dr. Hyun Shin and his associates at Johns Hopkins on C5 deficiency in the mouse. Studying the pneumococcus, Dr. Shin and his colleagues found that both *in vitro* and *in vivo* the C5-deficient mouse was at a disadvantage as far as the opsonic function was concerned. And that was a system where they did not have antibody present, as far as one could tell. The opsonic action seemed to depend entirely on what is called the heat-labile opsonin system, presumably the alternate complement pathway. Under those conditions, where the alternate complement pathway is presumably less efficient than the classic pathway in putting C3b on the particles, I am quite prepared to believe that C5b or some C5 product bound to the particle may improve opsonic function.

We went into this opsonic study of C5D human serum quite prepared to find that there was some requirement for C5. I still think there may be such an effect if you had a purely alternate pathway system available. In a serum that has antibody to the yeast or to the staphylococcus however (and these girls do have such heat-stable activities), the classic complement pathway would probably also be available. For both test organisms (yeast and staphylococci), heat-labile opsonic activity was about two-thirds of the total opsonic function of the C5D serum. Where this situation exists, i.e., where heat-stable opsonins are present along with the heat-labile opsonins, the classic pathway would probably be utilized. Perhaps this overcomes the need for any C5. So I would not want to rule out a role for C5 in opsonization; however, our data do demonstrate that C5 is not an absolute requirement.

Dr. Becker: I think it is worthwhile calling attention to the possible analogy between the genetic deficiency of complement component C5 and hereditary angioedema. The latter defect is also genetic, but nevertheless can be corrected or partially corrected by anabolic steroids.

That is especially relevant in C5-deficient patients where some protein is made. Therefore, the defect may not necessarily be a structural gene but may be secondary to something that is regulating the amount of synthesis.

Dr. Robert Clark: Even though the C5-deficient serum shows a profound defect in chemotactic factor generation, I think there are at least three lines of circumstantial evidence that suggest that it is not defective chemotactic or opsonic generation but a bactericidal defect in serum which may be responsible for clinical problems in these patients. (1) The first line of evidence is the occurrence of gonococcal and meningococcal infections in patients lacking the later complement components C6, C7, C8, where there is no problem with chemotactic factor generation. (2) The second relates to studies in our laboratory with C6-deficient rabbits. Dr. David Durack has been able to induce endocarditis with gonococci in the C6-deficient rabbits more easily than in normal rabbits. (3) The third is recently published evidence from Schoolnik and co-workers (*J. Clin. Invest.,* 58:1163, 1976) that strains of gonococci from disseminated infection have different growth requirements, different antibiotic sensitivities, and are resistant to the bactericidal activity of the normal human serum. Serum bactericidal activity appears to be very important for host defense against gonococci.

Dr. Leddy: That is very interesting. Our first C6 deficiency patient had two episodes of disseminated gonococcal disease with arthritis and microinfarcts. Since we do not have that highly virulent type of gonococcus in Rochester, her defect apparently allowed dessemination of a less virulent organism.

Dr. Stossel: Another word on the opsonic dysfunction of C5-deficient serum. We use an assay for opsonization which is entirely dependent on the alternative pathway, and when different dilutions are used, there is a small difference between serum samples with suspected C5 dysfunction and normal serum. The differences are small and read out as having normal opsonic activity. C5 and C3 are quite similar in structure. And I favor the idea that C5 may act as a C3 analog and have some opsonic activity of its own.

Dr. Leddy: We studied a C5 dysfunctional serum sent to us by Dr. Ulf Nilsson and that serum was in the lower range of normal in our laboratory. Our findings were similar to yours, Dr. Stossel. Another serum in the lowest range of normal was from a completely healthy medical student who was working in our laboratory for the summer. Activity in his serum was consistently lower than in any of those C5 dysfunction sera. We have analyzed this student's complement system backward and forward, and he is normal. He does not have a history of Leiner's syndrome or anything like that, and his family members are normal.

Leukocyte Chemotaxis, edited by Paul G. Quie
and John I. Gallin. Raven Press, New York
© 1978.

Overview

Peter A. Ward

*Department of Pathology, University of Connecticut Health Center, Farmington,
Connecticut 06032*

I would like to read a few sentences from an article written by Irving Page (*Perspectives in Biology and Medicine,* Autumn issue, 1976). Then, in the course of the overview, I would like to insert a few personal references. My reason for doing so, perhaps, may be reflected in Page's statements. He says: "It may well be asked what difference does it make in the long run who discovered what and when? My answer reflects my own deep biases and experiences with a particular discovery, in this case, serotonin. I believe that Science is best taught and remembered when it is humanized and thereby related to the people involved. This is simply good pedagogy—part fact—and often, part poetic license. How much of each, history will judge, but firsthand eyewitness report could provide substance for debate. This is the way it always has been in science and I hope the way it always will be. And there are many other reasons." This, perhaps, is or is not adequate justification for inserting a few personal notes, but I think that the perspectives which are gleaned over a period of 10 or 15 years are sometimes useful. For most of you whose entry into the chemotactic field has been of relatively recently, i.e., 1, 2, 5, or 10 years), I think it is useful to look back to the recent past and try to appreciate what happened in the last 20 or 30 years. Several advances occurring in tandem account for the rapid advancements in the field of chemotaxis. Much of the pioneering work was done upwards of 50 years ago by many men cited here in these chapters. Many others who have not been cited have also made contributions which appeared in the literature by the late 1940s. For the next 10 or 15 years, with only a few exceptions, not very much new information appeared in the literature. Valle Menkin, whose name has not been mentioned here, was probably the last of the old-line investigators, if one makes distinctions based on the classical (premicropore filter) methods for studying chemotaxis. Menkin departed the field, and departed this earth, in the late 1950s, but he had published a series of articles which suggested that when tissue damage occurs, the products of tissue breakdown are themselves chemotactic. These factors were presumably peptides, but their structures were relatively nonspecific; that is, breakdown from virtually any tissue would result in the release of small peptides, all of which had chemotactic activity.

Interest and enthusiasm in the field was brought to a rather abrupt halt by a review that Henry Harris published in the middle 1950s in *Physiological Reviews,* and in it Harris provided extremely encyclopedic coverage of what had been done in the field of chemotaxis. He went through all the various methodologies, pointing out the advantages and the disadvantages of each. The thrust, or message, and perhaps unintended result, of that review was almost a damnation of the biological meaning of chemotaxis. Harris came down hard in saying that chemotaxis was an *in vitro* phenomenon, which probably had no *in vivo* relevance. He pushed hard on the point that no one had conclusively shown that this phenomenon exists *in vivo.* A second review by Harris was published in 1962 in *Bacteriological Reviews.* It more or less reiterated the earlier theme. Being a relatively forceful and respected scientist, Harris's word was not taken lightly and I think it did have a definite impact and perhaps, to a lesser extent, tended to scare some younger investigators from the field.

My own involvement in the field occurred in late 1963 at La Jolla. Boyden had published an article in the *Journal of Experimental Medicine* the preceding year. In this article, he described the micropore filter method for studying chemotaxis. One of my tasks was to try to use the methodology that Boyden had described, to simplify it if necessary, and see if chemotactic principles could be identified, particularly in view of the fact that Hans Müller-Eberhard had just arrived on the scene from the Rockefeller Institute. It was anticipated that his expertise with complement might be useful.

In our early experiments, the blueprint plan for the Boyden chamber (which appeared in the *JEM* article) was a rather formidable description, and we turned to using a simple modification Sykes-Moore chamber. In those days, we had all of 15 chambers and one big experiment consisted of collecting data from 15 different setups. In some of the more active laboratories today (including our own), it is not uncommon to have a 200-or 300-chamber run in any given day. So, when one looks back, it is humbling to recognize that this start was very modest indeed.

The literature at that time (the mid 1960s) was also modest in terms of the contributions of various investigators to the field of chemotaxis. There were, on an average, perhaps two or three articles appearing in the literature a year. If one now goes to the *Index Medicus* and scans the frequency or the number of contributions, one finds contributions approaching half a thousand per year, so that there has been a veritable explosion of interest and progress in the chemotaxis field, and this has developed in ever-increasing intensity over the past 10 or 15 years.

As the work got underway in La Jolla, there was an important series of critical events, all of which came together. When I started working on chemotaxis, in the first few months, the C5 component of complement was not known. C5 had not yet been isolated and characterized by Nilsson and Müller-Eberhard, but they were in the process which soon would yield the critical information. By 1964, Nelson's group had just demonstrated that the C3 complex consisted of at least three or four activities, but these were only known by their hemolytic functions. With Cochrane and Müller-Eberhard, we were able to demonstrate that chemotactic activity could be generated by complement-activating agents and that intermediate complexes using sensitized erythrocytes, at some point beyond C3, but before C8,9, released a chemotactic principle.

At about the same time, there were several groups working on the question of the source of anaphylatoxin. Joerge Jensen was very actively involved in this work, as were many other groups (including Müller-Eberhard's laboratory, Lepow's, Voght's, and others). All these forces began coming together as it became recognized that the biological activities of the complement system, in large part, originated from the middle portion of that system. And not very long after that, it became appreciated that these various activities, as Jensen pointed out in his initial studies, could be generated not only by the convertases generated internally to the complement system, but also by external convertases, such as trypsin, and a variety of tissue proteases.

So, in very short order, the recognition and delineation of the biological activities of the complement system became a reality. In many respects, the middle and latter 1960s in La Jolla and elsewhere were the halcyon days of complement, certainly as far as excitement over the first gleanings of the origins of the complement-related biological activities.

After that time, most of the rest is history. My involvement then took the direction at the AFIP over a 6-year collaboration with Elmer Becker, in which our studies involved looking at the enzymatic activation mechanisms of leukocytes.

If one compares these historical developments with the events of the past decade, this latter pales in comparison, but it simply indicates that we have entered into an era of biology, and pathology, if you will, which is going to be exceedingly important and which will probably remake some of our basic concepts of disease and inflammation.

What I would like to do next is to emphasize some of the points which I think are obvious to most, and to point out some of the problems and questions that need to be answered. The list is far from inclusive. It represents some of my personal biases as to what I perceive are the more significant problems to be resolved.

We have heard a great deal about the methodologies for the measurement of chemotaxis and it is perfectly clear that, while very important advances have been made, we still do not know what parameters are most meaningful, nor do we know precisely the questions to which the results can be addressed. As an example, if one takes the investigations of clinical defects, it has become abundantly clear from our discussions here that defects in cell movement may or may not be uncovered, depending on the method employed in the chemotactic assay.

We know that one can measure the depth or the leading-front of migrating cells; one can measure numbers of migrating cells, either at the leading-front, or at various levels within the filter; one can measure the frequency of turns and the direction that cells take; one can measure less direct parameters of cell movement such as enzyme release, ion flux, changes in cell volume, and deformability. Whatever parameters are used we are still left with the problem that we do not know which one of these is most revealing and most relevant. We do not know which is most inclusive in terms of picking up defects. We do not know which one is most predictive of defects in the interactions of chemotactic factors with leukocytes.

So I think that we have much to learn and many questions to resolve concerning the fundamental approaches to the measurements of movement. In this regard, we have heard a good deal about the nomenclature and the concept of differentiating between directed and nondirected cell movement. These appear to be important questions which will have to be pursued vigorously in the future. For those who are particularly interested in looking at the paths of migrating cells, it might be useful to examine the work of the late Sumner Wood, Jr. There must be at least a million feet of film in which he very carefully recorded paths of migrations of leukocytes, and actually subjected the data to an extensive computerized approach. Unfortunately, Dr. Wood's untimely death recently has terminated those studies, but his archive of time-lapsed photography must still exist and might offer interesting and useful film-recorded data.

As far as current methodologies related to the micropore filter system, it has been our experience (and the experience of many others) that there is no predictable consistency between varying lots of filters. Even filters from the same lot number are erratic in the results obtained. The conventional parameters of filter characteristics used by industry (including intrusion of mercury vapor, water flow rate, etc.) are not predictive of whether the filters will be useful in chemotaxis. Our experience has been that one simply has to plough through the various batches of filters very carefully, testing each, and selecting useful batches. This becomes very time-consuming and a particularly expensive undertaking. If one is going to use filters at the present time, there seems to be no way around this.

There are problems with the cells. We have heard evidence that there may be a heterogeneity of leukocytes. We have no good systems, as far as I know, for separating cells on the basis of their possible functional heterogeneity. This is a very important question and I believe it is going to have to be resolved in order to try to bring some order to a lot of very confusing data.

What about the chemotactic factors? As I have indicated before, there used to be a widely held theory that these included any peptides derived from tissue breakdown. The studies many of us have been involved with, and particularly work with the synthetic peptides, point to the inescapable conclusion that primary structure is important for the associated chemotactic activity. While primary structure may not be the only essential parameter, it is certainly a critical one. So, any peptide, whether released from damaged tissues or resulting from hydrolysis of proteins by various enzymes, is not predictably chemotactic. If one goes through the spectrum of serum proteins and simply starts digesting them with trypsin, one finds out very quickly that the yields of chemotactic products are very slim indeed.

The synthetic peptides, as has been alluded to in this conference, have proved to be one of the most important and potent probes for the definition of interactions of chemotactic factors with cell surfaces and their putative receptors. I suppose the question can be asked: How will these data relate to the binding of the naturally occurring chemotactic factors with putative receptors on cell surfaces? This simply means we will have to proceed with the isolation of the naturally occurring peptides and go through the same drill as is now being used with the synthetic peptides. This is going to be an enormous task to try to isolate the factors in highly purified form, and in suitable quantities. The only naturally occurring peptides for which we have the structure are those which are chemotactic for the eosinophil and, as has been revealed here, it is possible, if not likely, that the peptides which have so far been described represent in fact the least important factors in a family of peptides with chemotactic activity for eosinophils. There may well turn out to be a spectrum of peptides chemotactic for eosinophils.

The lipids may represent another class of naturally occurring factors which could turn out to be important chemotactic factors, and perhaps we are much closer to resolving that structural question than we are for the naturally occurring peptides.

I think we have heard a great deal about regulation, both normal and abnormal, in the chemotactic system. Whenever one has vasoactive agents which are active in the neighborhood of 10^{-10} and 10^{-12} M concentration, it goes without saying that unless the inflammatory system is going to get out of order very quickly, there must be potent regulatory systems. We are beginning to see the evidence for this in human subjects as well as in animals.

Finally, just a few words about the perspectives of these findings as they relate to the *in vivo* situation. One of the very frustrating things in terms of working with human subjects is that we do not have a good way of measuring the inflammatory response. We can measure vasopermeability changes in man, but even that is difficult, because no one is going to be eager to have excisional biopsies of areas in which permeability has been carried out, or have body cavities intruded upon for the recovery of dyes or radioactive markers. The problem is even more difficult in looking at the cellular concomitants of the inflammatory response in humans because here we are in very deep trouble. There are two or three methods in which one can measure inflammation in the human, at least, the cellular aspects of inflammation. These include the skin window and several modifications of it. Also included is skin-testing of the delayed type, in which the focus has been on cell-mediated immune mechanisms. There is even a method that includes the induction of blisters in humans. On the latter point, I suspect that none of us is going to be terribly successful in convincing normal or diseased individuals to submit to the induction of blister formation just so we can see how many cells accumulate in the fluid. The delayed hypersensitivity skin reaction involving intradermal injection of various bacteriological and fungal products is a useful method, but it is a very poorly quantitative method, as I think everybody realizes. It might be pointed out that by so selecting the delayed skin reaction as the measure of testing one's ability to mobilize inflammatory cells, this has inadvertently created tunnel vision and has led people to conclusions about effects on inflammatory response which are not warranted. By this I mean that there has been a tendency in the past to say that if individuals do not develop the usual intensity of inflammatory reactions in the skin, these patients have a specific defect in the cellular immune mechanism. It has become increasingly clear that a defect in the effector limb of the lymphocyte-mediated inflammatory reaction is only one of many problems that can cause depression in mobilization of inflammatory cells in a cell-mediated immune type reaction. And it has also become increasingly clear that, as the regulatory defects of the inflammatory response are appreciated, one sees defects in these patients not only if one does skin-testing with fungal extracts, but if one takes the trouble to inject agents which do not demonstrably exert their activity via the lymphocyte system; defects in the mobilization of acute inflammatory cells are also found.

As stated above, the tendency to restrict studies of inflammatory reaction to skin-testing with antigens has tended to create a false impression in many cases about the nature of the defect in the inflammatory response.

We still do not know any good method to get around these problems in human subjects. No experimentation committee and no volunteer for a study is going to lie down and say, "I'd be happy to have you inject glycogen into my peritoneal cavity." And yet, we very much need to have some way to measure the mobilization of inflammatory cells without being too terribly invasive, to have a way to do this in a quantitative manner.

Technetium scanning has been employed in attempts to obtain quantitative estimates of cell mobilization in restricted locales. This depends upon the ability of circulating leukocytes to internalize this radiotag, which is a hard gamma emittor and can be scanned by external methods. The experience of using technetium over the past few years suggests that the technique is really not very useful. It probably only picks up large areas of on-going inflammatory reactions and it does not have the sensitivity to detect small, developing areas of accumulating inflammatory cells.

So, we still do not have a good method. There are even serious problems with the labeling of leukocytes. The chromium method provides low specific labeling of granulocytes and is a relatively insensitive method. Many attempts to label the neutrophil by the lactoperoxidase method (with ^{125}I) have been unsuccessful in our hands and in the hands of many other people, so that we are still groping for a good labeling method. The ^{32}P-DFP method seems to be a reasonably reliable one. The only caveat here is that in certain concentrations DFP will start to interfere with chemotactic function of leukocytes. But at the concentrations that have been used in the past for labeling, this reagent probably is useful. We still get around to the problem that we do not have a good way to measure quantitatively the inflammatory response in the human. And this is one of the biggest drawbacks in obtaining what necessarily must be good correlative studies *in vivo* with the *in vitro* correlates.

Subject Index

Note: In this index, page numbers in *italic* type refer to illustrations; page numbers followed by (t) refer to tables.

313
HL-A typing in, 326
incidence of, 314
levamisole in treatment of, 327
malignant histiocytic lymphoma in, 326
monocyte chemotactic defect in, 326
normal chemotaxis in, 324
principal infecting organisms, 326
Hypogammaglobulinemia, and abnormal
    neutrophil chemotaxis, 314
and neutrophil disorders, 309
Hypophosphatemia, defective chemotaxis
    in, 336, 339

Ichthyosis, defective chemotaxis in, 336,
    338
with subcutaneous abscesses and de-
    pressed neutrophil chemotaxis, 309
IgA, and abnormal chemotaxis, 319
circulating, in defective chemotaxis, 314
deficiency of, and inhibitory activity, 252
effective molar concentration of, 252
functional specificity of, for inhibition of
    chemotaxis, 243, *244*
inhibitory effect of, on various attractants,
    252
polymeric, dialysis and, 252
IgA M-components, and PMN luminescence,
    243–244
and PMN phagocytosis, 243–244
IgA myeloma, and defective chemotaxis,
    336, 342
serum chemotactic inhibition in, 241
IgE, high levels of, and defective neutrophil
    chemotaxis, 310
inhibition of leukocyte migration by, 253
IgG, and abnormal chemotaxis, 319
Immune response, effect of viruses on, 364
Immunoglobulin, deficiencies of, and
    granulocyte chemotaxis dysfunction,
    330, 334
Immunological reactions, subacute, 167–
    168
Infants, newborn, decreased chemotactic
    response in, 317
Infection(s), active, and defective chemo-
    taxis, 336, 339
increased serum chemotactic activity in,
    251
parasitic, eosinophil localization factors
    in, 196 (t)
recurrent, and defective chemotaxis, 314
and defective leukotaxis, 308

depressed neutrophil activity in, 308
Infectious agents, modulation of chemotaxis
    by, 362–367
Inflammation, cellular aspects of,
    measuring of, 409
Inflammatory responses, effect of neutro-
    phils on, 211
mechanisms for modulation of, 211–228
Influenza, chemotaxis in, effect of
    levamisole on, 365, 366 (t)
monocyte chemotaxis response in, 365,
    365, 366 (t)
Inhibitors, cell-directed, and defective
    chemotaxis, 336, 341
Insulin, and cGMP, effect of on diabetic
    patient's PMN chemotactic response
    to bacterial factor, 189 (t)
Interferon, 267
Intracellular elements, defects of, and
    defective chemotaxis, 344, 344 (t)
Iodacetate, in cell elastimetry studies, 380
Ion fluxes, defects of, and defective
    chemotaxis, 344, 344 (t)
Isoproterenol, effect of, on chemotaxis, 182
effect on PMN cGMP levels, 185

Job's syndrome, defective neutrophil
    chemotaxis in, 310, *311*, 312, *312*,
    313
typical features of, 311, 312
typical lesions of, *311*, *312*, *313*

K^+, effect of ouabain on, 114–115
external, in neutrophil movement, 113–
    115
extracellular, and locomotion of rabbit
    peritoneal neutrophils, 114–119
transport of, chemotactic factors and, 115
$K^+ Na^+$ pump, action of chemotactic peptide
    on, 117
KAF, 334
Kallikrein, 202
Kaolin, in experimental pleurisy study of
    chemotaxis factors, 301–302
Klinefelter's syndrome, deficiency of
    chemotactic factor in, 318
Kwashiorkor, delayed chemotactic response
    in, 317

Lamellepodia, characteristics of, 143
Lazy leukocyte syndrome, 308
abnormal chemotaxis in, 381
in chemotaxis disorders, 336, 337